Genetically Modified and Irradiated Food

Genetically Modified and Irradiated Food

Controversial Issues: Facts versus Perceptions

Edited by

Veslemøy Andersen, PhD

Global Harmonization Initiative (GHI)
Vienna, Austria

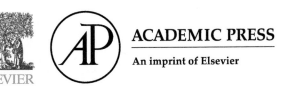

ELSEVIER

ACADEMIC PRESS
An imprint of Elsevier

Academic Press is an imprint of Elsevier
125 London Wall, London EC2Y 5AS, United Kingdom
525 B Street, Suite 1650, San Diego, CA 92101, United States
50 Hampshire Street, 5th Floor, Cambridge, MA 02139, United States
The Boulevard, Langford Lane, Kidlington, Oxford OX5 1GB, United Kingdom

Notices

Knowledge and best practice in this field are constantly changing. As new research and
experience broaden our understanding, changes in research methods, professional
practices, or medical treatment may become necessary.

Practitioners and researchers must always rely on their own experience and knowledge in
evaluating and using any information, methods, compounds, or experiments described
herein. In using such information or methods they should be mindful of their own safety
and the safety of others, including parties for whom they have a professional
responsibility.

To the fullest extent of the law, neither the Publisher nor the authors, contributors, or
editors, assume any liability for any injury and/or damage to persons or property as a
matter of products liability, negligence or otherwise, or from any use or operation of any
methods, products, instructions, or ideas contained in the material herein.

Library of Congress Cataloging-in-Publication Data
A catalog record for this book is available from the Library of Congress

British Library Cataloguing-in-Publication Data
A catalogue record for this book is available from the British Library

ISBN: 978-0-12-817240-7

For information on all Academic Press publications visit our website at
https://www.elsevier.com/books-and-journals

Publisher: Charlotte Cockle
Acquisition Editor: Patricia Osborn
Editorial Project Manager: Ruby Smith
Production Project Manager: Sreejith Viswanathan
Cover Designer: Alan Studholme

Typeset by TNQ Technologies

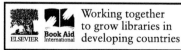

Working together
to grow libraries in
developing countries

www.elsevier.com • www.bookaid.org

Contents

Case studies

PART 2 Irradiated food

Contributors

Amos Oladimeji Adubi, MSc
Laboratory of Ecotoxicology, Genetics and Nanobiotechnology, Environmental
Biology Unit, Department of Pure and Applied Biology, Ladoke Akintola
University of Technology, Ogbomoso, Oyo State, Nigeria; Department of Biology,
School of Science, College of Education, Lanlate, Oyo State, Nigeria

Veslemøy Andersen
GHI Association, Global Harmonization Initiative, c/o University of Natural
Resources and Life Sciences (BOKU), Vienna, Austria

David Adedayo Animasaun, PhD
Department of Plant Biology, Faculty of Life Sciences, University of Ilorin, Ilorin,
Kwara State, Nigeria

Maria-Mihaela Antofie
Associate Professor at the University "Lucian Blaga" of Sibiu, Faculty of
Agricultural Studies, Food Industry and Environmental Protection, Sibiu,
Romania

Musibau Adewuyi Azeez, PhD
Laboratory of Ecotoxicology, Genetics and Nanobiotechnology, Environmental
Biology Unit, Department of Pure and Applied Biology, Ladoke Akintola
University of Technology, Ogbomoso, Oyo State, Nigeria

Joseph John Bevelacqua, PhD
Bevelacqua Resources, Richland, WA, United States

R. Blair, BSc, PhD, DSc
Faculty of Land & Food Systems, University of British Columbia, Vancouver,
Canada

Luc Bodiguel
Director of Research, National Center of Scientific Research (CNRS), UMR 6297
"Droit et Changement Social" (Law and Social Change) Associated Professor,
Faculty of Law of Nantes and IHEDREA (Paris), France

Moisés Burachik, PhD
Director, Regulatory Affairs, INDEAR, Rosario, Santa Fe Province, Argentina

Josias Correa de Faria, PhD, Plant Pathology
Embrapa Rice and Beans, Santo Antonio de Goiás, GO, Brazil

Felicia Adejoke Durodola, MSc
Laboratory of Ecotoxicology, Genetics and Nanobiotechnology, Environmental
Biology Unit, Department of Pure and Applied Biology, Ladoke Akintola
University of Technology, Ogbomoso, Oyo State, Nigeria

Andre Nepomuceno Dusi, PhD, Virology
Ministry of Agriculture, Livestock and Food Supply, Esplanada dos Ministérios, Brasília, DF, Brazil

Ronald F. Eustice
Tucson, AZ, United States

Deise Maria Fontana Capalbo, Bs, MSc, PhD, Food Engineering
Embrapa Environment, Jaguariúna, SP, Brazil

Jan-Hendrik Groenewald, BSc, BSc(Hons), MSc, PhD
Executive Manager-Biosafety South Africa, Somerset West, Western Cape, South Africa

S.M. Javad Mortazavi, PhD
Diagnostic Imaging Department, Fox Chase Cancer Center, Philadelphia, PA, United States

Kubiriba Jerome, PhD
National Agricultural Research Laboratories-Kawanda, National Agricultural Research Organisation, Kampala, Uganda

Tindamanyire Jimmy, PhD
National Agricultural Research Laboratories-Kawanda, National Agricultural Research Organisation, Kampala, Uganda

Namaganda Josephine, PhD
National Agricultural Research Laboratories-Kawanda, National Agricultural Research Organisation, Kampala, Uganda

Marie-Laurence Lemay, PhD
Département de biochimie, de microbiologie, et de bio-informatique, Faculté des sciences et de génie, Université Laval, Québec City, QC, Canada; Groupe de recherche en écologie buccale, Faculté de médecine dentaire, Université Laval, Québec City, QC, Canada

María Salomé Mariotti-Celis, PhD
Programa Institucional de Fomento a la Investigación, Desarrollo e Innovación, Universidad Tecnológica Metropolitana, Santiago, Chile

Endre Máthé, PhD
Associate Professor at the University of Debrecen, Faculty of Agricultural and Food Sciences and Environmental Management, Nutritional Genetics and Genomics Research Group, Debrecen, Hungary; Professor at the "Vasile Goldiş" Western University of Arad, Faculty of Medicine, Department of Life Sciences, Arad, Romania

Sylvain Moineau
Département de biochimie, de microbiologie, et de bio-informatique, Faculté des sciences et de génie, Université Laval, Québec City, QC, Canada; Groupe de recherche en écologie buccale, Faculté de médecine dentaire, Université Laval, Québec City, QC, Canada; Félix d'Hérelle Reference Center for Bacterial Viruses, Faculté de médecine dentaire, Université Laval, Québec City, QC, Canada; Professor, Biochemistry, Microbiology, & Bioinformatics, Université Laval, Quebec City, QC, Canada

Joseph Akintade Morakinyo, PhD
Department of Plant Biology, Faculty of Life Sciences, University of Ilorin, Ilorin, Kwara State, Nigeria

Jun Nishihira, MD, PhD
Department of Medical Management and Informatics, Hokkaido Information University, Ebetsu City, Hokkaido, Japan; Professor, Health Information Science Center, Hokkaido Information University, Ebetsu, Hokkaido, Japan

Wayne A. Parrott, BS, MS, PhD
Professor, Dept. of Crop and Soil Sciences, & Institute of Plant Breeding, Genetics, and Genomics, University of Georgia, Athens, GA, USA

Franco Pedreschi, PhD
Departamento de Ingeniería Química y Bioprocesos, Pontificia Universidad Católica de Chile, Santiago, Chile

Anuradha Prakash, PhD
Food Science Program, Schmid College of Science and Technology, Chapman University, One University Drive, Orange, CA, United States

Namanya Priver, PhD
National Agricultural Research Laboratories-Kawanda, National Agricultural Research Organisation, Kampala, Uganda

J.M. Regenstein
Professor, Emeritus of Food Science, Head of the Cornell Kosher and Halal Food Initiative, Cornell University, Ithaca, NY, United States; Department of Food Science, College of Agriculture and Life Sciences, Cornell University, Ithaca, NY, United States

Alan H. Schulman
Professor, Production Research, Natural Resources Institute (Luke), Helsinki, Finland; Institute of Biotechnology and Viikki Plant Science Centre, University of Helsinki, Helsinki, Finland

Buah Stephen, PhD
National Agricultural Research Laboratories-Kawanda, National Agricultural Research Organisation, Kampala, Uganda

Tushemereirwe Wilberforce, PhD
National Agricultural Research Laboratories-Kawanda, National Agricultural Research Organisation, Kampala, Uganda

Introduction

In the past 200 years, science has evolved with important discoveries that have an enormous influence on lifetime expectations, such as the discovery that microorganisms are the cause of diseases and food spoilage. As a result, methods have been and are continually developed to control the growth of these microorganisms or destroy them. Thanks to pasteurization, food could be preserved for a long time, avoiding famines in wintertime. Due to the discovery of antibiotics, people need not die of pneumonia anymore and vaccines took care of many, often deadly, viral diseases and eliminated pox (variola) completely (IRIS/PAHO, 1980). Science also resulted in the development of technologies that made possible to see, literally, what may be wrong in the body and save lives by increasingly precise surgery and even by replacing damaged parts by artificial ones. The result is that, on average, people live now twice as long as 200 years ago (Roser, 2018).

Regrettably, however, many people forget, never knew, or do not realize that they live happily beyond the age of 30, thanks to the application of scientific discoveries and developments. It is equally unfortunate that some people discovered that being negative about science can be a source of good income. Books that claim, without any evidence, that science is not the cure but the cause of many diseases sell well. There is tremendous media coverage every time that somebody claims that vaccines do not prevent diseases but make people ill, so that the pharmaceutical industry can sell more medicines. Without processing, much food would spoil before consumption. Nevertheless, when authors of popular books about food claim that processing of food is solely for the benefit of large food industries at the expense of the common people, these books receive much media attention and sell well. The same applies to improvement of crops. Governments are accused to allow all this because they have profitable relations with these companies. Barbara Peterson, the owner of the website "Farm Wars" who is leading a "revolution" against industry and government (Peterson, 2009), writes on her webpage: "We are already having to deal with food that is injected with foreign genes (GMOs), blasted with pesticides, irradiated beyond recognition, pasteurized, homogenized, scraped off a slaughterhouse floor, and making us sicker by the minute, ..." (Peterson, 2010).

This constitutes a challenge for decent scientists who must find ways to prevent too many people just believing what is claimed by somebody who looks good, has a high position, such as populist presidents or prime ministers in an increasing number of countries, or is a famous singer or movie star. These people often know that they are lying, but they are unscrupulous and have found out that the lying gives them more power, more money, or both. They state that there are chemicals in "normal" food and that therefore "organic" food is safer, thus using organic food prevents consumers from eating carcinogenic substances, ignoring that there are many natural carcinogens in any food, "organic" or not.

Consumers need to know that everything, including food, is chemistry and that chemicals are not, by definition, unhealthy. There is no life without chemicals and only if certain chemicals are consumed in too high amounts, they may cause harm. Not enough ingestion of vitamins and many minerals is also harmful and over time can be deadly. Too much, however, is harmful and can be fatal. Mankind (like everything that lives) has been exposed to an unbelievable variety of chemicals for millions of years. Thanks to evolution, the survivors—including mankind—learned to cope with those chemicals and often benefit from them. That is why we still live today. If we do not overload our body's protective system, which basically means that if we eat enough and varied, on average, we stay healthy.

Persistent misinformation, lacking any reference to truthful and verifiable published research, is also used to make consumers believe that irradiated food is radioactive and that food produced with genetically modified (GM) seeds changes the human genes. You will glow during the night and your progeny will be inhuman, beyond recognition.

Why is it that so many people believe misinformation? According to John Bargh, a professor in psychology at the Yale University in New Haven, Connecticut, USA, who studied the unconscious mind for decades, this is largely due to the brain that has learned over the ages that it is best to follow a leader and to follow the largest group, because it gives better protection against the enemy (Bargh, 2017). People who want to make their decisions consciously need more time but may come to different conclusions. Many people do not take that time nor have the interest to study available information; they follow the leader with the biggest mouth. While populations in poor countries will increasingly depend on GM food, organizations like Green Peace encourage people to destroy GM crops in test fields, sometimes even stimulated by the government (Various Sources, 2019).

The purpose of this book is to provide scientifically correct information on genetic modification and food irradiation, based on peer-reviewed articles published in high-quality scientific journals. That is why this book has many pages of references helping interested readers to verify statements and conclusions provided in the various chapters. These chapters are written by dedicated highly qualified expert scientists, from all continents. It is hoped that the book provides tools to help the readers to debunk misinformation, e.g., when teaching, presenting at conferences, and in debates with politicians.

Huub Lelieveld, Dr
Global Harmonization Initiative (GHI), Vienna, Austria

References

Bargh, J., 2017. Before You Know It: The Unconscious Reasons We Do What We Do. William Heinemann, London.

IRIS/PAHO, 1980. Smallpox Eradication. Epidemiological Bulletin 1 (1), 5—7.

Peterson, B.H., 2009. Farmwars.info. https://www.printfriendly.com/p/g/F9UNud.

Peterson, B.H., 2010. Farmwars.info. https://pdf.printfriendly.com/pdfs/1563219421_395f8b/download.

Roser, M., 2018. Twice as Long — Life Expectancy Around the World. Our World in Data blog. https://ourworldindata.org/life-expectancy-globally.

Various Sources. 2019. https://slate.com/technology/2013/08/golden-rice-attack-in-philippines-anti-gmo-activists-lie-about-protest-and-safety.html; https://www.independent.co.uk/hei-fi/news/scientists-plead-with-anti-gm-protesters-not-to-destroy-crop-7788322.html and https://www.abcplus.biz/GMO_6-26-13_Hungary_Torches_GM_Corn (all accessed 16 July 2019).

Genetically modified food

Why is genetic modification of interest or why can it be useful?

1

Endre Máthé, PhD [1,2], Maria-Mihaela Antofie[3]

[1]*Associate Professor at the University of Debrecen, Faculty of Agricultural and Food Sciences and Environmental Management, Nutritional Genetics and Genomics Research Group, Debrecen, Hungary; [2]Professor at the "Vasile Goldiş" Western University of Arad, Faculty of Medicine, Department of Life Sciences, Arad, Romania; [3]Associate Professor at the University "Lucian Blaga" of Sibiu, Faculty of Agricultural Studies, Food Industry and Environmental Protection, Sibiu, Romania*

The book is intended to inform a wide spectrum of readers, not only scientists and certainly not just geneticists, but anyone eager to survey the pros and cons of the proposed topics based on facts (peer-reviewed evidences) and to challenge the misinformation provided abundantly by fake scientists publishing views about how bad and dangerous genetically modified (GM) food is. It is the responsibility of scientists to explain the quintessence of such a research, as misinformation is more dangerous than ignorance.

Genetic modification is a term that captures the imagination of many people and has generated wide debate among many groups of interest, including life scientists, policy makers, and law and ethical specialists, while citizens from developed, developing, and underdeveloped countries are facing this issue from different perspective. The ongoing basic research aims to understand the genetic modification -specific cause-effect type of correlations and make use of the GMOs to study the function of genes. On the other hand, the heavily questioned applied research is meant to offer novel and efficient solutions for current problems like biomass production, food safety and security, treatment of human diseases, adaptation of plant and animal species to climatic changes, etc.

Can we stay impartial and face the reality with respect to genetic modifications? In order to address in a fairly comprehensive way the main issues related to GM food, we will present the major issues related to the natural occurrence and laboratory-made GM bacteria, plants, and animals. Next we will focus on GM food—specific major considerations and concerns. In this way, we will follow the implications of genetic modification across the whole food chain giving a much broader and a more carefully balanced picture of the applicability of such a powerful and promising life science—related research method.

The definition of genetic modification refers to a naturally and/or laboratory-assisted genetic material—/gene-/DNA-based phenomenon that would lead to

Genetically Modified and Irradiated Food. https://doi.org/10.1016/B978-0-12-817240-7.00001-2

3

some kind of modification(s) of the genome/DNA of the host organism, hence the term of genetically modified (recombinant) organism (GMO) emerges. It is also important to notice that initially the genetic modification term would cover both the naturally and laboratory condition—assisted genetic modifications, while currently it is more related to the laboratory-obtained transgenic organisms, containing a foreign piece of DNA (gene(s)) from other species.

How was the bacterial type of genetic modification discovered? Initially the phenomenon describing the formation of GMOs was named genetic transformation and was discovered accidently by Frederick Griffith in the 1920s as a natural phenomenon by which the host bacterial cell gains genetic material/genes from some molecules present in the culture media. At that time, we did not know much about the chemical nature and the subcellular localization of the hereditary material. Griffith was working with two *Streptococcus pneumonia* strains and showed that the nonvirulent strain got transformed into a virulent one when the sterilized virulent bacterial lysate was introduced into the media of the nonvirulent strain. Much later it has been demonstrated that such a genetic transformation implies the uptake of virulent DNA fragments by the host nonvirulent bacterial cell from the culture media, leading to a genetically recombined organism that acquires new trait(s). Moreover, it has also been demonstrated that the abovementioned genetic transformation among identical or different bacterial species is a seldom event as many bacterial cells are greatly restricted in taking up free DNA fragments from a liquid environment.

What is the competent cell—based bacterial transformation about? It is also interesting that since the 1970s, there have been developed novel laboratory methods by which the so-called competent host bacterial cells could take up circular DNA molecules like plasmids, and the efficiency of such bacterial transformations increased significantly in such conditions or controlled *ex situ* environments. Before transformation, the plasmid was cut open, and a foreign fragment of DNA, containing gene(s), could be incorporated by closing the plasmid back, resulting in a recombinant plasmid. It is worthwhile mentioning that Stephen Norman Cohen and Herbert Boyer published in 1973 the first scientific article proving an outstanding discovery for biology: obtaining a recombinant plasmid and ensuring the transfer from one living organism to another, laying the foundations of DNA/gene cloning that became one of the most powerful molecular methods (Cohen et al., 1973). We must specify that this is different from the implicated DNA uptaking mechanisms seen in the case of Griffiths competent host types of bacterial transformations. Moreover, the competent bacterial host strains were included into the molecular cloning methodologies so that the bacterial host cells could efficiently incorporate, replicate, and even express the plasmid-carried recombinant cloned gene(s) without getting integrated into the major bacterial DNA/genome. Thus, the trespassing of a biological barrier like the horizontal gene transfer (HGT, implying the movement of genetic material between different species) represents a remarkable achievement in the history of mankind, and it will open new challenging horizons accelerating the development of life sciences. Accordingly, high throughput basic research programs like genome projects (sequencing of the genomes of many species, including the human genomic DNA) were initiated, together with the ever-going quest, to understand the function(s) of genes. As a consequence, the humanity gained more knowledge than ever on the molecular and cellular aspects of life, so that today, we envision every life-related phenomena as an interplay between genomes/genes and the environment.

Once again, we must emphasize that the extraordinary development of our molecular and cellular knowledge explaining life related cause-effect type of correlations is very much built on the genetic transformation of bacteria using the competent bacterial host strains and recombinant plasmid techniques, though presently, the fundamental research makes use of the more efficient PCR (polymerase chain reaction) methods to operate with DNA molecules. On the other hand, the applied research activities in the field of biotechnology quite often rely on the GM bacteria to obtain some products that can be further processed by the pharma and food industries. So to give one such an example, until recently, the production of a biologically active insulin and its analogs in GM *E. coli* and yeast was preferred, but taking in consideration the obtained insulin biological activity and the increasing demand for insulin to treat diabetes, it was proposed to use GM plants and animals for such purposes (Baeshen et al., 2014).

Could the laboratory-obtained GM bacteria be a source of environmental safety hazard? In 1974 Paul Berg was the first to blow the whistle and raised ethical concerns about GM bacteria and molecular cloning during the early days of molecular biology and biotechnology (Berg et al., 1974). Through his involvement, *the Committee on Recombinant DNA Molecules* was founded in the United States that, together with the Assembly of Life Sciences, the National Research Council, and the National Academy of Sciences, organized the Asilomar Conference on Recombinant DNA in 1975. The scientific community recognized the outmost importance of biohazards that emerged due to the discovery and rapid advancement of knowledge in the field. At the meeting, more than 100 professionals (biologists, lawyers, and physicians) specified some voluntary guidelines to ensure the safety of GM bacteria—based molecular cloning and recombinant DNA technology. In modern times, this was the first momentum when the scientist demonstrated a strong spirit of responsibility for the benefits and costs of GM bacteria—promoted scientific progress, and they also showed determination to inform and engage large public into discussions.

Getting back to the initial question, it was obvious from the early days that the HGT-like phenomenon is a major concern, meaning that genetic sequences from a GM bacterium could be transferred to native bacterial species and modifying the latest genomes and subsequently their ecological niche (Heuer and Smalla, 2007). It is also possible that the GM bacteria released into the environment could capture mobile genetic elements from the natural environment living bacteria and through such mobile genetic elements—induced mutation(s) to acquire an extended ecological potential. Therefore, in laboratory and industrial conditions, several safety measures are applied in order to reduce hazards by limiting the possibility of escaping from controlled environment and by strictly controlling the expression of the inserted foreign DNA/gene. Again, we must admit that contrary to the abovementioned laboratory-made GM bacteria, in the case of naturally occurring bacterial transformation even if it is a very rare event, and most probably, existing ever since bacteria appeared on our planet, there is very little we can do about the monitoring and/or controlling of natural events as there are no such powerful research methods to globate all the Bacteria Kingdoms.

What would be the situation with the eukaryotic GMOs? Above all, we must notice that contrary to the prokaryotic bacteria, the DNA of a eukaryotic cell is integrated into chromosomes and the nucleus. Both the chromosomal and nuclear structures are ensuring a very special protective environment to keep intact the DNA or in other words to maintain the stability of the genome and to coordinate the genomic expression with the needs of cells. Keeping unaltered the genome in the life of a eukaryotic cell and a multicellular organism is absolutely crucial for the normal functioning and health. Cellular mechanisms like DNA repair, telomere capping, and RNA interference are meant to maintain chromosomal and genomic stability (for review see Chatterjee and Walker, 2017; Lu et al., 2013; Mello and Conte, 2004). Moreover, most of the eukaryotic species consist of multicellular individuals that are made of plethora of structurally and functionally differentiated cells being rendered into higher structures like organs and system of organs, and harmonized through integrative mechanisms to achieve a homeostasis type of integrity at the individual level. This higher structural and functional complexity of the eukaryotic genetic material/genome/cell/individual as compared to the bacterial genome/cell is considered the greatest impediment to the genetic modification of eukaryotic species.

We should also take into account the issue of eukaryotic soma and germline. A genetic modification that appears in a somatic cell cannot be propagated through sexual reproduction, as the somatic cells do not differentiate into sexual cells. Conversely to somatic cells, the genetic modifications occurring in the germline of females or males could be inherited to the offspring and perpetuated across several generations. Therefore, it seemed logic to increase research efforts to advance our knowledge on germline specific events, so that a better understanding of developmental cues during the differentiation of germline cells would provide novel opportunities to overcome the genomic integrity mechanisms and to generate efficiently GMOs in laboratory conditions.

How can we overcome the complexity of eukaryotic cells in order to produce GMOs across plant and animal species? Developing novel methods to introduce foreign piece(s) of DNA/gene(s) into the zygote or early embryonic cells became a reality through the combined efforts of molecular and developmental biologists. Currently, such a foreign piece of DNA could contain an entire gene or elements of a gene like the promoter, open-reading frame, suppressors and enhancers, or mutated versions of a gene, actually almost any DNA sequence a scientist desires. The successful integration of the abovementioned foreign piece of DNA (often called transgene) relies heavily on the transformation vector used to promote its insertion in host genome.

In 1980, the first genetic transformation of mouse embryos was carried out (Gordon et al., 1980), and in 1981, Franklin Costantini and Elizabeth Lacy successfully obtained GM mice by integrating the rabbit β-globin gene into the mouse germline cells (Costantini and Lacy, 1981). In 1982, Gerald Rubin and Allan Spradling reported the transposon-mediated genetic modification of the fruit fly (*Drosophila melanogaster*) (Rubin and Spradling, 1982). The idea to use a transposon as a vector to transfer genetic information seemed to be a great idea as the eukaryotic genomes do contain transposons. The transposons are mobile genetic elements that can move across the genome by cutting out and pasting back themselves in another genomic location aided through the action of their own transposase gene. The relevant transposon for *Drosophila* was a mutated P-element from which the transposase gene has been removed to restrict its genomic mobility. On the other hand, such an altered P-element (also called transformation vector) can be further modified through molecular cloning to make contain the preferred piece of DNA (transgene). The emerged modified P-element construct (carrying the transgene) is then injected into the *Drosophila* host embryo's firstly formed progenitor germline cells (pole cells), together with an additional plasmid that encodes for P-element transposase. The host fruit fly embryo is lacking any transposase activity so that the injected additional plasmid-encoded transposase is going to get expressed only during pole cell development, and through its activity will subsequently facilitate the random insertion of the transgene into the genome of the host embryo's germline cell. If the insertion event is successful, then the corresponding sexual cell(s) will contain the desired transgene so that when such a host individual is further propagated, some of the resulting offsprings would feature in their entire soma and germline the transgene, hence GM fruit flies emerge. The modified P-element is engineered in such a way that it contains next to the cloned transgene some other morphological marker genes like the wild type (w^+) or yellow (y^+), while the host embryos would lack the wild type (w^+) or yellow (y^+) allele, meaning that a successful P-element transformation would result in offsprings featuring the wild type (w^+) and yellow (y^+) phenotypes, making the transgenic GM flies easily recognizable.

The above mentioned modified P-element system presented some advantages like the increased transformation efficiency but did not allow to control the expression of a given transgene if only the gene in question was introduced into the transformation vector, together with its own regulatory 5′ and 3′ elements. To overcome this situation, special P-element-based transgenic vectors were obtained in which the transgene expression was put under somatic or germline control. Another outstanding achievement was the development of the Gal4-UAS transgenic binary expression system that allows the in vivo studying of gene expression in temporal and spatial fashion (for review see Duffy, 2002). This bipartite approach is based on the yeast-specific Gal4-UAS system that, being absent from the *Drosophila* genome, made possible the invention of a system by which the expression of the gene in question (the responder) is driven through the presence of the UAS element. It is important to notice that the binary system elements being separated from each other were placed in two different transgenic lines. In the absence of Gal4, the UAS responder remains transcriptionally silent. In order to activate the expression of a UAS responder, such transgenic lines must be crossed to fly strains expressing GAL4 in a given spatial and temporal pattern, termed the driver. The obtained progeny brings together the driver and the responder so that the responder will be expressed in a transcriptional pattern that reflects the GAL4 expression pattern of the applied driver. Several hundred of *Drosophila* type of organ/tissue/cell drivers were obtained that would guide the expression of the studied genes in the context of development, life cycle, every organ, and cell type. We have to admit that the *Drosophila* Gal4-UAS binary system is the most advanced and safe method to control the expression of a transgene in a GM organism.

Having seen some of the advantages of the modified transposons—assisted genetic transformation of *Drosophila,* an enormous number of transgenic mutant strains have been isolated affecting almost every single gene from the fruit fly genome. These GM strains that would allow the control of transgene either by reducing or by overexpressing it were deposited in several stock centers and lead to the discovery of many genes' function controlling important life-related events and the elaboration of transgenic disease models (corroborating even human pathological conditions), so that *Drosophila* emerges as the most versatile and detail-oriented model organism to study the genetic control of life. As a consequence, the fruit fly became the best known multicellular eukaryotic organism advancing significantly our knowledge in the fields of maternal effect, embryonic development, cell cycle regulation, cell fate specification and cellular differentiation, innate immunity, and circadian rhythm control.

Could the transgenic GM animals advance our knowledge further to basic research and bring other benefits to humanity? Next to *Drosophila,* representing an invertebrate species, the use of mice (*Mus musculus*), a mammalian vertebrate species, contributed substantially to the progress in the field of GM animals as novel genetic transformation techniques were introduced like the lentiviral infection of the zygote, microinjection of foreign DNA into the pronucleus of the fertilized egg, and genetic modification of embryonic (omnipotent) stem cells as followed by their microinjection into the blastocyst embryo. These transgenic methods were efficient in the transgene delivery and insertion, so they were applied to other vertebrate species from domestic livestock, poultry, and fish, though the spatial and temporal control of the transgene expression needed further improvements. In a very short period of time, many vertebrate GM animals were produced and used as models to recapitulate human diseases (like Alzheimer, Parkinson, cancer, diabetes, obesity, heart and coronary conditions, etc.) in laboratory conditions, shedding light on the genetic and environmental cues initiating and advancing the abovementioned clinical pathologies. Moreover, the vertebrate GM animals proved their usefulness for preclinical human drugs and vaccines testing, production of human antibodies and other proteins of pharmaceutical applications, etc (for review see Clark and Pazdernik, 2015). On the other hand, the application of genetic transformation to agriculturally important animal species could bring more benefits to farmers and consumers as theoretically any trait can be modulated through genetic modification. Reaching such a goal is rather challenging since we are short of knowledge related to the function(s) of the genes determining the so-called quantitative traits (like growth rate, yields of milk, egg, and meat) of domesticated livestock, poultry, and fish. Paradoxically, it is expected that the research on GMOs specific to vertebrate species would advance our knowledge regarding the quantitative traits—implicated genes and the interplay with environmental conditions. Most probably, the GMOs addressing quantitative traits would require bringing together several genes into one or fewer transgenes, while in case of wild type or normal animals' genomes, these genes are located onto different chromosomes. It is also important to mention that the GMOs specific for domesticated animal species could be envisioned like less prone to substantiate biohazards since their reproduction can be more tightly controlled due to the rigorous isolation from the natural environment.

Can genetic modifications occur in plant species under natural conditions? The answer is YES, but some characteristics of the genetic modifications are mainly specific to plants. The frequency of polyploidy type of genomic mutations is much higher among plants as compared to animals even under natural conditions, while by microtubule drugs, many plant species can be forced to undergo genetic modifications by doubling their genomes. It the case of animal and fungi cells, the prolonged activation of spindle assembly checkpoint (SAC) leads to the ultimate death of the affected cells, by overcoming abnormal chromosomal segregation and ensuring genomic stability. Contrary to animal and fungi cells, the prolonged activation of the plant-specific SAC does not necessarily lead to cell death, but it will be switched off, while the cell cycle is reset, and the cells will continue their life with duplicated genomes (Komaki and Schnittger, 2017). Further to SAC, it seems logic that the other structural and functional features of the acentrosomal plant cell spindles could have contributed to the successful perpetuation of duplicated genomes. Noticeably, during plant evolution, the angiosperms lost the centrosome, a highly efficient microtubule organizing center (MTOC) implicated in cellular growth and division (Sablowski, 2016). Accordingly, during interphase, flexible MTOCs would emerge on the plasma membrane, the nuclear envelope, and organelles depending on types of cells and organisms (for review see Lee and Liu, 2019). Moreover, during plant cell divisions, a two-stage acentrosomal spindle formation can be seen, as the bipolar prospindle gets transformed into a bipolar spindle with kinetochore microtubules having attached chromosomes (Yamada and Goshima, 2017). It is also possible that the movement of the sister chromatids (during mitosis and second meiotic division) or homologous chromosomes (first meiotic division) toward the spindle poles at anaphase relies on other mechanisms than the centrosome-assisted polar anchoring of spindle microtubules as suggested for some animal oocytes by Radford and colab (Radford et al., 2017). Therefore, it seems reasonable to hypothesize that bypassing the SAC-induced mitotic arrest, and resetting to normal the cell cycle control, together with the acentrosomal spindle—featured chromosome segregation, could ensure the faithful propagation of polyploidy type of genomic mutations across generations. Moreover, such polyploidy can arise not only through the duplication of the ancestral genome but by the fusion of genomes of closely related species. Several studies are suggesting that polyploidy played a crucial role in the genetic diversification and adaptive radiation of species across angiosperm lineages (De Bodt et al., 2005). From the prospect of natural evolution, the polyploid genome can acquire further genetic modifications reshaping the functions of individual genes and/or gene families (Soltis et al., 2009; Van de Peer et al., 2009). Therefore, the evolutionary edited polyploid genomes could confer some adaptive advantages to the more vigorous and plastic polyploid individuals for populating newer and extreme ecological niches (Fawcett and Van de Peer, 2010). So to give some examples, the diversity of species that belong to the mustard (Brassicaceae or Cruciferae) family (Franzke et al., 2011) and the bread wheat (*Triticum aestivum* L.) formation (Mirzaghaderi and Mason, 2017) was all put on the context of genome evolution following polyploidy. Taken together, all the abovementioned data are suggesting that the genetic modification of plants can take place even under natural conditions and are very much related to the polyploidy type of genomic mutations and as such, could have had an impact on plant species evolution, including domestication too.

What do we think in general about plant domestication? It is generally accepted that *plant evolution* is mainly due to spontaneous or induced mutations (of gene, chromosomal, and genomic types), while species are facing natural factors and need to adapt to ever-changing environmental conditions (Hancock, 2012). Accordingly, domestication as a process would imply the identification of mutations among crop species on which the main evolutionary forces would act, together with anthropic factors like empirical selection, the chance of the breeder to orientate the selection process, the need to explore new species relevant for diet, as well as the dissemination of crop species and agricultural practices. Today, it is considered that food crops domestication began some 10,000 years ago, after the last glaciation Era (i.e., Younger Dryas 12,900−11,700 years BP), as archaeological evidences are suggesting that wheat, rye, and lentils were first to become domesticated (Sonnante et al., 2009). The places and time of domestications in different centers of origin are still under debate, but some genetic crossing and cytogenetic data are indicating that lentils were domesticated at least in the same time, if not before cereals group for more than 10,000 years ago. Thus, humans started to control for the first-time domestication by devoting their work to propagate certain traits as part of a meditative and primitive empirical knowledge. As an example, they tried to maintain in the form of selected populations at least two distinct traits of lentils such as the pod dehiscence and seed dormancy (Ladizinsky, 1985; Ladizinsky and Abbo, 2015). Today, it is known that these traits are under simple genetic control, and therefore mutants must have been fixed in a relatively short time (Ladizinsky and Abbo, 2015).

Started from ancient to the beginning of modern times, the domestication of food crops evolved slowly as it was kept outside laboratory. In 1986, the theory of factorial heredity elaborated by Gregor Mendel would represent an important cornerstone by providing a new conceptual framework for the agriculture research based on the inheritance of gene-determined traits (Lee, 2005). It was the momentum when plant breeding was becoming less of an art and more of a science (Kloppenburg, 2005). In the 20th century, food crops cultivation and breeding was already an important asset for human civilization by combining the research results obtained in plant chemistry and physiology, together with soil fertilization. Thus, the mineral fertilization that started around 1880s became a common practice after the Great War and expanded on larger scale after World War II to increase the cereal yields from 2 tonnes/ha in 1900 to 7.5 tonnes/ha in 2000 in Europe (Roy et al., 2006). Later, based on the principles of the Mansfeld approach like high responsibility for field science (paying attention to genetic and ecosystem diversity), rational global thinking, and high ethical standards (Pistrick, 2003), it was suggested that humans might have domesticated around 7000 plant species (Hammer and Khoshbakht, 2015). Not all domesticated species exists today; some of them disappeared though supporting historical evidences do exist (Khoshbakht and Hammer, 2010). At the onset of the 21st century and with the advent of molecular biology, new horizons open, offering several opportunities to humanity to gain a better understanding of life-related phenomena, including plant breeding and domestication. It is now the era of the postgenomic plant research, and plant domestication is facilitated by genetic modifications carried out in laboratory conditions. Like never before, there is an urgent need to accurately define what a genetic modification is about or what the benefits and risks of modern time's domestication are. Clarifying the attributes of the laboratory-assisted genetic modifications in relation to present knowledge level would require mindful thinking by eliminating myths, constructing reasonable cause-effect type of correlations and reaching the highest ethical standards.

Can we control plant breeding in laboratory conditions? The answer is YES, and the story started to unfold in 1902, when Gottlieb Haberlandt, a plant physiology researcher, launched the concept of plant cell totipotency. Eventually a novel paradigm emerges, so that plant research will deliver unforeseeable results by laying the foundation of plant-specific developmental biology and biotechnology (Haberlandt, 1902). Therefore, at the beginning of the 20th century, the labs' doors got widely open for studying plants in aseptic conditions. Defining the methodology for somatic embryogenesis allowed us to regenerate a whole plant from a single cell and the clonal propagation of individuals with identical genomes and provided host cells/tissues for genetic transformation. It is also true that somatic embryogenesis greatly facilitated the elimination of viruses and the development of artificial seed technology. Moreover, thousands of in vitro micropropagation protocols (i.e., systems and methods) were elaborated, different plant explants and in vitro propagating tissues were analyzed, and explored to study differentiation of plant species (Gautheret, 1983). The plant breeding technology from laboratory level was massively transferred to industry during the second half of the last century, developing new innovative products and services. One great benefit of the micropropagation was the reduction of generation time with respect to the normal life cycle of angiosperm species. Over 100,000 plant varieties, species and genera have been micropropagated into laboratories in the Netherlands in the 1980s, and the seed industry was more than interested in the results of plant-based in vitro tools and technologies. The plant breeding became a serious business in a very short period of time, so to give an example; the turnover of the Dutch flower auctions was estimated at 2.556 million USD in 1989 (Pierik, 1991). Artificial seeds containing somatic embryos also gained a relevant place in the industrial research and business (Gosal and Grewal, 1991).

It is also true that during the 1950s and 1960s, as the number of successfully micropropagated plant species was increasing, the food crops breeders were preoccupied to improve the adaptation and resistance of cultivated plant species in order to ensure food security among the developing countries. The concept of Green Revolution was established with emphasis on the improvement of crops adaptation to environmental factors and resistance toward pests and diseases, together with the implication of state-directed economic and social mechanisms. As a consequence, starting with Mexico during 1950s, continuing in 1960s with India, Pakistan, and Philippines, the Green Revolution managed to alleviate substantially but failed to eradicate totally the famine (Borlaug, 2002). By the 1970s, scientists were realizing that the number of challenges the humanity was facing started to increase, so next to food security, new issues appeared like food safety, food market diversification, and global warming.

What would be the benefits of combining plant micropropagation with genetic modification? Most importantly, such a combination holds the promise of directed evolution on a reduced time scale. Everything started during the 1970s when the crops breeders' community was following with great interest the results of the bacterial type of genetic transformations by introducing foreign genetic material into the bacterial genome, through the use of molecular genetic (genetic engineering) technologies. They were also aware of the fact that the plant-specific applications of similar approaches would require some relevant discoveries and looking for answers regarding the future of GM plants. Experienced plant scientists in the micropropagation of plant cells/tissues did make use of novel molecular genetics techniques and managed to obtain *Streptomyces*-resistant GM plants originating from haploid tobacco callus (Maliga et al., 1973). Due to their totipotent ability and high reproducibility of the results, this haploid tobacco callus was used as a valuable instrument for reaching the goal of plant transformation by adding easily recognizable markers in order to evaluate the success of genetic transformation in plants (Paszkowski et al., 1984). Thus, the first successful genetic transformation of plants was reported by Zambryski and collaborators in 1984 (Zambryski et al., 1984), with the support of *Ti* plasmid of *Agrobacterium*, a pathogen bacterium discovered long time ago, known for infecting plants and producing galls (Smith and Townsend, 1907). This is the first such an attempt when plant scientists were accessing a natural infecting mechanism as real molecular portal to ensure the successful transfer and integration of a foreign piece of DNA in the host plant's genome that will be followed by the regeneration of a whole plant. Since then, new methods were developed to obtain GM plants and to control the expression of the inserted foreign genes or to reduce the expression of the host gene by the means of RNA interference (Zotti et al., 2018). Moreover, the latest genome editing by the CRISPR/Cas9 (clustered regularly interspaced short palindromic repeat) technologies opens unforeseen opportunities to develop novel plant varieties by deleting off detrimental and/or adding on beneficial traits determining genes (for review see Arora and Narula, 2017). The CRISPR/CAS9 technology is constantly advancing, and the genomic editing of cultivated plants is expected to bring about novel GM plant varieties to improve the plant-specific nutrition, disease resistance, and drought tolerance that all together would increase the sustainability of food production (for review see Bao et al., 2019; Liu et al., 2017).

What are the challenges regarding the field testing of GM plants? When the first GM plant was produced in the lab, it was also proposed to be moved from aseptic conditions to the field, and this issue generated a series of questions related to the monitoring procedures and the environmental risk assessment and management (Boyer, 1982). There were other puzzling questions too. Are they going to express the GM plants the corresponding transgene at the same level in all their cells or individuals among varying environmental conditions? Could the soil biota become affected? How can the putative environmental impact induced by the transfer of a GM plant–specific transgene through pollen to related plant species (an issue of HGT) be studied? What strategies must be applied to ensure safe level of transgene containment? Certainly there were many more questions to be answered, and it seemed reasonable to predict the emergence of a new science regarding the association of risks management with the field testing of GM plants. Initially the experiments were not totally conclusive, and scientists realized that there should be put in place some guidelines and regulations. 1986 was the year for the very first field trial in France and the United States of a GM tobacco plant carrying a transgene for herbicide resistance (James and Krattiger, 1996). Since then, across the world and denoting the consciousness of scientists, together with policy/law makers in many countries, the GMO studies should follow certain procedures. The field trials got fully regulated in the European Union based on the Directive 2001/18/EC. From 2001 onwards, an informal portal provides all the necessary information for the EU citizens related to the Deliberate Release and Placing on the EU Market of GMOs—GMO Register, under the supervision of the Joint Research Centre (JRC) (http://gmoinfo.jrc.ec.europa.eu/). Today, it is known that 5360 GMO plants corresponding to 82 species have been granted the permission to be tested into field conditions.

Countries like Spain (734) and France (615) obtained the highest number of grants related to field trials of GM plants at the European level. They were followed by Italy (303), Germany (273), United Kingdom (264), and the Netherlands (249). Countries like Bulgaria, Cyprus, Latvia, Luxembourg, and Malta have not filled any application for field trial for different reasons, while in Hungary there is a total ban on field trial or GM crop cultivation. Among the large multinational companies in terms of venture capital, we may cite the field testing interests of Pioneer Hi-Bred (181 notifications), Monsanto Europe (164 notifications), Syngenta Seeds (123 notifications) and Bayer CropScience (65 notifications), BASF Plant Science (32 notifications) and Dow AgroSciences (15 notifications).

The environmental relevance of field trials is obvious but it is equally important for the next stage of GM plant business like placing them onto the market in the form of feed and food. However, we have to admit that many of these field tests are meant to advance the GM plant—related basic knowledge without any immediate business purposes, while in the case of multinational companies, we have to presume that business objectives are also followed. We have to recognize that, in European terms, during the GM field trials, the DUS test (distinctiveness, uniformity, and stability) must be applied, and the new GM plant varieties should be registered into the European Catalog, following the guidelines agreed under the International Union for the Protection of New Varieties of Plants or UPOV treaty.

What are the major safety concerns related to GM plants? Today the GM plants are produced to bring benefices to the humanity, and based on such a rational, their classification distinguishes three categories (Magaña-Gómez and Calderón de la Barca, 2009; Gasser and Fraley, 1989). Thus, the first category of GM plants would include those that are referred to pest resistance such as Bt (*Bacillus thuringiensis*) resistance (Hutchison et al., 2010), herbicide tolerance such as glyphosate (Gaines et al., 2010), disease resistance such as powdery mildew resistance (Jørgensen, 1988), cold tolerance (Sanghera et al., 2011), drought tolerance, and salinity tolerance (Sinclair, 2011). The second category of GM plants are related to the improved nutritional and diet values designated for direct consumption such as the case of Golden Rice (Beyer et al., 2002) or food industry application such as an increased starch concentration (Jobling et al., 2002) and bioremediation (Macek et al., 2008). The third category of GM plants are represented by those that are relevant for the concept of molecular farming and do have pharmaceutical applications (Ma et al., 2003).

All these three GM plant categories raise concerns related to risks on environment and human health. Scientific evidences are suggesting that some GM crops could be considered potentially harmful to the environment (Tsatsakis et al., 2017a). Regarding the environmental implications of GM plants, one should pay attention to both direct and indirect consequences. The direct environmental impacts of GM plants could be related to phenomena like gene flow, transgene stacking, HGT, naked DNA fate, modification of crop pervasiveness or invasiveness, and emergence of herbicide-insecticide-pesticide toxicities. Among the indirect environmental impacts of GM plants, the effects on soil and water, biodiversity, efficiency of pest, disease and weed control, and evolution of herbicide-insecticide-pesticide and antibiotic resistance should be studied. It is also true that the assessment of environmental impacts associated with the GM plants is at an initial phase, when research strategies and methodologies are constantly improved, and while many of the results are disputable, it seems obvious that a much broader and more critical research is needed to reveal further facts about the modification of biodiversity.

Considering the GM crops—related human risks, due to the consumption of GM food, started from 1990s, toxicity tests are carried out on laboratory animals and human cell lines in order to analyze the possible toxicity effects. Even the FAO/WHO compelled a so-called Codex guidelines for the risk analysis of GM food. The accumulated evidences on toxicity studies this far do not suggest the need for applying restrictions on the use of GM crops as feed and food (Tsatsakis et al., 2017b).

Toxicity assessments of GM crops heavily rely on rats, broiler chickens, layer hens, dairy cows, monkeys, frogs, and pigs that were fed GM rice, soybean, maize, wheat, and potato, alone or in combination. Usually the experiments will last for 90 days, and multiple biological parameters are monitored, together with food intake. Such experiments showed minor to no adverse effects when GM- and non-GM-food—based diets were compared, so that the main results were not indicating direct toxicity risks to human or animal health.

What we hoped to achieve through the GM foods initially? The term GM food is in itself misleading because it creates the impression that during the manufacturing process by some genetic means, the food gets modified, while in reality, the primary materials, additives, or some microorganisms that have been used for food manufacturing could originate from GM plant, animal, or microorganism individuals with their species-specific genomes containing some extra genetic information. Accordingly, the GM foods are derived from GM organisms whose genetic material has been modified in a way that does not occur naturally. It is also true that many of the newly obtained GM plants or animals are harboring transgenes that are meant to improve the crop production technology and to ensure production stability across the food chain. The usefulness of plant and animal genomes modification to improve their nutritive values is still largely debated because such an objective could also be achieved by combining certain natural ingredients with proper manufacturing technologies in such a way that the final food product should meet all the envisioned nutritive parameters. Nevertheless, in some socioeconomic situations, the use of GM plants could be a more straightforward solution to obtain a fortified food. The Golden Rice is a GM variety of rice (*Oryza sativa*) that through the expression of its transgene acquired the capacity to synthesize β-carotene in the edible parts of the plant (Ye et al., 2000). The production and consumption of the Golden Rice in the Asian, African, and South American countries with severe vitamin A deficiency is expected to reduce the mortality among children and childhood blindness. Many other GM foods are related to intervention strategies to improve nutrition and health of consumers, but economic reasons are also considered. Here are some examples of GM plants that have reached the plate of consumers: (1) the pink GM pineapple producing the antioxidant lycopene, (2) the GM canola with modified oil composition or herbicide resistance, (3) the antibrowning GM apple, (4) the delayed ripening GM tomato and melon, (5) the virus-resistant GM squash, bean, potato, sweet pepper, zucchini, plum, and papaya, (6) the Bt maize, Bt potato, Bt eggplant, and Bt cotton all being pest resistant GMOs as they produce insecticides, (7) the late blight—resistant or insect-resistant or modified starch/carbohydrate GM potato, (8) the glyphosate-tolerant GM soybean, sugar beet, wheat, and alfalfa; (9) the GM maize resistant to the herbicides, and (10) the AquAdvantage salmon that would grow year-round instead of only during spring and summer (Zhang et al., 2016; Bawa and Anilakumar, 2013). The list of GM plants used as foods can be continued with the *Fusarium*-resistant GM bananas, the sweeter peach—flavored GM strawberries, the GM carrots that would increase calcium bioavailability, and spicy GM tomatoes in which the inactive genes for capsaicinoids got reactivated through the CRISPR-CAS9 genome-editing system (Naves et al., 2019). On the line with current trends, the diversification of food-oriented application of GM plants is expected to continue in the future, while the usage of GM animals for food production seems to await for the definition of applicative directions and innovative solutions, all based on advancing our knowledge related to the quantitative traits inheritance and genes' functions.

On the other hand, despite the fact that the laboratory-assisted genetic transformation of microorganisms has been intensively studied, the food industrial applications of the obtained GM microorganisms are lagging behind expectations. It is possible that the uncertainty about consumer reactions and/or the lower profit generating capacity are the impediment holding back the use of GM microorganisms for food production, though they can enter the food chain at several levels (Von Wright and Bruce, 2003). There were obtained GM lactic acid bacteria to improve the ripening and sensorial properties of cheese and yoghurt, while GM yeasts were intended to support the flavor development in the case of bakery products, beer, and wine (Zhang et al., 2014). Many of the microbial food processing enzymes are obtained through GM bacteria and yeast (Ray et al., 2016), while food additives like citric acid and amino acids could also be produced by specific GM bacteria (Kallscheuer, 2018; Willke, 2014). It is also important to pinpoint that many of the GM microorganisms implicated in food production due to the manufacturing technologies will not reach the final products so they cannot be considered GM foods.

Looking at the beginning of GM food story, we have to admit that the exceptional progress made in understanding how the genes are controlling traits and knowing the current challenges ahead of humanity urged researches to look for applicative solutions, so to transfer basic research data to applied research, and the concept of GMO-based food chain was promoted. By now, it is widely accepted among scientists that the GMOs can offer solutions for global challenges like the ever-growing population number and food consumption, together with the reduction of arable land, and the conventional breeding—associated bottleneck effect that reduces genetic diversity among life-stocks animals.

Where are the GM foods heading us? In the previous paragraph, we tried to describe through some examples what would be the rationale behind some GM foods, and we invoked nutritional and economic reasons. It is also true that, in recent years, an unforeseen role of GM foods emerged, as they were proposed to prevent food waste and spoilage. Paradoxically, humanity reached a stage of evolution when food production covered its entire needs, yet several hundred million people are still suffering from hunger and even more from poor diet, while at about one-third of the produced food is lost or wasted on a global scale, according to the United Nations Food and Agriculture Organization (FAO, 2015) Moreover, in the light of global warming, dealing with problems like food loss and waste would impose immediate preventive actions to reduce our impact on the environment. It seems obvious that having implicated so many players, there must exist multiple solutions for such a complex issue, and indeed, the introduction of the fair trade concept steered some responsible and meaningful collaborative actions among highly developed and developing countries. It is equally true that on a global level, we can reduce food waste and losses and especially in the case of fruit and vegetable commodities by using GMOs with longer self-life, like the delayed-ripening GM tomato (Mingchun et al., 2016) and bananas (Elitzur et al., 2016). On the other hand, the losses and/or waste of food commodities that are seen in the case of cereals (30%), oil seed and pulses (20%), and roots and tubers (45%) could be significantly diminished through GMOs that are resistant to extreme environmental conditions, crop diseases, weed competition, and pest attack (Zhang et al., 2016).

Undoubtedly, there is a lot of excitement around the beneficial prospects of GMOs, and for many of us seeing is believing, so reaching the immediate goals could be very convincing, but scientists have learned their lessons from the past and would only rely on evidence-based proofs, considering all implicated players and possible outcomes. Could there be some short- and long-lasting undesirable effects or collateral damages associated with GMOs? Are we facing a situation where we do a bit of good and create a much bigger problem? Does this remind us of the theory of thermodynamics and trying to reduce the entropy? These questions are all related to the issue of GMO safety that continuously creates debates, arguments and even fights among people. All this arise from uncertainties concerning the GM foods induced as potential human health and environmental hazards. It is important to emphasize that the public consumption of accessible GM foods has passed detailed risk assessments, including toxicity and allergenicity tests. The GM foods are consumed by millions of people across the world without any consistent reports of adverse effects (Tsatsakis et al., 2017b), but in some instances allergenicity was observed (for review see Lee et al., 2017). The Brazil-nut protein—expressing GM soybean caused an allergic reaction in human volunteers (Nordlee et al., 1996). In another experiment, the pea weevil—resistant GM bean induced an immune reaction in the lungs of the animals (Prescott et al., 2005), while the "Starlink" maize—specific transgene encodes for the Cry9c protein with insecticide property but unexpected strong allergenicity for humans (Sanchis, 2011). These GM crops did not get approved and were banned from the food market. These examples represent individual cases that are used to argument the harmful nature of GM foods to humans, while many other proofs supporting the healthy nature of GM foods are left aside, forgetting that a general and impartial conclusion would include both supporting and contradicting considerations.

How are the main actors in the unfolding genetic modification story? The ongoing genetic modification story should be envisioned not like a saga but an ongoing research project included in the conceptual frame of the sustainable food chain and circular economy. From this prospective, the traditional and genetic modification -based agriculture/food manufacturing and consumption are not meant to co-habituate in parallel socioeconomic dimensions and fiercely compete with each other, but by exchanging knowledge their reciprocal strengths could be further enhanced and altogether would advance efficiently food safety and security.

Earlier, we have emphasized several times the importance of the scientists participating in the genetic modification -based food chains, and besides them, we should underline the implication of business-oriented entrepreneurs and multinational companies, the political establishment and legislators setting the limits, together with the control exerting authorities and agencies, followed by governmental and nongovernmental agencies, civil associations, mass/electronic media and consumers preoccupied with the formulation and articulate presentation of opinions and the display or disclosure of any relevant information. Certainly we should not forget the importance of knowledge and technology transfer from basic to applied research and from highly developed to developing countries. All players should be aware of the responsibilities that they bear and the costs of compromises over any issue, including GM food safety.

The GM food chain has some critical points (quality control type of term) or bottleneck-prone stages (population genetics terminology) that could inflict decisive impacts on the whole system. In this respect, scientists are expected to come up with more versatile and validated testing systems to monitor the inflicted effects of GM foods on the health of consumers and the environment. Obviously, the implication of multinational companies is evident as they dispose of all the necessary human and financial resources to pursue their interests. The political establishment and legislators, together with the corresponding authorities and agencies, should gain a deep understanding of the benefits and concerns, in order to match legal regulations and controlling mechanisms with the relevant features of genetic modification technology and GM foods. In this respect, we are reaching a consensus by opting for total transparency based on the individual evaluation of every single GMO (case-to-case studies) and the mandatory labeling of every GM food. The relevance of mass and electronic media cannot be emphasized enough, as by being focused very much on negative news, they can provide the consumers a distorted image/meaning of GMOs. It would be of a crucial importance for the media to engage all the key actors of the genetic modification story in constructive evidence-based dialogs to address the GMO concerns. Finally, we have to talk about the responsibility of the consumer, whose knowledge level and attitude varies among individuals and on a large scale in every society, while no one should forget that despite many pros and cons, the choice between traditional and GM food remains to be decided exclusively by the consumers.

Concluding remarks

The laboratory-assisted genetic modification offers unprecedented opportunities, together with multiple challenges by acquiring the knowledge to manipulate the life warehouse that contains the genetic information. Quite interestingly, it is not the first time that we are facing life-changing situations, but like never before, the genomes of different species are becoming the subject of our interference with the Nature. Do we possess all the details for the safe manipulation of genetic information by crossing the naturally existing boundaries between species, and can we foresee all the consequences of such interventions?

The current progress of life sciences due to basic and applied research offers increasing number of opportunities to improve the quality of our life. As an example, the newly obtained knowledge allows humans to gain more insight into the mechanisms behind the initiation and progression of many chronic diseases, so that the efficiency of detection and therapeutic/preventive methods is steadily improving. However, when each of us has to face in person such a disease, we all realize that there are many more unknown details. Despite the progress we have made with respect to chronic diseases, we must admit that we are facing constantly threats and risks. Nevertheless, we move ahead treating such human diseases without disclosing that even if we fail, individually we would not pose much harm on a larger scale to the Nature, though socioeconomical and ethical issues can be evoked.

The situation with the GM organisms and food features similar aspects to many other humans' specific activities that interfere with the Nature. There are scientific, environmental, socioeconomic and political, ethical, and moral issues to be considered on local and global levels. From the very beginning of the genetic modification story, the scientists are facing with proper ethical conduit and professional dignity the boundaries of our knowledge. Moreover, they are totally aware of their responsibility to explain policy and legislation makers, business-oriented entrepreneurs, and the whole humanity what is the genetic modification about and what would be possible gains and losses.

Earlier in this chapter, we have shown that genetic transformation is a naturally occurring phenomenon that was discovered in bacteria, due to the bacterial cell structural and functional properties, while later by making use of molecular genetic (genetic engineering) tools (like plasmids, endonucleases, DNA ligases), scientists managed to introduce genes form other species (including humans) into the bacteria.

The genetic modification of eukaryotic organisms can also be considered a natural phenomenon, though in the context of multicellular eukaryotic species, would imply the unique combination of evolutionary factors, acting across several generations, and why not to say evolutionary linkages over very long period of time. The laboratory-assisted genetic modification of eukaryotic cells required solving the challenge of foreign gene delivery into the eukaryotic genome, identification of the integrated transgene, and the generation of whole multicellular GM plant and animal organisms from a totipotent undifferentiated cell. However, with the advent of the CRISPR/CAS9 technology, the targeted editing of eukaryotic genomes is becoming a reality and offers more powerful tools to control the foreign gene expression (Baliou et al., 2018).

In laboratory conditions, the genetic modification of animal species was based on the successful integration of the knowledge from embryology, genetics, and molecular biology. The genomes of the totipotent animal zygote and/or early embryonic cells were used to integrate foreign genes being carried by viral or transposon vectors. In the case of the eukaryotic plant species, the manipulation of zygote and early embryo proved to be an obstacle without solutions, and therefore the discovery of somatic embryogenesis, together with the micropropagation techniques, offered the chance to regenerate a whole multicellular plant from a few cells. Later on, the delivery vectors carrying the genetic information to be inserted into the host genome got diversified for both animal and plant species, so that more and more emphasis was put on the controlling of foreign gene expression in the host genome. Interestingly, the genetic transformation proved to be more efficient and reliable in the case of animal species with relatively short life cycle, geneticists realized that studying invertebrate GM animals could advance substantially our knowledge by defining the functions of genes. As a consequence, whole genome comprising gene-specific GM lines were obtained to study the cell-/tissue-/organ-specific expression and possible functions of the corresponding genes like in the case of *Drosophila melanogaster* that is followed by the mouse (*Mus musculus*) with a much longer life cycle and vertebrate species. This enthusiasm continues up to present days, and the obtained results help us to gain a better understanding of the way our genes, together with environmental factors, determine all our traits, including health, and help us to defeat diseases. It is also important to notice that these kinds of results made us to realize that many of the quantitative traits of animal species, including the domesticated ones, are determined through the interactions between several genes and environmental factors. Therefore, not being entirely sure on the genes implicated into the traits of economic importance of domesticated species, with a few exceptions, would explain the reason for producing not that many GM animals. Moreover, if we take into consideration the sexual reproduction, farming technologies, and safety control, then one can foresee that GM animals would represent a lower impact source for environmental hazards.

However, when it comes to the GM plants, the situation looks different. On pure scientific grounds, we have realized that the genetic modification of plants could have been a more likely natural event than in animals, and the domestication of plants is related to some such natural events. The laboratory-assisted development of a plant from a single seed was surpassed by acquiring the knowledge to regenerate a whole plant from somatic cells. The somatic embryogenesis combined with micropropagation, and defining vectors with methods to carry genetic information even across species, allowed us to obtain many GM plants not just for pure scientific but economic reasons too. The economic pressure was coming from somatic embryogenesis and micropropagation since these techniques have proved their usefulness for the advancement of biotechnology and business. It is important to notice that the rapidity by which the GM plants were produced to fulfill different socioeconomical purposes made people to develop a huge interest in the possible health and environmental risks associated with this powerful intervention regarding the natural evolution of life on our planet. To make things more complicated, we can put the GM bacteria, plants, and animals in the context of food chain so that the so-called GM feed and food have become a dietary component of livestock and humans. Specialists do agree that through proper geno- and cytotoxicity studies, including those that would refer to the epigenetic status, the health hazard issues can be thoughtfully addressed. However, the environmental issues are more complicated because as we move the GM plants to field testing, we would need to monitor the GMO-caused modifications on time and geographical scales, and we are not fully competent to face such a challenge. Safety regulations were put in place all over the world to control the GMO-based laboratory and field activities, including GMO food manufacturing and commercialization. Moreover, if any environmental hazard arises, we do not know precisely how to deal with it, and we have to admit that very little has been achieved with respect to the protection of endangered species or to restrict/eradicate invasive species, not mentioning the global warming. Being careful and paying attention to experimental details is the most rewarding cognitive attitude (including cognitive, affective, and behavioral levels) when we are facing unprecedented challenges. We would like to close this introductory chapter by admitting that scientists do deserve the trust of the society as their professional and ethical integrity stands at the basis of their existence, so that they will continue to do their best not just to fulfill their curiosity but they will keep awareness always at the highest level for the sake of Life on our planet Earth.

References

Arora, L., Narula, A., 2017. Gene editing and crop improvement using CRISPR-Cas9 system. Frontiers of Plant Science 8, 1932. https://doi.org/10.3389/fpls.2017.01932.

Baeshen, N.A., Baeshen, M.N., Sheikh, A., Bora, R.S., Ahmed, M.M., Ramadan, H.A., Saini, K.S., Redwan, E.M., 2014. Cell factories for insulin production. Microbial Cell Factories 13, 141. https://doi.org/10.1186/s12934-014-0141-0.

Baliou, S., Adamaki, M., Kyriakopoulos, A.M., Spandidos, D.A., Panayiotidis, M., Christodoulou, I., Zoumpourlis, V., 2018. Role of the CRISPR system in controlling gene transcription and monitoring cell fate. Molecular Medicine Reports 17 (1), 1421−1427.

Bao, A., Burritt, D.J., Chen, H., Zhou, X., Cao, D., Tran, L.P., 2019. The CRISPR/Cas9 system and its applications in crop genome editing. Critical Reviews in Biotechnology 39 (3), 321−336. https://doi.org/10.1080/07388551.2018.1554621.

Bawa, A.S., Anilakumar, K.R., 2013. Genetically modified foods: safety, risks and public concerns—a review. Journal of Food Science and Technology 50 (6), 1035−1046. https://doi.org/10.1007/s13197-012-0899-1.

Berg, P., Baltimore, D., Boyer, H.W., Cohen, S.N., Davis, R.W., Hogness, D.S., et al., 1974. Potential biohazards of recombinant DNA molecules. Science (New York, NY) 185 (4148), 303.

Beyer, P., Al-Babili, S., Ye, X., Lucca, P., Schaub, P., Welsch, R., Potrykus, I., 2002. Golden rice: introducing the β-carotene biosynthesis pathway into rice endosperm by genetic engineering to defeat vitamin A deficiency. The Journal of Nutrition 132 (3), 506S−510S.

Borlaug, N.E., 2002. The Green Revolution Revisited and the Road Ahead. Nobelprize. org, Stockholm, Sweden. https://www.nobelprize.org/prizes/peace/1970/borlaug/article/.

Boyer, J.S., 1982. Plant productivity and environment. Science 218 (4571), 443−448.

Chatterjee, N., Walker, G.C., 2017. Mechanisms of DNA damage, repair, and mutagenesis. Environmental and Molecular Mutagenesis 58 (5), 235−263. https://doi.org/10.1002/em.22087.

Clark, D.P., Pazdernik, N.J., 2015. Biotechnology, Applying the Genetic Revolution, second ed. Elsevier Inc. ISBN 978-0-12-385015-7.

Cohen, S.N., Chang, A.C., Boyer, H.W., Helling, R.B., 1973. Construction of biologically functional bacterial plasmids in vitro. Proceedings of the National Academy of Sciences of the United States of America 70 (11), 3240−3244.

Costantini, F., Lacy, E., 1981. Introduction of a rabbit beta-globin gene into the mouse germ line. Nature 294, 92−94.

De Bodt, S., Maere, S., Van de Peer, Y., 2005. Genome duplication and the origin of angiosperms. Trends in Ecology and Evolution 20, 591−597.

Duffy, J.B., 2002. GAL4 system in Drosophila: a fly geneticist's Swiss army knife. Genesis 34 (1−2), 1−15.

Directive 2001/18/EC of the European Parliament and of the Council on the deliberate release into the environment of genetically modified organisms and repealing Council Directive 90/220/EEC. Official Journal L 106, March 12, 2001.

Elitzur, T., Yakir, E., Quansah, L., Zhangjun, F., Vrebalov, J., Khayat, E., Giovannoni, J.J., Friedman, H., 2016. Banana MaMADS transcription factors are necessary for fruit ripening and molecular tools to promote Shelf-life and food security. Plant Physiology 171, 380−391.

FAO, 2015. Save Food: Global Inintiative on Food Loss and Wast Reduction. http://www.fao.org/save-food/resources/infographic/en/.

Fawcett, J.A., Van de Peer, Y., 2010. Angiosperm polyploids and their road to evolutionary success. Trends in Evolutionary Biology 2, e3 16−21.

Franzke, A., Lysak, M.A., Al-Shehbaz, I.A., Koch, M.A., Mummenhoff, K., 2011. Cabbage family affairs: the evolutionary history of Brassicaceae. Trends in Plant Science 16 (2), 108−116. https://doi.org/10.1016/j.tplants.2010.11.005.

Gaines, T.A., Zhang, W., Wang, D., Bukun, B., Chisholm, S.T., Shaner, D.L., et al., 2010. Gene amplification confers glyphosate resistance in *Amaranthus palmeri*. Proceedings of the National Academy of Sciences of the United States of America 107 (3), 1029−1034.

Gasser, C.S., Fraley, R.T., 1989. Genetically engineering plants for crop improvement. Science 244 (4910), 1293−1299.

Gautheret, R.J., 1983. Plant tissue culture: a history. The botanical magazine= Shokubutsu-gaku-zasshi 96 (4), 393−410.

Gordon, J.W., Scangos, G.A., Plotkin, D.J., Barbosa, J.A., Ruddle, F.H., 1980. Genetic transformation of mouse embryos by microinjection of purified DNA. Proceedings of the National Academy of Sciences of the United States of America 77, 7380−7384.

Gosal, S.S., Grewal, H.S., 1991. Tissue culture propagation: problems and potentials. In: Horticulture—New Technologies and Applications. Springer, Dordrecht, pp. 197−200.

Haberlandt, G., 1902. Uber die Statolithefunktion der Starkekoner. Berichte der Deutschen Botanischen Gesellschaft 20, 189−195.

Hammer, K., Khoshbakht, K., 2015. A domestication assessment of the big five plant families. Genetic Resources and Crop Evolution 62 (5), 665−689.

Hancock, J.F., 2012. Plant Evolution and the Origin of Crop Species, third ed. CABI. ISBN 978-1-84593-801-7.

Heuer, H., Smalla, K., 2007. Horizontal gene transfer between bacteria. Environmental Biosafety Research 6 (1−2), 3−13.

Hutchison, W.D., Burkness, E.C., Mitchell, P.D., Moon, R.D., Leslie, T.W., Fleischer, S.J., et al., 2010. Area wide suppression of European corn borer with Bt maize reaps savings to non-Bt maize growers. Science 330 (6001), 222–225.

James, C., Krattiger, A.F., 1996. Global Review of the Field Testing and Commercialization of Transgenic Plants, 1986 to 1995: The First Decade of Crop Biotechnology. ISAAA Briefs No. 1. ISAAA, Ithaca, NY, p. 31.

Jobling, S.A., Westcott, R.J., Tayal, A., Jeffcoat, R., Schwall, G.P., 2002. Production of a freeze–thaw-stable potato starch by antisense inhibition of three starch synthase genes. Nature Biotechnology 20 (3), 295.

Jørgensen, J.H., 1988. Genetic analysis of barley mutants with modifications of powdery mildew resistance gene Ml-a12. Genome 30 (2), 129–132.

Kallscheuer, N., 2018. Engineered microorganisms for the production of food additives approved by the European Union-a systematic analysis. Frontiers in Microbiology 9, 1746. https://doi.org/10.3389/fmicb.2018.01746.

Khoshbakht, K., Hammer, K., 2010. Threatened Crop Species Diversity. Shahid Behesti University Press, Teheran.

Kloppenburg, J.R., 2005. First the Seed: The Political Economy of Plant Biotechnology, second ed. Univ. of Wisconsin Press, p. 79. ISBN-10: 9780299192440.

Komaki, S., Schnittger, A., 2017. The spindle assembly checkpoint in arabidopsis is rapidly shut off during severe stress. Developmental Cell 43 (2), 172–185. https://doi.org/10.1016/j.devcel e5.

Ladizinsky, G., 1985. The genetics of hard seed coat in the genus Lens. Euphytica 34 (2), 539–543.

Ladizinsky, G., Abbo, S., 2015. The lens genus. In: The Search for Wild Relatives of Cool Season Legumes. Springer, Cham, pp. 1–28.

Lee, K., 2005. Biotic artefacts: mendelian genetics and hybridisation. In: Philosophy and Revolutions in Genetics. Palgrave Macmillan, London, pp. 83–111. ISBN 978-1-4039-4708-6.

Lee, T.H., Ho, H.K., Leung, T.F., 2017. Genetically modified foods and allergy. Hong Kong Medical Journal 23 (3), 291–295. https://doi.org/10.12809/hkmj166189.

Lee, Y.J., Liu, B., 2019. Microtubule nucleation for the assembly of acentrosomal microtubule arrays in plant cells. New Phytologist 222 (4), 1705–1718. https://doi.org/10.1111/nph.15705.

Liu, X., Xie, C., Si, H., Yang, J., 2017. CRISPR/Cas9-mediated genome editing in plants. Methods 121–122, 94–102. https://doi.org/10.1016/j.ymeth.2017.03.009.

Lu, W., Zhang, Y., Liu, D., Songyang, Z., Wan, M., 2013. Telomeres-structure, function, and regulation. Experimental Cell Research 319 (2), 133–141. https://doi.org/10.1016/j.yexcr.2012.09.005.

Ma, J.K., Drake, P.M., Christou, P., 2003. Genetic modification: the production of recombinant pharmaceutical proteins in plants. Nature Reviews Genetics 4 (10), 794.

Macek, T., Kotrba, P., Svatos, A., Novakova, M., Demnerova, K., Mackova, M., 2008. Novel roles for genetically modified plants in environmental protection. Trends in Biotechnology 26 (3), 146–152.

Magaña-Gómez, J.A., Calderón de la Barca, A.M., 2009. Risk assessment of genetically modified crops for nutrition and health. Nutrition Reviews 67 (1), 1–16.

Maliga, P., Sz-Breznovits, A., Márton, L., 1973. Streptomycin-resistant plants from callus culture of haploid tobacco. Nature: New Biology 244 (131), 29.

Mello, C.C., Conte, D., 2004. Revealing the world of RNA interference. Nature 431 (7006), 338–342.

Mingchun, L., Gomes, B.L., Mila, I., Purgatto, E., Peres, L.E.P., Frasse, P., Maza, E., Zouine, M., Roustan, J.-P., Bouzayen, M., Pirrello, J., 2016. Comprehensive profiling of ethylene response factor expression identifies ripening-associated ERF genes and their link to key regulators of fruit ripening in tomato. Plant Physiology 170, 1732–1744.

Mirzaghaderi, G., Mason, A.S., 2017. Revisiting pivotal-differential genome evolution in wheat. Trends in Plant Science 22 (8), 674–684. https://doi.org/10.1016/j.tplants.2017.06.003.

Naves, E.R., de Ávila Silva, L., Sulpice, R., Araújo, W.L., Nunes-Nesi, A., Peres, L.E.P., Zsögön, A., 2019. Capsaicinoids: pungency beyond capsicum. Trends in Plant Science 24 (2), 109–120. https://doi.org/10.1016/j.tplants.2018.11.001.

Nordlee, J.A., Taylor, S.L., Townsend, J.A., Thomas, L.A., Bush, R.K., 1996. Identification of a Brazil-nut allergen in transgenic soybeans. New England Journal of Medicine 334, 688–692.

Paszkowski, J., Shillito, R.D., Saul, M., Mandak, V., Hohn, T., Hohn, B., Potrykus, I., 1984. Direct gene transfer to plants. The EMBO Journal 3 (12), 2717–2722.

Pierik, R.L.M., 1991. Commercial aspects of micropropagation. In: Horticulture—new Technologies and Applications. Springer, Dordrecht, The Netherlands, pp. 141–153.

Pistrick, K., 2003. Mansfeld's encyclopedia of agricultural and horticultural crops and the Mansfeld phenomenon. Rudolf Mansfeld and plant genetic resources. Schriften zu Genetischen Ressourcen 22, 21–31.

Prescott, V.E., Campbell, P.M., Moore, A., Mattes, J., Rothenberg, M.E., Foster, P.S., Higgins, T.J., Hogan, S.P., 2005. Transgenic expression of bean alpha-amylase inhibitor in peas results in altered structure and immunogenicity. Journal of Agricultural and Food Chemistry 53, 9023–9030.

Radford, S.J., Nguyen, A.L., Schindler, K., McKim, K.S., 2017. The chromosomal basis of meiotic acentrosomal spindle assembly and function in oocytes. Chromosoma 126 (3), 351–364. https://doi.org/10.1007/s00412-016-0618-1.

Ray, L., Pramanik, S., Bera, D., 2016. Enzymes- an existing and promising tool of food processing industry. Recent Patents on Biotechnology 10 (1), 58–71.

Roy, R.N., Finck, A., Blair, G.J., Tandon, H.L.S., 2006. Plant nutrition for food security. A guide for integrated nutrient management. FAO Fertilizer and Plant Nutrition Bulletin 16, 368.

Rubin, G.M., Spradling, A.C., 1982. Genetic transformation of *Drosophila* with transposable element vectors. Science 218 (4570), 348–353.

Sablowski, R., 2016. Coordination of plant cell growth and division: collective control or mutual agreement? Current Opinion in Plant Biology 34, 54–60. https://doi.org/10.1016/j.pbi.2016.09.004.

Sanchis, V., 2011. From microbial sprays to insect-resistant transgenic plants: history of the biopesticide *Bacillus thuringiensis*. A review. Agronomy for Sustainable Development 31 (1), 217–231.

Sanghera, G.S., Wani, S.H., Hussain, W., Singh, N.B., 2011. Engineering cold stress tolerance in crop plants. Current Genomics 12 (1), 30.

Sinclair, T.R., 2011. Challenges in breeding for yield increase for drought. Trends in Plant Science 16 (6), 289–293.

Smith, E.F., Townsend, C.O., 1907. A plant-tumor of bacterial origin. Science 25 (643), 671–673.

Soltis, D.E., Albert, V.A., Leebens-Mack, J., Bell, C.D., Paterson, A.H., Zheng, C., Sankoff, D., Depamphilis, C.W., Wall, P.K., Soltis, P.S., 2009. Polyploidy and angiosperm diversification. American Journal of Botany 96, 336–348.

Sonnante, G., Hammer, K., Pignone, D., 2009. From the cradle of agriculture a handful of lentils: history of domestication. Rendiconti Lincei 20 (1), 21–37.

Tsatsakis, A.M., Nawaz, M.A., Kouretas, D., Balias, G., Savolainen, K., Tutelyan, V.A., Golokhvast, K.S., Lee, J.D., Yang, S.H., Chung, G., 2017a. Environmental impacts of genetically modified plants: a review. Environmental Research 156, 818–833. https://doi.org/10.1016/j.envres.2017.03.011.

Tsatsakis, A.M., Nawaz, M.A., Tutelyan, V.A., Golokhvast, K.S., Kalantzi, O.I., Chung, D.H., Kang, S.J., Coleman, M.D., Tyshko, N., Yang, S.H., Chung, G., 2017b. Impact on environment, ecosystem, diversity and health from culturing and using GMOs as feed and food. Food and Chemical Toxicology 107 (Pt A), 108–121. https://doi.org/10.1016/j.fct.2017.06.033.

Van de Peer, Y., Fawcett, J.A., Proost, S., Sterck, L., Vandepoele, K., 2009. The flowering world: a tale of duplications. Trends in Plant Science 14, 680–688.

Von Wright, A., Bruce, Å., 2003. 7. Genetically modified microorganisms and their potential effects on human health and nutrition. Trends in Food Science and Technology 14 (5–8), 264–276. https://doi.org/10.1016/s0924-2244(03)00068-2.

Willke, T., 2014. Methionine production–a critical review. Applied Microbiology and Biotechnology 98 (24), 9893–9914. https://doi.org/10.1007/s00253-014-6156-y.

Yamada, M., Goshima, G., 2017. Mitotic spindle assembly in land plants: molecules and mechanisms. Biology (Basel) 6 (1), E6. https://doi.org/10.3390/biology6010006.

Ye, X., Al-Babili, S., Klöti, A., Zhang, J., Lucca, P., Beyer, P., Potrykus, I., 2000. Engineering the provitamin A (beta-carotene) biosynthetic pathway into (carotenoid-free) rice endosperm. Science 287 (5451), 303–305. https://doi.org/10.1126/science.287.5451.303.

Zambryski, P., Herrera-Estrella, L., De Block, M., Van Montagu, M., Schell, J., 1984. The use of the *Ti* plasmid of *Agrobacterium* to study the transfer and expression of foreign DNA in plant cells: new vectors and methods. In: Genetic Engineering. Springer, Boston, MA, USA, pp. 253–278.

Zhang, G.C., Kong, I.I., Kim, H., Liu, J.-J., Cate, J.H.D., Jin, Y.-S., 2014. Construction of a quadruple auxotrophic mutant of an industrial polyploid *Saccharomyces cerevisiae* strain by using RNA-guided Cas9 nuclease. Applied and Environmental Microbiology 80 (24), 7694–7701. https://doi.org/10.1128/aem.02310-14.

Zhang, C., Wohlhueter, R., Zhang, H., 2016. Genetically modified foods: a critical review of their promise and problems. Food Science and Human Wellness 5 (3), 116–123. https://doi.org/10.1016/j.fshw.2016.04.002.

Zotti, M., Dos Santos, E.A., Cagliari, D., Christiaens, O., Taning, C.N.T., Smagghe, G., 2018. RNA interference technology in crop protection against arthropod pests, pathogens and nematodes. Pest Management Science 74 (6), 1239–1250. https://doi.org/10.1002/ps.4813.

Further reading

Ahmed, F.E., 2003. Genetically modified probiotics in foods. Trends in Biotechnology 21 (11), 491–497 (Review).

De Vos, C.J., Swanenburg, M., 2018. Health effects of feeding genetically modified (GM) crops to livestock animals: a review. Food and Chemical Toxicology 117, 3–12. https://doi.org/10.1016/j.fct.2017.08.031. Epub 2017 Aug 31. Review.

Dunfield, K.E., Germida, J.J., 2004. Impact of genetically modified crops on soil- and plant-associated microbial communities. Journal of Environmental Quality 33 (3), 806–815 (Review).

FAO, 2019. Save Food: Global Initiative on Food Loss and Waste Reduction. http://www.fao.org/save-food/resources/infographic/en/.

Gasson, M.J., 2000. Gene transfer from genetically modified food. Current Opinion in Biotechnology 11 (5), 505–508 (Review).

Venter, H.J., Bøhn, T., 2016. Interactions between Bt crops and aquatic ecosystems: a review. Environmental Toxicology and Chemistry 35 (12), 2891–2902. https://doi.org/10.1002/etc.3583. Epub. 2016 Sep 26 (Review).

A perspective on the evolution of genetic manipulation of biological materials, both plant and animal

J.M. Regenstein

Professor, Emeritus of Food Science, Head of the Cornell Kosher and Halal Food Initiative, Cornell University, Ithaca, NY, United States

GMOs are one of the most significant advancements in how the food supply and many other industries can address the needs of the future. Scientists have worked hard to develop and test these needed technologies for efficacy and safety. Then why is there such pushback on genetically modified organism (GMO) products in the food system? That is a complicated issue. One way to approach this is to look at the history of GMO itself, but also at a number of other issues that all have made for the perfect storm, a negative perception of GMO by consumers.

There seem to be four aspects to this story. The first is the lack of understanding of what GMOs are and how they came about, i.e., how they fit into a bigger picture of how we get our food supply and how it is or is not regulated. This chapter will focus on telling this story in broad strokes.

The second aspect is the dramatic change in the information age with the advent of computers, the internet, and social media. The whole way information has become more available but less reliable. A new world where what is fact, truth, perception, or reality are all much more fluid and varied. Thus, consumers are receiving a lot of information, and the negative information tends to be the ones that are easier to remember, scarier, and often wrong or misleading. The public's perception of GMOs seems to have been shaped by such information along with a failure of those able to provide positive information to even try to compete in the modern information age.

The third aspect is a change in how consumers interact with their purchases, particularly food, but also with many other purchases. The key word here is probably "transparency," although few actually know just what this means and what is a reasonable expectation? How much does one want to know about something other than everything, how much does someone really need to know, and how much will unnecessary information add to the cost of goods? Thus, the food industry has suffered at times because of a failure to tell consumers enough about product

Genetically Modified and Irradiated Food. https://doi.org/10.1016/B978-0-12-817240-7.00002-4

changes as they made them in a way that met consumer needs. Therefore, the consumers' trust of the food industry is lower than it ought to be, given the efforts that it has made to meet consumer expectations for a safe, high-quality food supply. Unfortunately, however, there are those in the food industry who feel they have something to gain by being misleading and even dishonest or by not doing the best job of assuring the quality and safety of food. Yet, the large number of recalls for food safety issues—much more publicized than any positive news—has also helped to erode consumer confidence in the food industry.

And the fourth aspect is the need to understand consumer motivation, values, and ethical beliefs. The assumption that everyone agrees on some fundamental values about food may be more complex and diverse than it appears at first. With globalization, polarization, and nationalism, many complex interactions emerge. For example, consumers in Europe have very different attitudes than Americans, and it is less clear how the rest of the world perceives many issues dealing with food. Again some of the "noise" on these issues comes from those most concerned about these issues often with a specific agenda, and they probably have the best access to having their voices heard. Thus, it is not clear where society may be heading and how moving forward consumer needs will be determined and then addressed. Certainly with globalization, there is a need to understand many more different consumers. Hopefully, scientists, communicators, industry, and the regulators will all listen to consumers but also take a leadership role in explaining in appropriate and respectful way what is happening that is new and possibly frightening for just that reason. Biotechnology and its resultant products such as GMO foods offer great potential, but only if the citizens of the world accept and, hopefully, support efforts to use this technology wisely. The industry has a responsibility to determine in consultation with the other stakeholders what is "responsible use."

To start the more detailed discussion, it may be helpful to look in very broad terms at how humankind got to where it is today. Human's earliest ancestors started the separation from their primate ancestors while still presumably being hunters/gatherers. At some point in time, they realized that they could grow certain crops, i.e., collect the seeds and plant them where they were more convenient, either closer to their camps or on land where they grew better or could be protected from other hunters/gatherers. And some of the animals could be captured alive and kept under their control. So began the long slow course of domestication (which might also be considered their loss of being natural—is anything that has been domesticated really natural?) of plants and animals.

Once they started along this line, at some point, they realized that they could start to select seeds or animals for the more beneficial traits by selecting those plants or animals that had the traits they found appropriate. These traits may have included better yield but may also have included many other factors like hardiness, i.e., the ability to survive the winter and possibly being docile for animals.

With these developments came new knowledge and a new realization. When they learned how plants and animals reproduced, they could begin to control this process. (With the suspicion that they learned how animals did reproduce a lot sooner than the plants!) They could decide which males to mate with which females among the animals, and they sometimes were able to control the mating of plants, which was took a lot more insight into empirical biology.

And then there were two other ideas that had to enter their understanding. The first was the idea that they could go beyond local to get a mate. They could bring plants and animals from other places and share good genetic traits. This also increased the risk, as they may not have been as familiar with the traits of the distant mate.

The second idea is that of hybridization. Keeping the male and female of the production species apart and breeding them separately until such time as they needed to be brought together to actually have the "food" version. This leads to what is now called "hybrid vigor." The modern poultry meat industry is based heavily on this fundamental biological principle.

While this was going on, humans were also becoming better and better farmers. So not only could they use breeding to improve the genetics, but they could do a better job of taking advantage of these materials. So all these improvements and the requirements needed to optimize these changes provided feedback to the breeder, working together with the farmer (who were often one and the same anyway at that time).

And supposedly starting with the famous monk, Mendel, humans were beginning the process of understanding the concepts of genetic, i.e., the ideas that eventually led to the understanding of chromosomes and genes, but starting first with simple observational work. They eventually learned that each species generally has a fixed number of chromosomes and they work in pairs. Sex then gets simplified down to dividing the entire set of chromosomes between two different cells (male and female) that only have one of each chromosome. The full set of chromosomes being randomly distributed into the male and female cells (i.e., sperm and egg). The randomness is important as it permits the diversity that is seen with siblings. Sex then brings the male and female cells, each with a single set of chromosomes, together to form the normal paired chromosomes of the next generation. Once fertilization occurs, the process of growth of cells with paired chromosomes takes place, i.e., each cell division gives each new cell a full set of paired chromosomes.

The genetic concepts were developed as part of the development of modern biology. To understand the chromosome is the start of understanding "molecular biology." Any one chromosome has many genes. Each gene codes for a protein. In a normal, nonreproductive cell, the genes on the two chromosomes will generally code for the same "gene product" but are not the same in their fine detail. So, if an animal has brown eyes, each chromosome's gene for eye color may be brown, but it also may be the case that one gene is for brown and the gene on the other chromosome is for blue. Remember that the pair of chromosomes represents one from the mother and one from the father. Even though both parents have brown eyes, the offsprings can still have another colored eye. If the animal has blue eyes and mates with a blue-eyed mate, then the offspring always has blue eyes. What does that suggest? That the blue-eye gene is recessive and the brown-eye gene is dominant. To get brown eyes, one only needs one of the genes on one of the chromosomes. But to get blue-eyes one needs to get the blue-eye gene from both parents. That is an oversimplified version of classical Mendelian genetics.

As the breeders came to learn, many traits are more complicated. (Some modern scientists and historians of science even questioned whether Mendel's results were just lucky and did he bury results that did not agree with his ideas?) Some genes are not so clearly dominant and recessive—and one can get a result somewhere in between. For example, the level of an enzyme might be higher with both genes able to produce a workable version while it would be lower if one had only one "working" gene or a less robust version.

As an aside, the issue of how a scientist views data is complicated. Early on Mendel might actually have helped progress by focusing on those results that he could at least understand. By burying data he did not understand, he moved the field forward. And eventually science rejected his approach and complicate things—but by then science and scientists were ready to deal with greater complexity that could be built on the foundation that Mendel and his early colleagues gave us. The path of scientific progress is not always straightforward.

Returning to the genes. Of course, with all this mixing and mingling, there is also the danger that one may have a "bad" gene that gets a chance to be expressed. For example, if both parents have a "recessive" gene for something bad, the bringing together of two relatively healthy parents (i.e., with respect to the trait under consideration) may lead to an offspring that is not healthy because the two recessive genes caused problems for the offspring. On the other hand, with luck (i.e., the randomness of the process), those two recessive genes might also be beneficial. And what is a "good" or "bad" gene may very much depend on the context of the overall animal or plant's genetics and of the needs of farmers/society at the time the selection decision is made. A human example is sickle cell anemia. It is viewed as a disease but in some circumstances, it is lifesaving.

Therefore, there are a lot of genes that breeders ideally would like to keep track of. Until very recently for many different reasons, this was essentially impossible. First, no one knew what all the genes were and certainly had no way to keep tract of them. With whole genome sequencing, it is possible to identify all the genes, but this has also led to the understanding that not every gene codes for a protein and the functions associated with the protein. Scientists actually expected that there would be more genes than actually found. Computers, artificial intelligence and big data are all rather recent technologies, and the breeders in the past could only deal with improving key traits. Sometimes because the gene is part of a larger chromosome, it was not possible to breed only for a single trait; the other traits on that chromosome came along at the same time. And sometimes the impact of those other genes and the changes they caused were subtle, while the selected trait made measureable improvements. Thus, the new seed or animal was "accepted" in the system for growing and breeding. But over time that slightly changed trait might cease to be subtle, i.e., when matched with its "paired" gene from other sources of that trait, the results might become obviously negative (or positive). At other times, the trait may not have changed but the changes due to the genes that were being selected for might make the "normal" trait inadequate. For example, as the weight of a broiler (meat) chicken increased, mainly as increased breast muscle (white meat), their legs were not able to support the birds' body. This meant that the animal was no longer able to function well.

Through all this new knowledge, the breeders also began to learn that they could breed for "less objective" traits including issues such as calmness or sociability. So the breeders could really make a lot of progress. And, of course, as the world got smaller, breeders could share parent genetic stocks (i.e., animals and seeds) around the world. And thus traits that had been developed in various parts of the world could be shared.

Important note: Although the discussion is focusing on "a" gene, it should be understood that many traits involve complex interactions between multiple genes. This complicates the process but does not have a major impact on the bigger picture issues that this chapter is trying to address.

And then, in fairly recent times, the scientists were ready for a major shift in their thinking. The first was the idea that they could "interfere" with the genetic process. That is, breeders could, for example, treat seeds with mutagens (chemicals) or radiation to intentionally mutate genes. Mutations occur naturally and they have been a source of both good and bad genes. They were always the wild card in all the breeding taking places. Natural genes would sometimes change. Whether good or bad, it made the breeder's job more difficult because it was a "rules" change in the middle of the game. Most times mutations are a "disaster," but sometimes they are just great. Those changes that were useful were a key to understand evolution as started as a subject within biology by Charles Darwin. What followed, i.e., the natural selection process would take advantage of these mutations and adjust plants and animals to their environment was a powerful and in its time (and to some extent still is) a very controversial idea. The selection of the best genes and the decision of what to do with a mutation were critical to how plants and animals naturally coped with their environment and gained a competitive advantage. The competitive advantage allowed those plants or animals with that new trait to better compete with both other plants/animals of the same species and often with other plants and animals. Eventually scientists realized that overall mutations (even though very few were positive) were extremely important in making new traits possible. Through all of this, it could be argued that genetics has from the beginning been allowing humans to be "playing G-d." As a concept this has been going on for a long time, long before the modern controversy over GMO. This will need further discussion later in the essay.

But what happens when chemicals and radiation are used to speed up the natural rate of mutations? Like natural mutations, most of these mutations are bad. However, the issue of statistics needs to be introduced. Although only one in a thousand or some other really bad odds are involved, an occasional gene would modify a trait in a positive way. With lots of seeds, those odds could be acceptable. The one positive trait could often more than justify the costs associated with finding it. Again, plants that were annuals and were easily grown in large numbers were most successfully used in this process. Trees and animals are harder to intentionally mutate. But now the bad news. The mutations may be anywhere along the chromosome. So what if one had one good mutation on a gene that was part of the genes the breeder was selecting for and you also had a less obvious (i.e., not lethal or obviously noticed) change in another trait. That "bad" gene as was already pointed out might eventually express itself in a way that is detrimental to the plant when it finds itself in new circumstances not studied by the breeder and the breeder was unaware of this. It is now in the "gene pool" and, in fact, is heavily promoted because it is free riding with a gene that was desirable. The plant (or animal) may become very vulnerable, and if it has been a widely promoted cultivar, it could have very serious negative implications. As all of this was happening, the scientists were working on trying to understand more and more about what was going on "underneath the hood." This reached an important step with the discovery of the genetic code and the structure of DNA by James Watson and Francis Crick along with work that was done by Rosalind Franklin although she did not get as much credit! And from that start, scientists have learned a great deal about the make up of genes and chromosomes and all the complications that go with making these systems work properly. That is, how a DNA gene codes for a protein (and how proteins sometimes get modified after they are first made), how to turn genes on and off, and how both reproduction of cells with both chromosomes going together and with the two chromosomes separating happens. And they have learned how to remove pieces of a chromosome and reproduce that in a test tube. So if they cut a chromosome in the right place, they can have a gene in a test tube and can make lots of copies. The simplest technique is called PCR (polymerase chain reaction). So you can have lots of a single gene to work with, i.e., many, many copies.

The next step was to figure out how to get that gene into another organism, one that does not have that gene but might benefit from it, i.e., the plant or animal might be able to do something it cannot do and would take a long time to get to happen with traditional breeding. In other cases, it is only of benefit to humans without harming the organism. Examples include when a microbe is used to produce a desirable chemical, such as chymosin. Another example is to have a banana or tobacco leaf produce a human vaccine. It should be noted that to the surprise of many scientists, microbes have been swapping genes all along without human help. So, the scientists were able to piggyback on these natural processes, but with time they also discovered new ways to get genes into microbes. And so, companies began to make a lot of different and interesting chemicals (including medicines) cheaper and faster by letting the microbes do the work. The first such product for the food industry was the cheese-clotting enzyme chymosin, mentioned above, which was the first of many food enzymes now being made in bacteria factories, i.e., microbial fermenters. Other enzymes are used by other industries and some are used by the medical profession. So lots of exciting developments. And interestingly enough, most of these materials have not been questioned. This, in part, may be due to the fact that the compounds produced are purified before they are used. And for food use, all of the microbes have to be ones with a long history of safe use by humans.

But the harder challenge was to figure out how to get new genes into plants and animals, where the scientists had to get it in, but they also had to sometimes get the new gene in the right place. Scientists work on these kinds of problems until they solve them. And they did. So, they learned to add traits to plants. And the companies doing this work were already heavily involved in agriculture, often in the area of dealing with all the other organisms that wanted to eat our human food before humans could harvest and process it, i.e., the broad area of pesticides. And these companies realized that they would have to first convince farmers to use these modified crops, which meant they have to address agricultural issues. Therefore, the first products generally did not resonate with consumers (and were not meant to). However, the agricultural companies did not always realize the need to bring consumers along as they did these marvelous things on the farm. They were focused on communicating with the farmers. And so others, mostly those with an unfavorable view of these processes (often with an agenda that opposes these technologies to fit their bigger agenda) got to tell the story and it was to their advantage to tell negative stories. Many organizations, often referred to as nongovernmental organizations or NGOs need to constantly raise money to pay for themselves: their salaries, pensions, offices, etc. They have to convince some number of people to share their hard-earned funds with these folks. And negative stories are so much more interesting and often scary and definitely help with fund raising. Unfortunately, a great deal of misinformation was communicated to consumers by these people and the level of misinformation accepted by consumers is rather high, strengthening the anti-GMO sentiment.

But returning to the main story, over time the scientists moving genes started to look at all sorts of other things, beyond the emphasis on using the new technology for biological pest control, recognizing that they could do many other beneficial things with the technologies at hand. And so slowly but surely, more and more traits are being added to plants (and animals, but that is a separate story) that will make consumers' life better in ways that they can observe: The prevention of spoilage, better flavor, more nutrients, and other good stuff for all of us. A few of these consumer-oriented traits in some products have been developed, but consumers remain reluctant to use them, even if it makes the product safer for consumers. For example, potatoes and other starchy foods when heated to higher temperatures (often with frying) will produce a possibly toxic compound called acrylamide. But a potato that was designed to produce less acrylamide during use has so far been rejected by enough consumers that the industry is not adopting this technology.

It should also be noted that even though the biological control of pests has been controversial, it has also been shown that the use of these crops has cut down the amount of pesticide being used in food production. There is a trade-off between chemical and biological compounds. And even when pesticides are used, the plants-modified genes allow these pesticides to be used more efficiently and less often. It has been pointed out that the strong anti-GMO sentiment in Europe means that they are continuing to use more pesticides. There are real trade-offs, and the failure to adopt GMO technology comes with its own price, especially environmentally.

It is worth noting that over time it is to be expected that some of the first generation of pesticide/plant systems will lead to pest-resistance developing among the pest being targeted. By careful management of the systems, e.g., adding a small area of nontreated crops gives the pest food so that the selection for resistance is less. Thus, the speed of the process can be slowed, but it is happening and the seed companies and pesticide companies (often one and the same) are working on the next generation.

At the same time farmers in the developing world have come to realize that these modified products are really good for them too. A key point is that pesticides are expensive and hard to handle, and buying modern farm equipment is very expensive. But buying better seeds, especially ones that replace more expensive pesticides, is a good thing and actually might be affordable by the small farmers around the world. So currently (2019), over half of the modern genetically modified products are used in the emerging economies. And in some countries the farmers are actually protesting that their governments are too slow to accept these technologies. Farmers are trying to address the need for more food and thus recognize the benefits of many new developments in agricultural sciences. But they need access to these technologies in an affordable way.

And as climate change continues to increase with all its potential challenges, more and more crops are being genetically modified to deal with the issues that plants may face in the future: warmer temperatures, more storms, more salinity in the soil, and new and different pests. As humans, it is important to recognize that a number of other creatures want to eat our food. So the issue is not whether pesticides are needed, but how the farmers will protect their crops. One commentator pointed out that most of the world's farmers are organic, not by choice but by necessity. And the system is not producing enough food to feed the people of their country.And in recent years, science has taken one more step. It is called CRISPER (sp) and it is the ability to actually modify the gene where it is, that is to make changes in situ. This science is just on the cusp of explosive growth and new opportunities. It is also presenting new regulatory challenges, because it does not "mix" species, which has been the premise of the regulations for current GMO products. And this new technology will also bring new ethics questions along the lines of if scientists can do something, do they do it. The issue of "playing G-d" continues to require the attention of ethicists, scientists, policy-makers, and consumers. The recent apparently unauthorized use of this technology to modify two babies before birth has certainly highlighted this concern. But again, the use of a technology and the specific applications need to be separated. The new technologies are powerful, but it is humans that make the decision as to what is good and what is bad.

At the same time, the first animal product has had a very complex path in its coming to market. AquaBounty has developed a salmon that grows faster because of the addition of a growth hormone gene from a different salmon species. The salmon are sterile and production is done indoors to avoid the possibility of release of living animals into the wild. The AquaBounty salmon are now available in Canada (and being used mainly for sushi [i.e., eaten raw so the modified genes are not being destroyed by heat] according to trade reports).

Although the US FDA finally approved the use of these salmon after a lot of political hesitation, it insisted that the fish be raised in the United States if it is to be sold in the United States. The company is, therefore, now building/adapting facilities to make this possible. Hopefully, that is coming soon. The author is looking forward with total confidence to try the product. So, in rather a short span of time, the entire history of agriculture has been covered. But what does it all mean?

The first and main lesson of this chapter is that what is happening in genetics is really the natural progression of science and that each new technology is more sophisticated and more powerful than the technologies before it. But, as already indicated, how it is used is up to us. (As people are learning, the Internet and the globalization of connectivity is leading to unanticipated problems from a change in social behavior to the hacking of all types of information to the world of "alt-facts.") So with all of these technologies, it will require a lot of people working together to define the parameters for the use of new technology in conjunction with the scientists and the government. Ideally these processes will be transparent and respectful of multiple opinions but also hopefully will not be poorly done because of fear and a lack of understanding of the technology. It must be recognized that policy-making is the art of compromise and that everyone will, hopefully, recognize the legitimate concerns of the many different stakeholders. It also needs to be understood that regular breeding is not going away. Not is seed mutation using chemicals. All of these technologies will be needed to address climate change and food insecurity as population increases. So which cultivars and even which crops will be planted and grown needs to be adjusted to allow humans to continue to thrive.

Sometimes what seems like improvements can themselves lead to new challenges. For example, irrigation has made it possible to grow crops in many places where it would not otherwise be possible, but all natural water has a little bit of "salts" in it. Thus, over time the salt level in soils increases and, therefore, salt-tolerant crops are necessary.

A few other specific examples of how GMO and CRISPER technology are being applied to help show the scope of what is possible. There are now some crop diseases where traditional pesticide treatments are simply not working. An example is papaya, which can only be grown in America (mainly Hawaii) with a gene resistant to the disease. Currently citrus fruits and possibly even the current Cavendish banana have diseases that have the capability according to the scientists to wipe out these commodities. Given the shortage of time to solve the problem and the long time needed with trees to do traditional breeding, these problems may only be solved with gene modification. Therefore, possibly in the near future the only choice for consumers may be to accept the use of a gene-modified product or eliminate these fruits from their diet. Also, note that as populations increase, they need more land to live. Often that means the available land for agriculture is actually decreasing. The only way to deal with this is to increase, probably dramatically, the productivity per acre/hectare of farmland. All of the breeding methods along with a lot of other technologies, will be needed to meet this challenge.

The second area that is worth considering is to present a few more examples from the food point of view of products that are being designed to meet specific needs of certain populations. Because rice is deficient in vitamin A, and many people depend on rice as their staple carbohydrate, creating golden rice was an initial high priority effort, i.e., a vitamin A—enriched rice. But the work also highlights the challenges that new food products face that go beyond the technical. Golden rice is called "Golden" because it now has a lovely yellow color—but rice is supposed to be white. So it will take a lot of education to get very traditional rice consumers to make the change.

Other efforts are going on to create products with easily identifiable traits that consumers relate to. In addition to the previous potato example, other efforts include apples that do not brown after cutting. And long-term work is being done to bring back the stronger, more traditional tasting tomato while retaining all the traits needed for it to be used commercially—either with long supply chains needed to reach consumers at retail all year around or to the many fast food dishes that include a sliced tomato. Other applications of these technologies depend only on the vision of consumers working with scientists. Beyond foods, of course, the same technology can be used to make drugs and medicines. Thus, the opportunities really are almost infinite.

So this brings us back to the issue of consumer acceptance. Very few of us have not eaten products that are produced using modern technology, including GMO. The safety of such products are well established as seen in Chapter 6 written by my colleague Robert Blair and myself, and elsewhere in this book.

On the other hand, I do criticize the scientific community, including food scientists, for not having done more to prepare consumers for this new technology, but rather try to bring it into the food supply (and other places) under the radar screen. There are too many examples in the food industry where that approach just does not work. Hopefully, with the new emphasis on transparency, the industry will provide consumers with more information about the great things they are doing. But in the new age of information overload, it is important to understand that all the information consumers wish for cannot be put on the product label. Hopefully, the government will work to have the appropriate symbols and QR codes for companies to provide the actual information at various levels of detail for different consumers without resorting to a label that is punitive and will be resisted by the industry. The idea is to use modern communications technology to inform and not to slow progress with negative information of questionable substance.

Religious viewpoints

As reported by Blair and Regenstein (2015), the Catholic Pontifical Academy of Sciences and 33 outside experts made a passionate endorsement in 2009 of GMOs for global food security and development. Their report (Meldolesi, 2011) stated that *"there is a moral imperative"* to make the benefits of genetic engineering technology *"available on a larger scale to poor and vulnerable populations who want them,"* urging opponents to consider the harm that withholding this technology will inflict on those who need it most. *Technology, in this sense, is a response to God's command to till and to keep the land (cf. Gen 2:15) that he has entrusted to humanity, and it must serve to reinforce the covenant between human beings and the environment, a covenant that should mirror God's creative love.'*

GM crops are being grown by Amish farmers in the United States, a group that follows a very traditional lifestyle.

Finally I would like to talk about the kosher and halal issues with respect to the Jewish and Muslim faiths, respectively. In the United States, approximately 40% of supermarket packaged goods are kosher, and more and more products are becoming halal. And around the world about a one-fourth of the world's population is directly impacted by the need of Muslims for halal food, either as a dietary need of the individual or by living in a country where these laws are an inherent part of the food system. In both cases, the general attitude of the religious leaders has been that these are allowable technologies and they have been accepted, and in some cases welcomed because it made possible new or better foods that were not previously available. The only exception for now of GMO materials seems to be that halal will not accept genes from porcine sources while kosher will. A brief summary of the kosher and halal laws can be found in Regenstein et al., (2003).

A consequence of this acceptance has had some interesting outcomes. One of these changes is the status of whey, the by-product of cheese making when milk is separated into Miss Muffet's "curds and whey." The use of chymosin, the microbially produced cheese-clotting enzyme that has already been discussed, was originally produced using a gene from a milk-fed calf. This has led to most whey to be kosher and thus has increased its marketability, i.e., using whey as a high-quality protein is not precluded commercially in kosher products although in the past whey could not be used in such products. (Note: whey is a "dairy" product and thus its use in kosher products is limited to products that are "dairy.")

In halal, there is also the question of tayyab, generally translated as wholesomeness. In fairness, a few Muslim leaders are raising issues with respect to this issue.

And some folks in the other religious communities are also raising some issues, often based on pushes by the antiactivists. The Animal Agricultural Alliance has undertaken to look at the issue from a Christian point of view (Jamieson et al., 2018).

In summary, the use of gene insertion technology and gene editing technology is part of the natural and continuous progression of the scientific understand of biological systems and the attempt by humans to use their skills to provide more and better appropriate foods for everyone.

References

Blair, R., Regenstein, J.M., 2015. Genetic Modification and Food Quality: A Down to Earth Analysis. Wiley-Blackwell, Oxford, UK, 276 pp.

Meldolesi, A., 2011. Vatican panel backs GMOs. Nature Biotechnology 29, 11.

Jamieson, W., Copan, P. (Eds.), 2018. What Would Jesus Really Eat. Castle Quay Books, Burlington, Ont., Canada, p. 130.

Regenstein, J.M., Chaudry, M.M., Regenstein, C.E., 2003. The kosher and halal food laws. Comparative Reviews in Food Science and Food Safety 2, 111−127.

How are genes modified? Crossbreeding, mutagenesis, and CRISPR-Cas9

Marie-Laurence Lemay, PhD[1,2]**, Sylvain Moineau**[1,2,3,4]

[1]*Département de biochimie, de microbiologie, et de bio-informatique, Faculté des sciences et de génie, Université Laval, Québec City, QC, Canada;* [2]*Groupe de recherche en écologie buccale, Faculté de médecine dentaire, Université Laval, Québec City, QC, Canada;* [3]*Félix d'Hérelle Reference Center for Bacterial Viruses, Faculté de médecine dentaire, Université Laval, Québec City, QC, Canada;* [4]*Professor, Biochemistry, Microbiology, & Bioinformatics, Université Laval, Quebec City, QC, Canada*

Glossary/abbreviations

5′-NRG	PAM recognized by SpCas9, where N = A, C, G, or T and R = A or G
5′-TTN	PAM recognized by FnCpf1, where N = A, C, G, or T
A	adenine
AAV	adeno-associated viral vector
C	cytosine
Cas gene	gene coding for Cas protein
Cas protein	CRISPR-associated protein
Cas9	a specific signature Cas protein, a nuclease used for genome editing
CjCas9	Cas9 of *Campylobacter jejuni*
Cpf1	CRISPR-associated nuclease in *Prevotella* and *Francisella*
CRISPR	clustered regularly interspaced short palindromic repeats
CRISPR-Cas9	gene-editing tool using Cas9
crRNA	CRISPR RNA dictating the specificity of the CRISPR-Cas9 tool
dCas9	catalytically dead Cas9
DNA	deoxyribonucleic acid
DSB	double-strand break
FnCpf1	Cpf1 from *Francisella novicida*
G	guanine
GMO	genetically modified organism
HDR	homology-directed recombination
HGT	horizontal gene transfer
HNH	Cas9 nuclease domain cleaving the strand complementary to the spacer
MMEJ	microhomology-mediated end joining
nCas9	Cas9 nickase cleaving only one strand of the DNA double helix
NHEJ	nonhomologous end joining
NmCas9	Cas9 of *Neisseria meningitidis*

Genetically Modified and Irradiated Food. https://doi.org/10.1016/B978-0-12-817240-7.00003-6

Nuclease	enzyme acting as molecular scissors
PAM	protospacer adjacent motif (two to six base pair DNA sequence)
PEG	polyethylene glycol
phages	bacterial viruses
RNA	ribonucleic acid
RNP	ribonucleoprotein
RuvC	Cas9 nuclease domain cleaving the strand noncomplementary to the spacer
SaCas9	Cas9 of *Staphylococcus aureus*
sgRNA	single-guide RNA, combination of crRNA and the tracrRNA
SpCas9	Cas9 of *Streptococcus pyogenes*
T	thymine
T-DNA	transferred DNA
TALEN	transcription activator-like effector nuclease
Ti	tumor-inducing
tracrRNA	trans-activating CRISPR RNA
ZFN	zinc finger nuclease

Introduction

At the beginning of agriculture, farmers promptly started to domesticate plants to produce crops with more desirable characteristics than their wild-type counterparts. Without any theoretical knowledge of genetics, they crossbred plants with different traits to produce improved hybrids. It was only in the mid-19th century that Gregor Mendel described his theory of heredity using a series of pea plant hybridization experiments (Mendel, 1866). His laws of inheritance explained how traits (phenotypes) were passed on from parents to offspring in a nonrandom fashion through defined elements (genes). It took over 3 decades for the scientific community (and the general public) to acknowledge his work, thus hindering advancements in modern genetics. In the 20th century, Mendel's discoveries transformed conventional breeding into an applied science positively correlated with the improvements in agricultural performance and quality (Hossfeld et al., 2017). While unequivocally successful, traditional plant breeding has its limitations. For example, it is constrained by fertilization incompatibility between plant species, the long generation time of crops, the extensive backcrossing required, and the lack of efficient methods of selection. Moreover, when plants are crossed, undesirable traits can also be transferred along with the trait of interest (Breseghello and Coelho, 2013).

Mutations have also been exploited for crop improvement. These mutations can naturally occur spontaneously at a very slow rate, but they can also be induced by chemicals or by physical methods. For instance, mutagenesis methods such as irradiation (X-rays and gamma-rays) of seed and plant germplasm have been exploited to generate random mutations to obtain desirable phenotypes for crop improvement. Interestingly, plant varieties generated by random mutagenesis are exempt from regulatory restrictions, licensing costs, and societal prejudice framing genetically modified organisms (GMOs) since the induced mutations could occur naturally. However, mutation breeding also has its limitations. It causes highly unpredictable DNA damage, and selection of an agronomically relevant crop mutant is an extremely laborious and time-consuming process (Georges and Ray, 2017).

As the world's population continues to rise, a new revolution in agriculture is urgently needed to reverse the declining trend in global food security. New targeted mutagenesis technologies could offer more reliable means to accelerate the pace of agricultural research and innovation (Liu et al., 2013). The groundbreaking discovery of site-directed nucleases, or molecular scissors, and the ability to deliver foreign genes into the nucleus of plant cells led to the development of powerful gene modification techniques. Meganucleases, zinc finger nucleases (ZFNs), and transcription activator-like effector nucleases (TALENs) have all proven useful for site-directed gene modification. More recently, clustered regularly interspaced short palindromic repeats (CRISPR, pronounced "crisper") and CRISPR-associated (Cas) genes coding for proteins working together with CRISPR were recognized as a powerful asset to the genetic toolbox due to their increased efficiency, versatility, and accessibility (Wright et al., 2016). Modern sequencing and genome assembly technologies as well as big data analyses also enable rational crop improvement and testing. The characterization of genetic variations and their association with agronomically relevant traits are now feasible at an unprecedented level (Bevan et al., 2017). The CRISPR-Cas9 (with CRISPR-associated protein 9) gene-editing tool offers an important alternative for overcoming the limitations of traditional breeding techniques. It has proven useful for rapidly creating desirable phenotypes in plants, but its adoption has been controversial.

According to the US Department of Agriculture (USDA), plant varieties developed using precise gene-editing technologies like CRISPR-Cas9 can be commercially grown without being regulated as GMO (USDA, 2018), whereas these crops are subjected to GMO laws in the European Union (Callaway, 2018). A negative emotional response is associated with the GMO label although scientific evidences demonstrate the safety and positive impact of GMOs. For example, they have reduced chemical pesticide use, boosted crop yields, and increased farmer profits significantly, including in developing countries (Klumper and Qaim, 2014). The opposition to GMO is often driven by fear and misinformation. This chapter explains how genes are modified, and we hope the readers will gain knowledge to form their own opinions and speak out on the issue in an informed way. Of note, in the next paragraphs, we will explain the concepts behind the CRISPR-Cas9 technology. For readers not highly familiar with this branch of biology, we encourage you to read the text while simultaneously glancing at the figures and the abbreviation list.

The microbial origin of CRISPR-Cas9

About half of the known bacteria possess a segment of genomic material consisting of a CRISPR region and *cas* genes (Burstein et al., 2016; Haft et al., 2005; Jansen et al., 2002; Mojica et al., 2005). In these microbes, CRISPR-Cas act as a natural defense mechanism against invading nucleic acids, such as DNA or RNA from bacteriophages (bacterial viruses called "phages" for short) and plasmids (mobile genetic elements). These systems are highly diverse. To-date, there are two classes, six types, and various subtypes of CRISPR-Cas systems classified according to their associated Cas genes/proteins (Makarova et al., 2015; Shmakov et al., 2017). Recent analyses of CRISPR-Cas systems in uncultivated microbes suggest that the currently known systems are just the tip of the iceberg and a vast number likely remain to be discovered (Burstein et al., 2017). Class 1 systems employ a multisubunit cleavage complex composed of numerous Cas proteins whereas class 2 systems are much simpler and employ a single multidomain Cas protein. One of the class 2 systems, type II CRISPR-Cas, is characterized by the presence of the signature protein Cas9, the widely used genome-editing enzyme (Koonin et al., 2017).

The first experimental demonstration of the adaptive immunity provided by CRISPR-Cas systems in bacteria was reported just over a decade ago (Barrangou et al., 2007). *Streptococcus thermophilus*, a bacterium used by the dairy industry to make cheese and yogurt, was shown to naturally respond to phage infection by incorporating a short DNA fragment (named a spacer) from the invading phage genome into its CRISPR region. Transcription and maturation of the CRISPR region lead to the production of several small CRISPR RNAs (crRNAs) that, individually, form a duplex with a trans-activating CRISPR RNA (tracrRNA) (Deltcheva et al., 2011). The RNA duplex becomes a tracking device as any given crRNA can bind a sequence-matching DNA (Brouns et al., 2008). Because the RNA duplex also binds to the nuclease Cas9, the tracking device can bring the molecular scissors to its matching DNA target. As such, this "surveillance/interference complex" (crRNAs + Cas9) arms the microbes to defend against subsequent invasion by foreign DNA containing a region matching the crRNA.

Interestingly, Cas9 was reported to be the only protein required for the interference process (on-target DNA cleavage) of the *S. thermophilus* type II CRISPR-Cas system (Garneau et al., 2010; Sapranauskas et al., 2011). It is the spacer in the crRNAs that dictates the specificity of the system by annealing to the corresponding sequence (protospacer) on a DNA target. Moreover, a very specific and short motif (PAM; protospacer adjacent motif) is required next to the protospacer for Cas9 to cut (Bolotin et al., 2005; Deveau et al., 2008; Mojica et al., 2009). If these requirements are met, both strands of the DNA target will be cleaved by the two catalytic domains of Cas9; HNH and RuvC. The HNH domain, named for characteristic histidine (H) and asparagine (N) residues, cleaves the strand complementary to the spacer and the RuvC domain, named after a bacterial protein involved in DNA repair, cleaves the noncomplementary strand (Nishimasu et al., 2014) (Fig. 3.1).

The acquisition of a spacer in the CRISPR region, called adaptation, is akin to immunization, although hereditary in nature. Typically, during cell division, each daughter cell inherits an identical copy of the parent cell's DNA, including the CRISPR region. This heredity means that the daughter cells can defend themselves against viruses they have not yet encountered (Fineran and Charpentier, 2012). Today, biotech industries leverage CRISPR immunization by exposing relevant

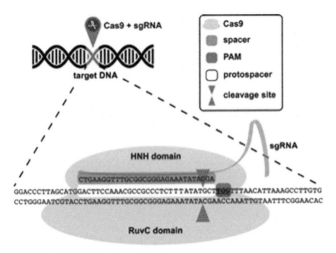

FIGURE 3.1 Cas9 site-directed nuclease.

Cas9 is the molecular scissors programmed to cleave a precise genomic region when paired with a sgRNA. The interchangeable spacer in the sgRNA dictates the specificity of the system by annealing to the corresponding sequence (protospacer) on the target DNA if that sequence is adjacent to a PAM. The catalytic domains of Cas9, HNH, and RuvC cleave both DNA strands, three nucleotides upstream of the PAM. *PAM, protospacer adjacent motif.*

Credit: Marie-Laurence Lemay.

bacterial strains to specific phages, making them more robust. This "vaccination" can even be improved by exposure to defective phages (Hynes et al., 2014). Across the globe, people have been consuming CRISPR-enhanced fermented dairy products for years as this natural system protects the "good" dairy bacteria from their natural predators, namely phages. This microbial system can now be harnessed to ensure sustainable and climate-compatible food systems.

Programmable DNA cleavage

Guided by a crRNA-tracrRNA duplex, Cas9 proteins naturally scan DNA for a specific PAM and bind their target protospacer through complementary base pairing with the spacer. Interestingly, Cas9 can be customized to target any DNA sequence upstream of a PAM by modifying the 20-nucleotide spacer sequence in the crRNA (Gasiunas et al., 2012). To make the system even simpler, the crRNA and the tracrRNA have been fused together to generate a single-guide RNA (sgRNA) (Jinek et al., 2012) (Fig. 3.1). Additionally, several sgRNAs with different spacers can be coexpressed to target multiple genes simultaneously (Cong et al., 2013). The possibility of multiplexing the CRISPR-Cas9 system is an important advantage over meganucleases, ZFNs and TALENs. For example, only a single CRISPR-Cas9 construct was needed to mutate 14 different genes at once in the model plant *Arabidopsis thaliana* (Peterson et al., 2016).

Only a few years after CRISPR-Cas9 was reported to function in several bacterial species (Sapranauskas et al., 2011), the system was successfully repurposed to edit the genome of eukaryotic cells (Cong et al., 2013; Mali et al., 2013). Currently, Cas9 from *Streptococcus pyogenes* (SpCas9) is the most intensely studied Cas protein and the most widely used for gene modification in many different plant species (Demirci et al., 2018). A key feature of SpCas9 is that it requires a 5′-NRG (where N = A, C, G, or T and R = A or G) PAM to target a sequence (Fig. 3.1). Targeting of a specific genomic region is limited by the stringency of PAM recognition.

Specificity

The PAM is a strict requirement for Cas9 targeting. Even though the PAM associated with SpCas9 (5′-NRG) is abundant in most genomes, its location might not be adequate for a specific gene modification. Target sites must be close to the genomic region to be modified. SpCas9 derivatives with altered and improved PAM specificities can address this constraint. The nuclease has been evolved to recognize a variety of less restrictive PAMs without compromising its specificity (Hu et al., 2018; Kleinstiver et al., 2015). Moreover, many Cas9 orthologues that naturally require different PAM sequences have been characterized, expanding the reach of the CRISPR-Cas9 technology. Some of these Cas9 orthologues have additional useful features. For instance, Cas9 from *Staphylococcus aureus* (SaCas9) (Ran et al., 2015), *Campylobacter jejuni* (CjCas9) (Kim et al., 2017), and *Neisseria meningitidis* (NmCas9) (Lee et al., 2016) are significantly smaller than SpCas9, so they can be packaged into adeno-associated viral vectors (AAVs) for delivery to mammalian cells.

Off-target events (Cas9 cutting an unintended target) can arise in genomic regions with high sequence similarity to the DNA target sequence. In human cells, such unpredictable mutations represent a serious concern due to the potentially unwanted damage they can induce. In plants, off-target mutations caused by CRISPR-Cas9 seem rare (Mohanta et al., 2017) and should not be a source of concern—irradiation causes far more off-target mutations. Still, the frequency of off-target events can be decreased by using different promoters or mutated versions of Cas9 (Zhang et al., 2018). As such, SpCas9 has been engineered to increase the energy of activation required for DNA cleavage and therefore limit off-target activity (Kleinstiver et al., 2016; Slaymaker et al., 2016). *In silico* prediction of potential off-target sites can inform the design of sgRNA to help avoid such off-target mutations. Mismatches in the PAM and in the seed sequence (7−12 nucleotides close to the PAM) generally prevent Cas9 interference, but some mismatches can be tolerated (Hsu et al., 2013). Additionally, NmCas9 was reported to have a lower off-target activity than wild-type SpCas9, making it an appealing alternative for precise gene modification (Lee et al.,

2016). The recent discovery of viral proteins that specifically inhibit Cas9 activity *in vivo,* thereby allowing phages to bypass the CRISPR-Cas system, offers a novel application as a backup safety measure to limit off-target effects (Stanley and Maxwell, 2018). These off-switches, called anti-CRISPR proteins, could be harnessed to restrict editing activity to particular tissues or developmental stages.

The discovery of non-Cas9 nucleases from other types of CRISPR-Cas systems has further enriched the genome-editing toolbox. Cpf1 from *Francisella novicida* (FnCpf1) is an important alternative to SpCas9 for plant gene modification (Endo et al., 2016). It generates a staggered double-strand break (DSB) on its target DNA, generating sticky ends rather than the blunt ends created by the various Cas9. This creates the possibility for directional gene integration. Moreover, FnCpf1 requires a 5′-TTN PAM, making it more suitable for modifying AT-rich genomes (Zetsche et al., 2015). Similar to Cas9, the RuvC domain of Cpf1 is required for DNA cleavage of the target strain. However, Cpf1 has a novel putative nuclease domain responsible for cleavage of the nontarget strain (Yamano et al., 2016).

Repairing the cut

Nucleases, such as Cas9, generate DSBs, in which both strands of the DNA double helix are cleaved. If not repaired, the induced break will lead to cell death. Fortunately, cells can rely on several distinct DNA repair pathways to survive (Fig. 3.2). Nonhomologous end joining (NHEJ) and microhomology-mediated end joining (MMEJ) are important repair systems, but they are also error-prone mechanisms due to the lack of fidelity, thereby resulting in the loss of genetic information (Manova and Gruszka, 2015). NHEJ is the most active repair mechanism in plants (Puchta and Fauser, 2014), and it directly stitches the broken DNA ends together. Normally, it results in perfect repair, but in some cases, such as a nuclease repetitively targeting a specific DNA sequence, this pathway creates DNA insertions or deletions (indels). Providing that the indels involve a number of base pairs that are not a multiple of three, the triplet reading frame of the gene will be disturbed, leading to a so-called frameshift mutation (Manova and Gruszka, 2015).

DNA end resection is a process that inhibits the NHEJ repair pathway by catalyzing the 5′ to 3′ degradation of DSB ends, which triggers either MMEJ or homology-directed recombination (HDR) (Huertas, 2010). During MMEJ, the DSB ends are resected until microhomologous DNA sequences are found on either side of the DSB and the ends can be rejoined to repair the break (Fig. 3.2). MMEJ often generates larger DNA deletions but can occasionally produce insertions and chromosomal rearrangements (Villarreal et al., 2012). Both NHEJ and MMEJ can be exploited as a means for generating loss-of-function mutants and for inserting exogenous donor templates into a targeted plant locus. Conversely, HDR is usually

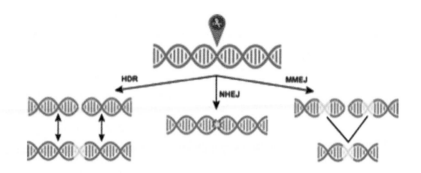

FIGURE 3.2 DNA repair mechanisms.

The two strands of the DNA double helix are cleaved by Cas9. This damage activates several DNA repair mechanisms. During HDR, a DNA template containing long DNA homologous regions at or near the breakpoint recombines with the damaged DNA. In this example, the red target sequence is replaced by the yellow sequence to avoid further cleavage by Cas9. Repair by NHEJ rejoins broken DNA ends by direct ligation and often leads to random mutations. During MMEJ, digestion of DNA strands beside the break leads to exposure and annealing of microhomologous sequences (yellow). In this example, the DNA target (red) and the regions flanking the original break are deleted. *HDR*, homology-directed recombination; *MMEJ*, microhomology-mediated end joining; *NHEJ*, nonhomologous end joining.

Credit: Marie-Laurence Lemay.

an error-free mechanism and can lead to gene modification, given that a suitable DNA template is provided (Jiang et al., 2013; Mali et al., 2013) (Fig. 3.2). Templates for HDR are designed to contain not only a desired mutation and homologous flanking arms to allow recombination, but also to lack the motif targeted by nucleases to prevent further interference. However, the efficiency of HDR is reduced due to the large proportion of DSBs repaired by NHEJ. Inactivating one of the Cas9 nuclease domains (RuvC or HNH) has been shown to increase the HDR to NHEJ ratio (Mali et al., 2013).

Both NHEJ and MMEJ repair systems impede the efficiency of HDR by competing to repair DSBs, thereby reducing the rate of precise gene modification. Still, the outcomes are highly dependent on cell type, genome site, and nuclease (Miyaoka et al., 2016). Base editing is a good alternative to rewrite specific letters in the genome. It does not require the introduction of DSB or a foreign DNA donor for HDR, but instead a mutated version of Cas9 is used. Indeed, a Cas9 nickase (nCas9) or a catalytically dead Cas9 (dCas9) is fused to an enzyme, a cytidine deaminase. While nCas9 retains the ability to cleave one DNA strand, dCas9 contains mutations that inactivate both the RuvC and HNH domains. The n/dCas9-cytidine deaminase fusion protein is programmed with a guide RNA to a target DNA locus and mediates the irreversible conversion of a cytosine (C) into a thymine (T) or a guanine (G) into an adenine (A) within a window of approximately five nucleotides

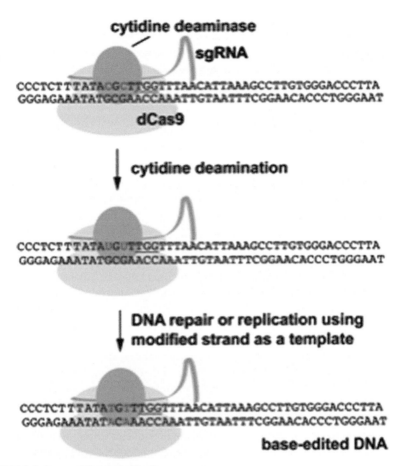

FIGURE 3.3 Base editing with dCas9.

The protein complex dCas9-cytidine deaminase is guided to a specific sequence by a sgRNA. The two C's (red) upstream of the PAM (*underlined*) are converted to U's at the target site without DSB. The U:G mismatches are then modified by the cell and result in C → T (or G → A) substitutions. *DSB*, double-strand break; *PAM*, protospacer adjacent motif.

Credit: Marie-Laurence Lemay.

(Komor et al., 2016) (Fig. 3.3). Similarly, an n/dCas9-adenosine deaminase fusion protein can convert T to C or A to G (Gaudelli et al., 2017), expanding the precise genome-editing possibilities. With this approach, single nucleotides can be modified to produce early STOP codons to inactivate genes, without DSB involvement (Billon et al., 2017). Base editing has been successfully adapted for the introduction of point mutations in rice, tomato, wheat, maize, and potato (Li et al., 2018, 2017; Ren et al., 2018; Shimatani et al., 2017; Yan et al., 2018; Zong et al., 2018, 2017).

Plant transformation

Horizontal gene transfer (HGT) is a nonsexual transfer of genes between organisms that are not in a parent-offspring relationship. It is a natural process that drives evolution of organisms and has been adapted by plant scientists to develop controversial genetically modified crops. Sweet potatoes have been eaten by humans for millennia and are one of the world's most consumed foods. Yet, they are naturally transgenic (Kyndt et al., 2015). Genome analysis revealed evidence of an ancient HGT between *Agrobacterium* and an ancestor of sweet potatoes. Remarkably, the majority of transgenes identified are still intact and their expression was detected in different plant tissues. Some transgenes were detected in all cultigens examined but not in close wild-type relatives, suggesting their involvement in traits selected for during domestication by humans.

The lack of universal, efficient, and simple transformation methods is probably among the most significant bottleneck to implementing gene editing in crops. Nevertheless, *Agrobacterium*-mediated transformation is one of the most popular methods for transferring genes into plant cells. *Agrobacterium tumefaciens* is a plant parasite naturally found in soil. This bacterium induces abnormal growths on roots upon the delivery, integration, and expression of oncogenes encoded by the T-DNA (transferred DNA) region found on the tumor-inducing (Ti) plasmid (Joos et al., 1983). Biotechnologists leveraged this ability to transfer DNA into plant cells to generate transgenic plants. For plant transformation, *A. tumefaciens* are disarmed (oncogenes are removed) but retain their ability to mediate T-DNA delivery. The T-DNA can be modified to contain the genes to be transferred, such as *cas9* and sgRNA. The engineered bacteria are incubated with plant cells, and, during infection, they deliver the gene-editing machinery that can alter the plant's genome (Fig. 3.4). The T-DNA can either integrate into the plant's genome, or it can remain extrachromosomal for transient gene expression. In these cells, the genome-editing tools do not become part of the plant's genome but just do the work of gene editing. Cas9 and the sgRNA are naturally lost, and the resulting plant can be crossed with the original one. The modified DNA is passed on through seeds, similar to traditional breeding, with no permanent introduction of foreign DNA. Many protocols have been developed and optimized for *Agrobacterium*-mediated transformation in crops, but they are limited by the bacteria's host range (Nam et al., 1997) and regeneration capacity of modified cells (Altpeter et al., 2016). Moreover, the technique is poorly suited to drive HDR since the level of DNA template delivered is often insufficient (Baltes et al., 2017).

Aside from *Agrobacterium*, the other main tools for introducing heterologous DNA into plant cells include electroporation, polyethylene glycol (PEG)-mediated transformation, and biolistics (Fig. 3.4). All three techniques can help circumvent the host-range limitations sometimes encountered with *Agrobacterium*. During electroporation, plant cells are made transiently permeable to molecules through exposure to a high-voltage electric field pulse. Subjecting membranes to such stress results in the reversible formation of pores large enough to allow macromolecules (such as DNA) to enter the cell. Generally, plant cells need to be stripped of their

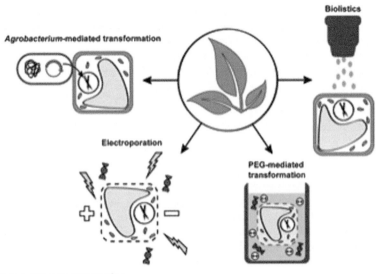

FIGURE 3.4 Plant transformation.

During *Agrobacterium*-mediated transformation, the bacterium infects a plant cell and delivers the T-DNA (*red arrow*), originally on the Ti plasmid. For electroporation and PEG-mediated transformation, plant cells are deprived of their cell walls and the protoplasts are either exposed to an electric field or incubated in a solution of PEG and divalent cations. In both cases, the membrane is destabilized and permeable to the surrounding DNA, which can be brought into the cell. Alternatively, plant cells can be bombarded (biolistic) with gold particles coated with DNA to be delivered to plant cells. *PEG*, polyethylene glycol.

Credit: Marie-Laurence Lemay.

cell walls (protoplasts) before DNA can be introduced (Potter and Heller, 2018). PEG-mediated transformation is similar to electroporation. In the presence of divalent cations, such as calcium ions (Ca^{2+}), exposure to PEG stimulates endocytosis by protoplasts (Kao and Michayluk, 1974). Gene transfer using electroporation or PEG is highly efficient, and multiple plasmids can be delivered at the same time. However, both techniques are time-consuming, labor intensive, and not all species of plant are amenable to regeneration from protoplasts.

Biolistics, or gene guns, do not require protoplast preparation. For this approach, gold particles are coated with the desired donor genes and shot at plant cells using high-pressure gas. Once inside the nucleus, the gold particles dissolve and the donor DNA can be integrated into the plant genome or transiently expressed (Sanford et al., 1993). The protocol is simple but expensive to perform. Even though multiple DNAs can be efficiently delivered concomitantly into many different tissues and cell types, the DNA integration patterns are unpredictable and the cellular target (nucleus, cytoplasm, mitochondria, or plastid) cannot be controlled (Baltes et al., 2017).

The choice of delivery method is important for plant gene modification, especially for governmental authorities since the introduction of new DNA into a cell is a red flag. Some concerns with DNA transformation include random transgene integration and imprecise levels of gene expression. Approaches for modifying plant genomes that do not require DNA delivery would prevent unwanted DNA integration and would have value in both commercial and academic settings. Precomplexed Cas9-sgRNA ribonucleoproteins (RNPs), rather than the plasmid DNAs that encode these components, can also be delivered into plant cells (Woo et al., 2015).

Conclusion

Although naturally occurring homologous recombination can be co-opted to generate mutations in a plant genome, recombination rates are very low and the selection of a specific mutant requires time-consuming large-scale screening. Site-directed gene modification offers an efficient short-cut to conventional breeding. The most popular nuclease is now Cas9 due to its simplicity and versatility, as well as its more achievable success rates at low cost. It is very likely that the CRISPR-Cas9 technology will have a significant and positive impact on food supplies across the globe. It could be harnessed to develop crops resistant to common pathogens. Ripening genes could be turned off in fruits and vegetables to slow down deterioration and reduce food waste. The first CRISPR-Cas9-modified food product to reach supermarkets (outside of the US regulatory authority) was a non-browning button mushroom (*Agaricus bisporus*) with an extended shelf life (Waltz, 2016). In the European Union, such improved foods must pass GMO legislation before they can be commercialized (Callaway, 2018), which will likely lead to lost opportunities for several farmers, the environment, and society in general. Different strategies to increase public awareness and understanding of genetic modification should be adopted and could lead to thoughtful amendments to the law.

References

Altpeter, F., Springer, N.M., Bartley, L.E., Blechl, A.E., Brutnell, T.P., Citovsky, V., et al., 2016. Advancing crop transformation in the era of genome editing. Plant Cell 28, 1510−1520.

Baltes, N.J., Gil-Humanes, J., Voytas, D.F., 2017. Genome engineering and agriculture: opportunities and challenges. Progress in Molecular Biology and Translational Science 149, 1−26.

Barrangou, R., Fremaux, C., Deveau, H., Richards, M., Boyaval, P., Moineau, S., et al., 2007. CRISPR provides acquired resistance against viruses in prokaryotes. Science 315, 1709−1712.

Bevan, M.W., Uauy, C., Wulff, B.B.H., Zhou, J., Krasileva, K., Clark, M.D., 2017. Genomic innovation for crop improvement. Nature 543, 346−354.

Billon, P., Bryant, E.E., Joseph, S.A., Nambiar, T.S., Hayward, S.B., Rothstein, R., et al., 2017. CRISPR-mediated base editing enables efficient disruption of eukaryotic genes through induction of STOP codons. Molecular Cell 67, 1068−1079.

Bolotin, A., Quinquis, B., Sorokin, A., Ehrlich, S.D., 2005. Clustered regularly interspaced short palindrome repeats (CRISPRs) have spacers of extrachromosomal origin. Microbiology 151, 2551−2561.

Breseghello, F., Coelho, A.S.G., 2013. Traditional and modern plant breeding methods with examples in rice (*Oryza sativa* L.). Journal of Agricultural and Food Chemistry 61, 8277−8286.

Brouns, S.J., Jore, M.M., Lundgren, M., Westra, E.R., Slijkhuis, R.J.H., Snijders, A.P.L., et al., 2008. Small CRISPR RNAs guide antiviral defense in prokaryotes. Science 321, 960−964.

Burstein, D., Harrington, L.B., Strutt, S.C., Probst, A.J., Anantharaman, K., Thomas, B.C., et al., 2017. New CRISPR-Cas systems from uncultivated microbes. Nature 542, 237−241.

Burstein, D., Sun, C.L., Brown, C.T., Sharon, I., Anantharaman, K., Probst, A.J., et al., 2016. Major bacterial lineages are essentially devoid of CRISPR-Cas viral defence systems. Nature Communications 7, 10613.

Callaway, E., 2018. CRISPR plants now subject to tough GM laws in European Union. Nature 560, 16.

Cong, L., Ran, F.A., Cox, D., Lin, S., Barretto, R., Habib, N., et al., 2013. Multiplex genome engineering using CRISPR/Cas systems. Science 339, 819−823.

Deltcheva, E., Chylinski, K., Sharma, C.M., Gonzales, K., Chao, Y., Pirzada, Z.A., et al., 2011. CRISPR RNA maturation by *trans*-encoded small RNA and host factor RNase III. Nature 471, 602−607.

Demirci, Y., Zhang, B., Unver, T., 2018. CRISPR/Cas9: an RNA-guided highly precise synthetic tool for plant genome editing. Journal of Cellular Physiology 233, 1844−1859.

Deveau, H., Barrangou, R., Garneau, J.E., Labonté, J., Fremaux, C., Boyaval, et al., 2008. Phage response to CRISPR-encoded resistance in *Streptococcus thermophilus*. Journal of Bacteriology 190, 1390−1400.

Endo, A., Masafumi, M., Kaya, H., Toki, S., 2016. Efficient targeted mutagenesis of rice and tobacco genomes using Cpf1 from *Francisella novicida*. Scientific Reports 6, 38169.

Fineran, P.C., Charpentier, E., 2012. Memory of viral infections by CRISPR-Cas adaptive immune systems: acquisition of new information. Virology 434, 202−209.

Garneau, J.E., Dupuis, M.E., Villion, M., Romero, D.A., Barrangou, R., Boyaval, P., et al., 2010. The CRISPR/Cas bacterial immune system cleaves bacteriophage and plasmid DNA. Nature 468, 67−71.

Gasiunas, G., Barrangou, R., Horvath, P., Siksnys, V., 2012. Cas9−crRNA ribonucleoprotein complex mediates specific DNA cleavage for adaptive immunity in bacteria. Proceedings of the National Academy of Sciences of the United States of America 109, E2579−E2586.

Gaudelli, N.M., Komor, A.C., Rees, H.A., Packer, M.S., Badran, A.H., Bryson, D.I., et al., 2017. Programmable base editing of A*T to G*C in genomic DNA without DNA cleavage. Nature 551, 464−471.

Georges, F., Ray, H., 2017. Genome editing of crops: a renewed opportunity for food security. GM Crops and Food 8, 1−12.

Haft, D.H., Selengut, J., Mongodin, E.F., Nelson, K.E., 2005. A guild of 45 CRISPR-associated (Cas) protein families and multiple CRISPR/Cas subtypes exist in prokaryotic genomes. PLoS Computational Biology 1, e60.

Hossfeld, U., Jacobsen, H.-J., Plass, C., Brors, B., Wackernagel, W., 2017. 150 years of Johann Gregor Mendel's "Versuche uber Pflanzen-Hybriden". Molecular Genetics and Genomics 292, 1−3.

Hsu, P.D., Scott, D.A., Weinstein, J.A., Ran, F.A., Konermann, S., Agarwala, V., et al., 2013. DNA targeting specificity of RNA-guided Cas9 nucleases. Nature Biotechnology 31, 827–832.

Hu, J.H., Miller, S.M., Geurts, M.H., Tang, W., Chen, L., Sun, N., et al., 2018. Evolved Cas9 variants with broad PAM compatibility and high DNA specificity. Nature 556, 57–63.

Huertas, P., 2010. DNA resection in eukaryotes: deciding how to fix the break. Nature Structural and Molecular Biology 17, 11–16.

Hynes, A.P., Villion, M., Moineau, S., 2014. Adaptation in bacterial CRISPR-Cas immunity can be driven by defective phages. Nature Communications 5, 4399.

Jansen, R., Embden, J.D., Gaastra, W., Schouls, L.M., 2002. Identification of genes that are associated with DNA repeats in prokaryotes. Molecular Microbiology 43, 1565–1575.

Jiang, W., Bikard, D., Cox, D., Zhang, F., Marraffini, L.A., 2013. RNA-guided editing of bacterial genomes using CRISPR-Cas systems. Nature Biotechnology 31, 233–239.

Jinek, M., Chylinski, K., Fonfara, I., Hauer, M., Doudna, J.A., Charpentier, E., 2012. A programmable dual-RNA-guided DNA endonuclease in adaptive bacterial immunity. Science 337, 816–821.

Joos, H., Timmerman, B., Montagu, M.V., Schell, J., 1983. Genetic analysis of transfer and stabilization of *Agrobacterium* DNA in plant cells. The EMBO Journal 2, 2151–2160.

Kao, K.N., Michayluk, M.R., 1974. A method for high-frequency intergeneric fusion of plant protoplasts. Planta 115, 355–367.

Kim, E., Koo, T., Park, S.W., Kim, D., Kim, K., Cho, H.-Y., et al., 2017. *In vivo* genome editing with a small Cas9 orthologue derived from *Campylobacter jejuni*. Nature Communications 8, 14500.

Kleinstiver, B.P., Pattanayak, V., Prew, M.S., Tsai, S.Q., Nguyen, N.T., Zheng, Z., et al., 2016. High-fidelity CRISPR-Cas9 nucleases with no detectable genome-wide off-target effects. Nature 529, 490–495.

Kleinstiver, B.P., Prew, M.S., Tsai, S.Q., Topkar, V.V., Nguyen, N.T., Zheng, Z., et al., 2015. Engineered CRISPR-Cas9 nucleases with altered PAM specificities. Nature 523, 481–485.

Klumper, W., Qaim, M., 2014. A meta-analysis of the impacts of genetically modified crops. PLoS One 9, e111629.

Komor, A.C., Kim, Y.B., Packer, M.S., Zuris, J.A., Liu, D.R., 2016. Programmable editing of a target base in genomic DNA without double-stranded DNA cleavage. Nature 533, 420–424.

Koonin, E.V., Makarova, K.S., Zhang, F., 2017. Diversity, classification and evolution of CRISPR-Cas systems. Current Opinion in Microbiology 37, 67–78.

Kyndt, T., Quispe, D., Zhai, H., Jarret, R., Ghislain, M., Liu, Q., et al., 2015. The genome of cultivated sweet potato contains *Agrobacterium* T-DNAs with expressed genes: an example of a naturally transgenic food crop. Proceedings of the National Academy of Sciences of the United States of America 112, 5844–5849.

Lee, C.M., Cradick, T.J., Bao, G., 2016. The *Neisseria meningitidis* CRISPR-Cas9 system enables specific genome editing in mammalian cells. Molecular Therapy 24, 645–654.

Li, C., Zong, Y., Wang, Y., Jin, S., Zhang, D., Song, Q., et al., 2018. Expanded base editing in rice and wheat using a Cas9-adenosine deaminase fusion. Genome Biology 19, 59.

Li, J., Sun, Y., Du, J., Zhao, Y., Xia, L., 2017. Generation of targeted point mutations in rice by a modified CRISPR/Cas9 system. Molecular Plant 10, 526–529.

Liu, W., Yuan, J.S., Stewart, C.N.J., 2013. Advanced genetic tools for plant biotechnology. Nature Reviews Genetics 14, 781–793.

Makarova, K.S., Wolf, Y.I., Alkhnbashi, O.S., Costa, F., Shah, S.A., Saunders, S.J., et al., 2015. An updated evolutionary classification of CRISPR-Cas systems. Nature Reviews Microbiology 13, 722–736.

Mali, P., Yang, L., Esvelt, K.M., Aach, J., Guell, M., DiCarlo, J.E., et al., 2013. RNA-guided human genome engineering via Cas9. Science 339, 823–826.

Manova, V., Gruszka, D., 2015. DNA damage and repair in plants - from models to crops. Frontiers of Plant Science 6, 885.

Mendel, G., 1866. Versuche über Pflanzenhybriden. Verhandlungen des naturforschenden Vereines Brunn 4, 44.

Miyaoka, Y., Berman, J.R., Cooper, S.B., Mayerl, S.J., Chan, A.H., Zhang, B., et al., 2016. Systematic quantification of HDR and NHEJ reveals effects of locus, nuclease, and cell type on genome-editing. Scientific Reports 6, 23549.

Mohanta, T.K., Bashir, T., Hashem, A., Abd Allah, E.F., Bae, H., 2017. Genome editing tools in plants. Genes 8, 399.

Mojica, F.J.M., Diez-Villasenor, C., Garcia-Martinez, J., Almendros, C., 2009. Short motif sequences determine the targets of the prokaryotic CRISPR defence system. Microbiology 155, 733–740.

Mojica, F.J.M., Diez-Villasenor, C., Garcia-Martinez, J., Soria, E., 2005. Intervening sequences of regularly spaced prokaryotic repeats derive from foreign genetic elements. Journal of Molecular Evolution 60, 174–182.

Nam, J., Matthysse, A.G., Gelvin, S.B., 1997. Differences in susceptibility of *Arabidopsis* ecotypes to crown gall disease may result from a deficiency in T-DNA integration. Plant Cell 9, 317–333.

Nishimasu, H., Ran, F.A., Hsu, P.D., Konermann, S., Shehata, S.I., Dohmae, et al., 2014. Crystal structure of Cas9 in complex with guide RNA and target DNA. Cell 156, 935–949.

Peterson, B.A., Haak, D.C., Nishimura, M.T., Teixeira, P.J.P.L., James, S.R., Dangl, J.L., et al., 2016. Genome-wide assessment of efficiency and specificity in CRISPR/Cas9 mediated multiple site targeting in *Arabidopsis*. PLoS One 11, e0162169.

Potter, H., Heller, R., 2018. Transfection by electroporation. Current Protocols in Molecular Biology 121, 9.3.1–9.3.13.

Puchta, H., Fauser, F., 2014. Synthetic nucleases for genome engineering in plants: prospects for a bright future. The Plant Journal 78, 727–741.

Ran, F.A., Cong, L., Yan, W.X., Scott, D.A., Gootenberg, J.S., Kriz, A.J., et al., 2015. *In vivo* genome editing using *Staphylococcus aureus* Cas9. Nature 520, 186–191.

Ren, B., Yan, F., Kuang, Y., Li, N., Zhang, D., Zhou, X., et al., 2018. Improved base editor for efficiently inducing genetic variations in rice with CRISPR/Cas9-guided hyperactive hAID mutant. Molecular Plant 11, 623–626.

Sanford, J.C., Smith, F.D., Russell, J.A., 1993. Optimizing the biolistic process for different biological applications. Methods in Enzymology 217, 483–509.

Sapranauskas, R., Gasiunas, G., Fremaux, C., Barrangou, R., Horvath, P., Siksnys, V., 2011. The *Streptococcus thermophilus* CRISPR/Cas system provides immunity in *Escherichia coli*. Nucleic Acids Research 39, 9275–9282.

Shimatani, Z., Kashojiya, S., Takayama, M., Terada, R., Arazoe, T., Ishii, H., et al., 2017. Targeted base editing in rice and tomato using a CRISPR-Cas9 cytidine deaminase fusion. Nature Biotechnology 35, 441–443.

Shmakov, S., Smargon, A., Scott, D., Cox, D., Pyzocha, N., Yan, W., et al., 2017. Diversity and evolution of class 2 CRISPR-Cas systems. Nature Reviews Microbiology 15, 169–182.

Slaymaker, I.M., Gao, L., Zetsche, B., Scott, D.A., Yan, W.X., Zhang, F., 2016. Rationally engineered Cas9 nucleases with improved specificity. Science 351, 84−88.

Stanley, S.Y., Maxwell, K.L., 2018. Phage-encoded anti-CRISPR defenses. Annual Review of Genetics 52, 445−464.

USDA, 2018. Secretary Perdue Issues USDA Statement on Plant Breeding Innovation. Press release No. 0070.18. URL: https://www.usda.gov/media/press-releases/2018/03/28/secretary-perdue-issues-usda-statement-plant-breeding-innovation.

Villarreal, D.D., Lee, K., Deem, A., Shim, E.Y., Malkova, A., Lee, S.E., 2012. Microhomology directs diverse DNA break repair pathways and chromosomal translocations. PLoS Genetics 8, e1003026.

Waltz, E., 2016. Gene-edited CRISPR mushroom escapes US regulation. Nature 532, 293.

Woo, J.W., Kim, J., Kwon, S.I., Corvalan, C., Cho, S.W., Kim, H., et al., 2015. DNA-free genome editing in plants with preassembled CRISPR-Cas9 ribonucleoproteins. Nature Biotechnology 33, 1162−1164.

Wright, A.V., Nunez, J.K., Doudna, J.A., 2016. Biology and applications of CRISPR systems: harnessing nature's toolbox for genome engineering. Cell 164, 29−44.

Yamano, T., Nishimasu, H., Zetsche, B., Hirano, H., Slaymaker, I.M., Li, Y., et al., 2016. Crystal structure of Cpf1 in complex with guide RNA and target DNA. Cell 165, 949−962.

Yan, F., Kuang, Y., Ren, B., Wang, J., Zhang, D., Lin, H., et al., 2018. Highly efficient A.T to G.C base editing by Cas9n-guided tRNA adenosine deaminase in rice. Molecular Plant 11, 631−634.

Zetsche, B., Gootenberg, J.S., Abudayyeh, O.O., Slaymaker, I.M., Makarova, K.S., Essletzbichler, P., et al., 2015. Cpf1 is a single RNA-guided endonuclease of a Class 2 CRISPR-Cas system. Cell 163, 759−771.

Zhang, Q., Xing, H.-L., Wang, Z.-P., Zhang, H.-Y., Yang, F., Wang, X.-C., et al., 2018. Potential high-frequency off-target mutagenesis induced by CRISPR/Cas9 in *Arabidopsis* and its prevention. Plant Molecular Biology 96, 445−456.

Zong, Y., Song, Q., Li, C., Jin, S., Zhang, D., Wang, Y., et al., 2018. Efficient C-to-T base editing in plants using a fusion of nCas9 and human APOBEC3A. Nature Biotechnology 36, 950−953.

Zong, Y., Wang, Y., Li, C., Zhang, R., Chen, K., Ran, Y., et al., 2017. Precise base editing in rice, wheat and maize with a Cas9-cytidine deaminase fusion. Nature Biotechnology 35, 438−440.

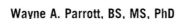

Can genetic modification go wrong, and what if it does?

Wayne A. Parrott, BS, MS, PhD

Professor, Dept. of Crop and Soil Sciences, & Institute of Plant Breeding, Genetics, and Genomics, University of Georgia, Athens, GA, USA

Images of genetic modification going wrong

To get a mental image of genetic modification gone awry, one only has to look at Hollywood. To this day, the name, Frankenstein, still evokes visions of science gone awry. Yet, by the time the novel became a movie in 1931, the public surely was already too familiar with electricity to feel threatened by it. Hollywood needed a more powerful and mysterious force than electricity and more believable than magic. In 1954, the answer came from Japan. The film, *Gojira,* featured a creature that while not technically a mutation was somehow associated with nuclear bombs and linked to radiation. The discovery of radioactivity as a mutagen was a boon for scriptwriters in Hollywood. It provided a way to obtain monsters that was just plausible enough for audiences to suspend their disbelief. Two years later, Gojira was reincarnated as Godzilla in Hollywood. Monsters and mutations have been inextricably linked since then.

Occasionally, radioactivity could have effects that, while not negative, were still dramatic. The Fantastic Four acquired their powers after being exposed to cosmic rays in 1961. A year later, a radioactive spider was able to transfer its spidery qualities to Peter Parker by biting him, thus transforming him into Spider-Man. Although Superman had been around since 1938, it was not until 1963 that the cause of his strength was revealed—radiation, in the form of yellow sunlight. The message remained clear: radiation is a powerful thing that leads to unexpected results, often negative. Case in point, radiation became the explanation for kryptonite's detrimental effects on Superman.

The advent of genetic engineering opened a new era for Hollywood. Hollywood writers find genetic engineering and now, gene editing, to be useful precisely for the same reason that plant geneticists do: these technologies provide a way to bypass the randomness of mutagenesis and provide results that are more predictable. Genetic engineering in the hands of arrogant scientists invariably makes for easy scripts.

Hence, the 2002 reincarnation of Godzilla was created by genetic engineering, not radiation. Also in 2002, the spider that gave Peter Parker his Super-Man powers was genetically engineered. Engineered animals in movies range from 1999s engineered sharks in *Deep Blue Sea* to 2010s *Mega Piranha.* The most notable of these is 1990s *Jurassic Park*'s tale of engineering gone wrong, which has been repeated in several sequels since then.

But as genetic engineering become passé in science with the advent of gene editing, so it goes in Hollywood (or is it the other way around?). The 2018 film, *Rampage,* featured monstrous animals obtained using CRISPR gene editing.

The precursor to all the engineering movies may well be 1951s *Day of the Triffids.* Triffids are a fictional invasive, toxic plant species that wreaks havoc. The novel's protagonist explains he thought that triffids resulted from "ingenious biological meddlings—and very likely accidental, at that." By the time the book and movie became a TV series in 1981, the triffid's creation was blamed on Lysenko and the Soviets. Lysenko himself is forever identified with his unconventional view of genetics.

But Hollywood depictions of genetic modification have little basis in reality. Inasmuch as Hollywood does not need to abide by the laws of physics or any other biological constraints, real-world genetic biology does. Nevertheless, for a public not familiar with the laws of physics and other biological constraints, there is no clear demarcation between Hollywood fantasy and the wonders of science. Inasmuch as it is possible to split the atom and put a man on the moon, engineering a shark can seem equally possible.

The best indication of what modification of any type can and cannot do comes from taking a look at past modifications and their subsequent effects. The hazards associated with genetic modification are in two broad categories: food and feed safety, and environmental safety. The former is addressed through a series of compositional, toxicological, and allergenicity studies (Kuiper and Kleter, 2003). The latter tends to be context-specific and centers on evaluating the potential effects of the modification on environmental components that have been targeted for protection, as will be discussed later.

Modification and food safety

Although the genetic modification of crop plants tends to garner the most attention, microorganisms are modified as well. The modification and use of microorganisms tends to go unnoticed by the public at large, primarily due to an absence of problems associated with their modification.

The one exception is an outbreak of eosinophilia—myalgia syndrome that took place in 1989. Patients had taken L-tryptophan supplements manufactured by Showa Denko K.K. An investigation showed that the company had switched to a genetically engineered strain of *Bacillus amyloliquefaciens* right before the health incidents began. Although users of L-tryptophan from nonengineered bacteria had occasionally come down with the syndrome, critics were quick to blame genetic engineering per se as the cause of eosinophilia—myalgia syndrome outbreak. Conceivably, metabolic shifts from the overproduction of L-tryptophan could be leading to the production of toxic byproducts.

Further investigation showed that the L-tryptophan contained another compound detected through high performance liquid chromatography and referred to as "peak E" and that this compound seemed to be responsible for the syndrome. However, at the same time, the company had also cut in half the amount of activated carbon it was using to remove impurities. In the end, it was the change in the manufacturing process that was singled out as the most probable cause of the syndrome outbreak (Belongia et al., 1990; Mayeno and Gleich, 1994), as opposed to the use of a genetically engineered strain.

In the absence of further issues with modified microorganisms, plants dominate the discussion. Many plants contain toxins that are commonly known, and many poisons have been derived from plants, such as pyrethrum, strychnine, and rotenone. Socrates committed suicide by drinking hemlock, while Nancy Hanks Lincoln, mother of Abraham Lincoln, died after she drank milk from a cow that had eaten white snakeroot.

Accordingly, many crop plants are known to contain toxins, ranging from phytohemagglutinin in common bean to solanine in potato to linamarin in cassava and lima beans, thereby precluding the consumption of these in their raw or unprocessed form (Stewart, 2009). In 2019, almost 280 persons became ill in Sweden after eating improperly cooked legumes (Food Safety News, 2019). While the presence of given toxins tends to be specific to given plant families, the range of toxins in crop plants is diverse, encompassing toxic amino acids, lectins, glucosinolates, and diverse alkaloids (D'Mello et al., 1991; Beier, 1990). In addition to toxins present in levels that can cause illness or death, food plants also have a multitude of other toxins present at low levels (Ames et al., 1990). It is the possibility of inadvertently increasing the levels of toxins during genetic modification that leads to concerns over food safety.

Since many of these toxins have a bitter or undesirable taste associated with them, it is commonly assumed that high toxin levels have been bred out of most of the common crops (Drewnowski and Gomez-Carneros, 2000). Nevertheless some crops can still exceed desirable levels if handled inappropriately (Sinden and Webb, 1972). Case in point, six people have died from solanine glycoalkaloid poisoning over the past 160 years after eating raw potatoes, fruit, or foliage. Numerous others have fallen ill after eating meals prepared from green tubers (Friedman et al., 1997). These incidents are all due to the fact that many crops can be dangerous if not prepared properly (Fig. 4.1), and not the result of modification.

Unusual environmental conditions also can lead to elevated toxin levels. The case of the "Magnum Bonum" potato from Sweden illustrates the point. This variety had been widely grown throughout Sweden for 50 years without any incidents. Then in 1986, consumption of Magnum Bonum led to complaints of bitter taste and intestinal discomfort. Magnum Bonum planted throughout Sweden was found to have glycoalkaloid levels elevated beyond the safe level, though there were no serious adverse consequences as a result. It is not clear what it was about the 1986 growing conditions that caused Magnum Bonum to have elevated glycoalkaloid levels when most other potato varieties did not (Hellenäs et al., 1995).

Another reported example is that of 11 workers who developed dermatitis because the 1991 Gulf War delayed harvest in southern Israel, so the celery was

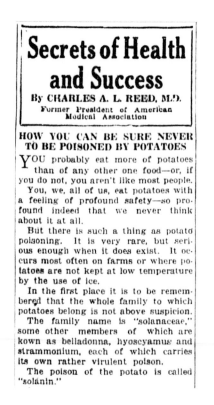

Secrets of Health and Success

By CHARLES A. L. REED, M.D.
Former President of American Medical Association

HOW YOU CAN BE SURE NEVER TO BE POISONED BY POTATOES

YOU probably eat more of potatoes than of any other one food—or, if you do not, you aren't like most people.

You, we, all of us, eat potatoes with a feeling of profound safety—so profound indeed that we never think about it at all.

But there is such a thing as potato poisoning. It is very rare, but serious enough when it does exist. It occurs most often on farms or where potatoes are not kept at low temperature by the use of ice.

In the first place it is to be remembered that the whole family to which potatoes belong is not above suspicion.

The family name is "solanaceae," some other members of which are known as belladonna, hyoscyamus and strammonium, each of which carries its own rather virulent poison.

The poison of the potato is called "solanin."

FIGURE 4.1

The start of an advice column, from *The Minneapolis Star* 15 Nov 1924. It acknowledges that potatoes can be risky if handled improperly.

Credit: The Minneapolis Star *November 15, 1924.*

more mature than normal at harvest time (Finkelstein et al., 1994). Thus this example is not related to breeding but to the harvest of plants older than optimal.

The point is that issues unrelated to modification are frequently to blame for cases of intoxication from plants, even if modification gets the blame. Nevertheless, there are rare examples of modification that led to the unintentional increase of toxicants in crop cultivars.

Almost 50 years ago, "Lenape," a potato variety developed from a cross to a wild species and tested as "B5141-6" and finally released in 1969, was found to have twice as many glycoalkaloids as other commercial varieties and was withdrawn prior to being marketed (Anonymous, 1970). The tip-off was an unusually bitter taste (Zitnak and Johnston, 1970).

The only other documented incident associated with plant breeding is that of a disease-resistant variety of celery, in which the resistance was apparently due to elevated levels of furanocoumarins. This variety caused dermatitis among supermarket personnel who handled the celery and who subsequently used tanning beds (Berkley et al., 1986; Seligman et al., 1987).

The report that conventional breeding raised toxin levels in cucurbits (Kirschman and Suber, 1989) does not appear to be correct. Bitter taste once again alerted to the rare presence of elevated levels of cucurbitacin E in squash fruits found in California and Alabama. Fruits from two varieties of zucchini poisoned 22 people in Australia who ate the fruit between 1981 and 82 despite the bitter taste. These bitter fruits occurred among the widely grown cultivars, "Blackjack" and "Castle Verde" (Herrington, 1983). Other incidences of cucurbit poisoning have led to hair loss (Assouly, 2018). Because bitter fruit are only rarely produced by widely grown varieties, these toxins cannot be due to breeding but could be due to spontaneous mutations, or perhaps to cross-pollination with undomesticated (Rymal et al., 1984) or ornamental squash varieties (Le Roux et al., 2018), both of which maintain their toxicity.

Given that there are literally hundreds of thousands of crop varieties developed and released by plant breeders, it is remarkable that only two varieties developed since World War II have presented any health-related problems related to the breeding process: one led to dermatitis and the second was intercepted before it could cause harm. The situation has been summed up as follows (Stevens, 1974):

> *The array of naturally occurring toxins in vegetables and fruits is great. However, absence of health problems caused from eating these crops, coupled with the lack of any attempt to limit toxins by breeding, indicate that the potential for problems is small.*

A concern was expressed early on that the physical insertion of DNA in the form of a transgene into a genome could activate genes involved in toxin production (Kessler et al., 1992). This concern led to the current food safety-testing paradigm for transgenic crops (König et al., 2004; Cellini et al., 2004). Since then, it has become evident that natural DNA insertions are common in genomes, without any ensuing safety consequences (Weber et al., 2012; Schnell et al., 2015). To wit, the US Food and Drug Administration has reviewed 161 transgenic crops as of this writing (https://www.accessdata.fda.gov/scripts/fdcc/?set=Biocon, accessed 31 Dec 2018). In every case, the FDA found that the engineered crop was "not materially different in composition, safety, and other relevant parameters" from its conventional counterpart. The inference is that DNA insertions in and of themselves have little, if any, ability to elevate toxins to levels of toxicological concern.

Since the Lenape potato, breeders always check for the presence of elevated levels of known toxicants in new varieties before they are released. However, such safety testing depends on the knowledge of the toxin being evaluated. If a new and unexpected type of toxin were to arise, testing would probably miss it. There is one such report, whereby an interspecific hybrid obtained via protoplast fusion between potato and *Solanum brevidens* produced demissin, a toxin not found in either parent (Laurila et al., 1996). However, this toxin is well known in close relatives within the genus (Friedman et al., 1997) and was previously known to exist in potato itself (Jadhav et al., 1981). Thus the claim that demissin is a novel toxin in a potato hybrid had more to do with unfamiliarity with the literature than with any biological reality. In the end, there has not been a single substantiated report of a completely novel toxin or allergen appearing in a genus as a result of conventional breeding.

While elevated toxins appear not to be an issue, genetic engineering can transfer an allergen into plants that previously do not produce this allergen (Nordlee et al., 1996). This concern appears to be unique to modification by genetic engineering, and an extensive protocol is in place to ensure allergens are not inadvertently transferred into plants (Ladics, 2018).

A final concern is that a point mutation can convert an otherwise-harmless protein into a toxic or allergenic one. Thus so far, point mutations can take a toxin and inactivate it, but there are no examples of the reverse being true. Likewise, there are no examples of point mutations turning harmless proteins into allergens. The reason is that acquisition of new biochemical function is an evolutionarily slow process. Each mutation cannot negatively affect the proper folding of the novel protein, and the biochemical function must provide an advantage to the organism, or at least, not be deleterious (Weber et al., 2012).

In conclusion, certain toxins are associated with certain crops and their relatives, and genetic modification of any type can raise them to harmful levels, as can improper use or adverse growing conditions. Whenever the presence of elevated toxins in crops has occurred, the effects have been reasonably local. Individuals who ate inedible parts (e.g., potato leaves) or ignored the bitter taste were not so fortunate. Regardless, it is prudent to keep toxin levels down as low as possible. Thus the levels of known toxins should always be monitored, as has become customary, regardless of whether the modification is done with recombinant DNA or otherwise. In contrast to known toxins, the probability that new, unexpected toxins or allergens could arise during modification is too low to measure over the historical record.

Environmental concerns

The *Day of the Triffids* mentioned earlier may be fictional, but it does exemplify many of the environmental concerns that can come from any type of genetic modification. These have been succinctly categorized as the ability to become weedy or invasive, the ability to cross with wild relatives to produce more weedy or invasive progeny, the ability to become a pest that affects plants, the ability to impact biodiversity, and the ability to affect nontarget species, i.e., species not intended to be affected by the modified organism (Canadian Food Inspection Agency, 1994).

The greatest environmental damage outside of agriculture can come from invasive species (Lowry et al., 2013; Marbuah et al., 2014; David et al., 2017). There are thousands of examples, mostly due to humans transporting species into new habitats, sometimes on purpose, sometimes accidently. At times, the results can be spectacular, such as the kudzu vines that anyone driving through the American South can see growing along roadsides (Fig. 4.2).

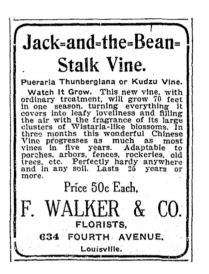

FIGURE 4.2

Advertisement from *The Courier-Journal*, 5 May 1906, highlighting kudzu's attributes that today would be recognized as giving kudzu invasiveness potential.

Credit: The Courier-Journal, *May 5, 1906.*

Can genetic modification lead to invasiveness? It is worth noting that most invasive species involve no genetic modification of any type. There are however notable examples, such as the Africanized honeybee (Schneider et al., 2004), which is a hybrid between two subspecies. Most recently, the invasive marbled crayfish also was shown to be a hybrid (Gutekunst et al., 2018). These examples represent naturally occurring hybrids. As such, they represent the fusion of two genomes, which is a modification totally unlike the much more limited modifications done during editing, engineering, or mutagenesis.

So, historically, hybridization can lead to the creation of invasive species. It also can lead to new weeds and contribute to the extinction of other species (Ellstrand et al., 2013). In addition, hybridization is the first step for gene flow. If gene flow happens, and genes from one group of organisms eventually get established in another, then introgression has taken place. In agriculture, introgression under a breeder's direction is an important tool for the development of improved crop varieties. In other settings, genes have flowed without human intervention between crops and their weedy relatives. In most cases, the introgression has been very difficult to detect (Ellstrand et al., 2013), suggesting that any accompanying environmental effects are minor. But, there are exceptions that have been problematic, such as the transfer of herbicide tolerance from rice to red rice or the creation weed beets (Ellstrand et al., 2013). All these examples are from conventional modification.

Regardless of their origin, invasive species can be troublesome. For example, Africanized bees are more likely to defend their nests (Collins et al., 1982), thus resulting in multiple stings. The amount of venom delivered via multiple stings can result in renal failure and death, even for persons not allergic to bee venom (Mejia et al., 1986). Deaths aside, estimates of the damage losses and costs of mitigation and control of invasive species are as high as 12% of the US gross domestic product (Marbuah et al., 2014).

Modified plants can have, at least theoretically, unintended and undesired effects on desirable species, referred to as nontarget species. The claim that pollen from corn engineered to resist insect pests could kill monarch butterfly larvae (Losey et al., 1999) is an example. Although this study was later shown not be valid under field conditions (Hellmich et al., 2001), the point is made that there could be harm if a desirable organism is exposed to a plant modified to be toxic.

Anytime one organism is modified to resist another, the unmodified organism must adapt to survive. This reality has driven evolution (Dawkins et al., 1979) and plagued efforts to control pests in agriculture, as a long string of resistance genes and pesticides have lost their effectiveness over time. As an example, weeds that become resistant to herbicides have been a long-term problem in agriculture (Délye et al., 2013) ever since the first report of an herbicide-resistant weed (Ryan, 1970).

Most recently, the trend has been to engineer crops to resist broad-spectrum herbicides. The first of these traits to reach the market was tolerance to glyphosate. Soon glyphosate-tolerant crops became widespread, followed by the emergence of glyphosate-tolerant weeds (Powles, 2008). Though glyphosate-tolerant weeds account for only about 9% of all herbicide-tolerant weeds (http://weedscience.com accessed 30 Dec 2018), they dominate the headlines and rhetoric under the name of "superweeds," even though the weeds themselves are not modified by humans. The term evokes images of overgrown plants (Fig. 4.3). In reality, and in the absence of herbicide, they look just like their susceptible counterparts.

For these reasons, organisms modified by recombinant DNA are subject to an environmental risk assessment (U. S. Environmental Protection Agency, 1992; European Food Safety Agency, 2010). The assessment is carried out case by case, as the hazards posed are unique to each crop, gene, and environmental combination. In the earlier example on kudzu (Fig. 4.1), its proponents noted its rapid growth, hardiness, and adaptability in the American South. Today, those attributes would be immediately identified as being attributes of invasive species. In other words, an environmental risk assessment can identify adverse impacts before they occur. It can also identify management and mitigation measures to prevent or minimize any adverse effects.

Nevertheless, the more subtle or tenuous relationships between modification and adverse effects can be difficult to predict and harder to prove. For example, because glyphosate is so efficient at controlling milkweed, the food for monarch butterfly larvae, the domination of the agricultural landscape by glyphosate-tolerant crops may be having other effects as well. Glyphosate-tolerant crops have been both blamed (Pleasants and Oberhauser, 2013) and exonerated (Inamine et al., 2016; Boyle et al., 2019) for the decline of the monarch butterfly.

Nevertheless, organisms modified using conventional methods do not undergo environmental safety assessments in most parts of the world, though they can have the same consequences as those modified using recombinant DNA. The lesson

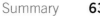

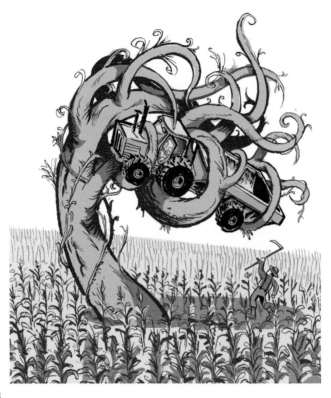

FIGURE 4.3

Genetically modified organisms make for dramatic fiction. In reality, GMOs are usually hard to distinguish from their unmodified counterparts.

Credit: Paul Hoppe, and used with permission.

is that if modification is to cause problems, it is the modified trait that would cause them; the method used for the modification is irrelevant.

In the end, if a future-modified species is to have adverse effects on the environment, it is difficult to envision a negative outcome that is worse than what has been caused by current-day invasive or weedy species. These effects can wan over time, as people and the environment adapt to the presence of the new organism. Thus, even Africanized honeybees have faded away from public attention as the scenarios that were depicted in such movies as *The Swarm* from 1978 and *Killer Bees* in 2002 failed to materialize.

Summary

The genetic modification of plants and animals by humans is an ancient practice, going back at least to the beginnings of agriculture. The human modification of other organisms has become widespread as well. Over the span of thousands of years, there have been multiple opportunities to observe the effects of modification on both food safety and the environment.

When it comes to food safety, the main role of modification has been to make food safer, and it will take further modification to overcome remaining food safety issues, such as environmentally induced elevated levels of toxins. Adverse effects from human-mediated modification have not gone beyond the production of a skin rash, or perhaps a stomachache. This review recognizes that of all the modification technologies in use today, engineering poses a unique risk in that it is possible to transfer the capacity to produce an allergen to foods where it is unexpected. Hence, strict evaluation criteria are employed to ensure such a transfer does not happen. Environmentally, the effects of modification have been greater, though usually, have been rather localized and manageable, regardless of whether the modification was natural or made by humans using conventional technologies. Other than the cost of mitigation, these issues are sufficiently low key that the public and media hardly ever notice them.

Over the years, modification has become more deliberate, scientific, and precise. Regardless, what is clear is that effects on food safety or the environment come from the trait modified, not the way in which the trait was modified. It does not matter if the modification occurred naturally or was driven by humans. Hollywood style disasters caused by genetic modification have failed to become reality. For that matter, so have all of Hollywood's other monsters, whether mutated, engineered, or otherwise.

References

Ames, B.N., Profet, M., Gold, L.S., 1990. Dietary pesticides (99.99% all natural). Proceedings of the National Academy of Sciences of the United States of America 87 (19), 7777−7781.

Anonymous, 1970. Name of potato variety Lenape withdrawn. American Journal of Potato Research 47, 103.

Assouly, P., 2018. Hair loss associated with cucurbit poisoning. JAMA Dermatology 154 (5), 617−618.

Beier, R.C., 1990. Natural pesticides and bioactive components in foods. In: Ware, G.W. (Ed.), Reviews of Environmental Contamination and Toxicology. Springer-Verlag, New York and Heidelberg.

Belongia, E.A., Hedberg, C.W., Gleich, G.J., White, K.E., Mayeno, A.N., Loegering, D.A., Dunnette, S.L., Pirie, P.L., MacDonald, K.L., Osterholm, M.T., 1990. An investigation of the cause of the eosinophilia−myalgia syndrome associated with tryptophan use. New England Journal of Medicine 323 (6), 357−365.

Boyle, J.H., Dalgleish, H.J., Puzey, J.R., 2019. Monarch butterfly and milkweed declines substantially predate the use of genetically modified crops. Proc. National Acad. Sci. 116 (8), 3006−3011.

Canadian Food Inspection Agency, 1994. Assessment Criteria for Determining Environmental Safety of Plants with Novel Traits.

Cellini, F., Chesson, A., Colquhoun, I., Constable, A., Davies, H.V., Engel, K.H., Gatehouse, A.M.R., Kärenlampi, S., Kok, E.J., Leguay, J.J., Lehesranta, S., Noteborn, H.P.J.M., Pedersen, J., Smith, M., 2004. Unintended effects and their detection in genetically modified crops. Food and Chemical Toxicology 42 (7), 1089−1125.

Collins, A.M., Rinderer, T.E., Harbo, J.R., Bolten, A.B., 1982. Colony defense by Africanized and European honey bees. Science 218 (4567), 72−74.

D'Mello, J.P.F., Duffus, C.M., Duffus, J.H. (Eds.), 1991. Toxic Substances in Crop Plants. The Royal Society of Chemistry, Cambridge.

David, P., Thébault, E., Anneville, O., Duyck, P.F., Chapuis, E., Loeuille, N., 2017. Chapter One - impacts of invasive species on food webs: a review of empirical data. In: Bohan, D.A., Dumbrell, A.J., Massol, F. (Eds.), Advances in Ecological Research. Academic Press.

Dawkins, R., Krebs, J.R, 1979. Arms races between and within species. Proceedings of the Royal Society of London. Series B. Biological Sciences 205 (1161), 489−511.

Délye, C., Jasieniuk, M., Le Corre, V., 2013. Deciphering the evolution of herbicide resistance in weeds. Trends in Genetics 29 (11), 649−658.

Drewnowski, A., Gomez-Carneros, C., 2000. Bitter taste, phytonutrients, and the consumer: a review. American Journal of Clinical Nutrition 72 (6), 1424−1435.

Ellstrand, N.C., Meirmans, P., Rong, J., Bartsch, D., Ghosh, A., de Jong, T.J., Haccou, P., Lu, B.-R., Snow, A.A., Stewart Jr., C.N., Strasburg, J.L., van Tienderen, P.H., Vrieling, K., Hooftman, D., 2013. Introgression of crop alleles into wild or weedy populations. Annual Review of Ecology, Evolution, and Systematics 44 (1), 325−345.

European Food Safety Agency, 2010. Guidance on the environmental risk assessment of genetically modified plants. EFSA Journal 8 (11), 1879.

Finkelstein, E., Afek, U., Gross, E., Aharoni, N., Rosenberg, L.E., Halevy, S.H., 1994. An outbreak of phytophodermatitis due to celery. International Journal of Dermatology 33, 116−118.

Food Safety News, 2019. https://www.foodsafetynews.com/2019/10/tomatoes-linked-to-salmonella-outbreak-in-sweden-71-infected/. Accessed on 15 Oct 2019.

Friedman, M., McDonald, G.M., Filadelfi-Keszi, M.A., 1997. Potato glycoalkaloids: chemistry, analysis, safety, and plant physiology. Critical Reviews in Plant Sciences 16 (1), 55−132.

Gutekunst, J., Andriantsoa, R., Falckenhayn, C., Hanna, K., Stein, W., Rasamy, J., Lyko, F., 2018. Clonal genome evolution and rapid invasive spread of the marbled crayfish. Nature Ecology and Evolution 2 (3), 567−573.

Hellenäs, K.-E., Branzell, C., Johnsson, H., Slanina, P., 1995. High levels of glycoalkaloids in the established Swedish potato variety Magnum Bonum. Journal of the Science of Food and Agriculture 68 (2), 249−255.

Hellmich, R.L., Siegfried, B.D., Sears, M.K., Stanley-Horn, D.E., Daniels, M.J., Mattila, H.R., Spencer, T., Bidne, K.G., Lewis, L.C., 2001. Monarch larvae sensitivity to *Bacillus thuringiensis*- purified proteins and pollen. Proceedings of the National Academy of Sciences 98 (21), 11925−11930.

Herrrington, M.E., 1983. Intense bitterness in commercial zucchini. Cucurbit Genetics Cooperative Report 6, 75−76.

Inamine, H., Ellner, S.P., Springer, J.P., Agrawal, A.A., 2016. Linking the continental migratory cycle of the monarch butterfly to understand its population decline. Oikos 125 (8), 1081−1091.

Jadhav, S.J., Sharma, R.P., Salunkhe, D.K., 1981. Naturally occurring toxic alkaloids in foods. CRC Critical Reviews in Toxicology 9 (1), 21−104.

Kessler, D., Taylor, M., Maryanski, J., Flamm, E., Kahl, L., 1992. The safety of foods developed by biotechnology. Science 256 (5065), 1747−1749.

Kirschman, J.C., Suber, R.L., 1989. Recent food poisonings from cucurbitacin in traditionally bred squash. Food and Chemical Toxicology 27, 555−556.

König, A., Cockburn, A., Crevel, R.W.R., Debruyne, E., Grafstroem, R., Hammerling, U., Kimber, I., Knudsen, I., Kuiper, H.A., Peijnenburg, A.A.C.M., Penninks, A.H., Poulsen, M., Schauzu, M., Wal, J.M., 2004. Assessment of the safety of foods derived from genetically modified (GM) crops. Food and Chemical Toxicology 42 (7), 1047−1088.

Kuiper, H.A., Kleter, G.A., 2003. The scientific basis for risk assessment and regulation of genetically modified foods. Trends in Food Science and Technology 14 (5−8), 277−293.

Ladics, G.S., 2018. Assessment of the potential allergenicity of genetically-engineered food crops. Journal of Immunotoxicology 1−11.

Laurila, J., Laakso, I., Valkonen, J.P.T., Hiltunen, R., Pehu, E., 1996. Formation of parental-type and novel glycoalkaloids in somatic hybrids between *Solanum brevidens* and *S. tuberosum*. Plant Science 118 (2), 145−155.

Le Roux, G., Leborgne, I., Labadie, M., Garnier, R., Sinno-Tellier, S., Bloch, J., Deguigne, M., Boels, D., 2018. Poisoning by non-edible squash: retrospective series of 353 patients from French Poison Control Centers. Clinical Toxicology 56 (8), 790−794.

Losey, J.E., Rayor, L.S., Carter, M.E., 1999. Transgenic pollen harms monarch larvae. Nature 399, 214.

Lowry, E., Rollinson, E.J., Laybourn, A.J., Scott, T.E., Aiello-Lammens, M.E., Gray, S.M., Mickley, J., Gurevitch, J., 2013. Biological invasions: a field synopsis, systematic review, and database of the literature. Ecology and Evolution 3 (1), 182−196.

Marbuah, G., Gren, I.-M., McKie, B., 2014. Economics of harmful invasive species: a review. Diversity 6 (3), 500−523.

Mayeno, A.N., Gleich, G.J., 1994. Eosinophilia-myalgia syndrome and tryptophan production: a cautionary tale. Trends in Biotechnology 12 (9), 346−352.

Mejia, G., Arbelaez, M., Henao, J.E., Sus, A.A., Arango, J.L., 1986. Acute renal failure due to multiple stings by Africanized bees. Annals of Internal Medicine 104 (2), 210−211.

Nordlee, J.A., Taylor, S.L., Townsend, J.A., Thomas, L.A., Bush, R.K., 1996. Identification of a Brazil-nut allergen in transgenic soybeans. New England Journal of Medicine 334 (11), 688−692.

Pleasants, J.M., Oberhauser, K.S., 2013. Milkweed loss in agricultural fields because of herbicide use: effect on the monarch butterfly population. Insect Conservation and Diversity 6 (2), 135−144.

Powles, S.B., 2008. Evolved glyphosate-resistant weeds around the world: lessons to be learnt. Pest Management Science 64 (4), 360−365.

Ryan, G.F., 1970. Resistance of common groundsel to simazine and atrazine. Weed Science 18 (5), 614−616.

Rymal, K.S., Chamblis, O.L., Bond, M.D., Smith, D.A., 1984. Squash containing toxic cucurbitacin compounds occurring in California and Alabama. Journal of Food Protection 47 (4), 270−271.

Schneider, S.S., DeGrandi-Hoffman, G., Garnier, R., Smith, D.R., 2004. The African honey bee: factors contributing to a successful biological nvasion. Annual Review of Entomology 49 (1), 351−376.

Schnell, J., Steele, M., Bean, J., Neuspiel, M., Girard, C., Dormann, N., Pearson, C., Savoie, A., Bourbonnière, L., Macdonald, P., 2015. A comparative analysis of insertional effects in genetically engineered plants: considerations for pre-market assessments. Transgenic Research 24 (1), 1−17.

Seligman, P.J., Mathias, C., O'Malley, M.A., et al., 1987. Phytophotodermatitis from celery among grocery store workers. Archives of Dermatology 123 (11), 1478−1482.

Sinden, S.L., Webb, R.E., 1972. Effect of variety and location on the glycoalkaloid content of potatoes. American Potato Journal 49, 334−338.

Stevens, M.A., 1974. Breeding for safety in vegetables and fruits. In: Hanson, C.H. (Ed.), The Effect of FDA Regulations (GRAS) on Plant Breeding and Processing. Crop Science Society of America, Madison, Wisconsin.

Stewart, A., 2009. Wicked Plants: The Weed that Killed Lincoln's Mother & Other Botanical Atrocities, Chapel Hill. Algonquin Books of Chapel Hill, North Carolina.

U. S. Environmental Protection Agency, 1992. Framework for Ecological Risk Assessment. U. S. Environmental Protection Agency, Washington, DC).

Weber, N., Halpin, C., Hannah, L.C., Jez, J.M., Kough, J., Parrott, W., 2012. Crop genome plasticity and its relevance to food and feed safety of genetically engineered breeding stacks. Plant Physiology 160 (4), 1842−1853.

Zitnak, A., Johnston, G.R., 1970. Glycoalkaloid content of B5141-6 potatoes. American Potato Journal 47, 256−260.

GM food and human health

5

R. Blair, BSc, PhD, DSc [1], J.M. Regenstein[2]

[1]*Faculty of Land & Food Systems, University of British Columbia, Vancouver, Canada;*
[2]*Department of Food Science, College of Agriculture and Life Sciences, Cornell University, Ithaca, NY, United States*

Introduction

It is very difficult to determine the effects of any food on the health of human populations, because of many interacting factors. Therefore, the approach taken in this review is to assess whether the health of humans is at risk by eating GM foods, using data from animal testing. Blair and Regenstein (2015) conducted a review of the available data from peer-reviewed scientific investigations and from reports by regulatory authorities and scientific bodies and concluded that the safety and nutritional composition of approved GM food and feeds are similar to their related, non-GM counterparts. This chapter summaries the results in question, reviews more recent findings, and provides an overall assessment of the safety of GM foods and feeds together with assessments provided by other researchers, scientific bodies, and regulatory authorities.

A criticism made of the current situation regarding the official approval process for GM foods is that the relevant data are not published in peer-reviewed journals. Thus they are not available for review by other scientists. One explanation for this apparent lack of openness is that the policy relating to GM organisms is similar to that which has existed for many years for drug approvals: a positive decision based on submitted data resulting in the granting of a patent and giving the applicant company the right to market the product in question for its intended use.

In spite of the claim about a lack of data on the safety of GM foods, reports providing peer-reviewed data have been published in the scientific literature, as described below.

Evidence on safety

Plants and animals can be altered in genetic makeup by:

1. Traditional selection and crossbreeding techniques
2. Exposure to chemicals or radiation (mutagenesis)

Genetically Modified and Irradiated Food. https://doi.org/10.1016/B978-0-12-817240-7.00005-X

3. Genome editing: the process of changing the genetic makeup by altering, removing, or adding nucleotides to the genes
4. Introduction of a gene from one species into another species (genetic modification, transgenesis)

Generally it is method 4 that receives most attention with regard to possible effects on human health, requiring assessment before the GM plant or animal can be accepted as human or animal food. Also, it is the most controversial. Our review therefore concentrates on the safety aspects of foods derived in this way. In total these foods comprise over 80 worldwide, ranging from insect-resistant maize to yeasts that improve the quality of wines.

In 2018 the European Union ruled that products from crops plant modified by gene-editing (category 3 above) would be subject to EU regulations governing GM foods.

Although mutation breeding (2 above) has relevance to our review, it will not be included since by tradition it is considered a conventional breeding technique, the products being excluded from the regulatory assessment applied to those produced by method 3. Some organic farming systems even permit food from mutated varieties to be sold as organic (Wikipedia, 2013). The Joint Food and Agriculture Organization (FAO)/International Atomic Energy Agency (IAEA) Mutant Variety Database (2014) lists more than 3218 cultivars of various plant species worldwide that have been developed using induced mutagenic agents, including ionizing irradiation and ethyl methane sulfonate.

Some GM foods (such as fruit) are eaten directly by consumers, whereas others are fed to poultry and livestock and their products (meat, milk, and eggs) are eaten by consumers.

It is logical, therefore, to review the relevant evidence separately.

GM foods likely to be eaten directly by consumers
Fruits and vegetables

Fruit and vegetable crops have to compete for nutrients with weeds and are subject to attack by viruses and insects; therefore GM cultivars have been developed with resistance to these pests and reduce or avoid the need for pesticide treatment. All of these improved crops have received regulatory approval in the United States and Canada following a nutritional and safety assessment by the US Department of Agriculture (USDA), the US Food and Drug Administration (FDA), the Canadian Food Inspection Agency (CFIA), and Health Canada and in other countries by relevant agencies.

The list of GM fruit includes cultivars of apple, cantaloupe, melon, papaya, and plum.

Papaya is susceptible to papaya ringspot virus (PRV), the main factor limiting commercial papaya production throughout the world and responsible for a decline of 40% of the Hawaiian papaya industry in the early 1990s. A control method adopted was to develop cultivars modified by insertion of a coat protein from the virus into the DNA of papayas, thus conferring resistance to the virus. There was no alternative method of control. Other countries have adopted a similar approach to dealing with the problem. In 2011 Japan approved the importation of GM papaya from Hawaii for food use. Consequently, papaya is regarded as the first commercialized GM fruit crop.

Several independent studies on GM papaya have been reported. Fermín et al. (2011) investigated whether the GM papayas could cause allergies and reported that they did not possess the sequence of eight amino acids found in known allergens. They also reported that the coat protein from the virus was degraded in simulated gastric and intestinal conditions and various heat treatments under which allergenic proteins are stable.

Powell et al. (2008) conducted a 90-day feeding study in which male and female rats received diets formulated to contain GM or parent-line (non-GM) papayas at twice (100 g per kg) the equivalent of the average daily human consumption of fresh papayas. No significant differences in body and organ weights or activities of important enzymes in liver and kidney were observed, and cholesterol levels in the plasma and liver of all animals were comparable. Also, the livers and kidneys of all the rats showed normal morphological structure.

Similar findings were reported on a GM papaya line that is resistant to both PRV and papaya leaf distortion mosaic virus (PLDMV) on immune responses in mice (Chen et al., 2011). On the other hand, inclusion of the GM fruit markedly increased serum total IgM levels, suggesting that the GM fruit had a protective effect on immunity. Lin et al. (2013) tested the potential toxicity of three GM PRV-resistant papaya cultivars relative to the parent-line non-GM cultivar. Results confirmed that the coat protein was rapidly broken down in simulated gastric fluid and that no fragments were detected in organs (brain, heart, liver, spleen, lung, kidneys, and testes) or in the stomach contents, cecal contents, colon contents, urine, whole blood, and serum of rats fed the ground fruit. No deaths or abnormalities were observed in any of the groups, and no biological or toxicological significances between groups fed the conventional or GM papaya were recorded.

Some fruits have been genetically modified to improve their ripening characteristics. Two cultivars of cantaloupe with a reduced production of ethylene in the fruit and slower ripening properties have been approved. Another approach with apples has been a modification to prevent or reduce the amount of browning after slicing. When the protective skin of apples (or potatoes) is damaged or removed and the tissues exposed to air, there is usually a rapid production of melanin, activated by the enzyme polyphenol oxidase (PPO). This gives the tissues a brown tint and a reduced flavor. The modified apples, which have been approved by the regulatory authorities in Canada and the United States, produce less than 10% of the PPO produced by conventional apples and therefore do not turn brown when sliced.

The list of approved GM cultivars of vegetables includes lucerne (alfalfa), potatoes, squash, sugar beet, sweet corn (maize), and tomatoes. Safety studies related to the development of GM potatoes have led to much of the controversy about GM foods in general. Dr. Arpad Pusztai of the Rowett Research Institute in Aberdeen, Scotland, reported in a TV interview in 1998 that GM potatoes he was testing had a deleterious effect on growth, organ development, and immune function in rats (Blair and Regenstein, 2015). The cultivar had been modified to contain a protective protein (Galanthus nivalis agglutinin [GNA], a lectin) and make it resistant to insects and nematodes, as had been done with other crop plants. In response to a question, he is reported to have stated that he would not eat GM food and that he found it "very, very unfair to use our fellow citizens as guinea pigs." The announcement made headlines in the news media around the world. The most important aspect of the pronouncement by Pusztai was that not only was the GM potato that he was studying unsafe to eat, but that GM food in general was unsafe. This was the first major criticism of GM foods to be made by a respected scientist.

An audit committee appointed at the Institute later concluded that the findings did not support his claims. The Royal Society UK (1999) reviewed all the relevant material and issued a summary statement concluding that the experiments had been poorly designed, the statistical analysis inappropriate, and the results inconsistent. Their recommendation was that the experiments be repeated and the results published.

Pusztai subsequently published a paper in a medical journal The Lancet (Ewen and Pusztai, 1999) as a Research Letter, summarizing data on the effects of diets containing the parent-line conventional potatoes, GM potatoes, or the parent-line potatoes supplemented with 25.4 µg/g of the purified GNA on the gut histology of rats. Analysis confirmed that the content of GNA in raw GM potatoes was 25.4 µg/g dry matter and was 4.9 µg/g dry matter after boiling for 1 h. The data showed that mean crypt length (µm) in the jejunum section of the small intestine was 75, 78, and 78, respectively, with boiled potatoes and was 57, 90, and 64, respectively, with raw potatoes ($P < 0.041$). Therefore, the authors suggested that "the promotion of jejunal growth was the result of the transformation of the potato with the GNA gene, since the jejunum of rats was shown to be stimulated only by GM potatoes but not by dietary GNA." That conclusion is debatable since the stimulatory effect was seen only with raw potatoes, the practical significance being that potatoes are never eaten raw by humans. Overall mean values for the caecum were 95, 70, and 98, respectively, and for the colon were 146, 139, and 177, respectively, suggesting no stimulatory effect of the boiled GM potatoes in these organs. Mean lymphocyte counts per 48 villi were stated to be 7.6 in rats fed on boiled parent-line potatoes, compared with 10.3 in rats fed diets containing boiled GM potatoes ($P < 0.01$). No data supporting the earlier claim of stunted growth were presented.

This was a relatively small trial, and it seems clear that no firm conclusions can be made from the data presented, either as to the safety for the human consumer of the specific GM potatoes in question or GM foods in general. A fact that appears to have been omitted in the discussions related to this whole matter is that consumers were never exposed to any possible dangers from consuming the GM potatoes in question. These potatoes were at the testing stage and had not been approved for release to the public by any regulatory authority. Any alarm at the possible exposure of consumers to the GM potatoes was, therefore, unfounded and premature. The subsequent introduction of GM potatoes has occurred successfully.

An important GM crop being grown in several countries is sugar beet, as a source of sugar for human use. As with oilseeds, all of the GM DNA is removed from the sugar (or oil) during processing and remains in the residue which is used in animal feeding.

Cereal crops

Several GM cultivars of cereal crops have approved, but maize (including sweet corn) is the only GM cereal being grown internationally in commercially significant quantities. A large body of data published in peer-reviewed scientific journals shows that no established human safety concerns have emerged with approved cultivars of GM maize. The data suggest a lower level of mycotoxins in GM maize possessing the trait for insect resistance, which is beneficial to animals and humans consuming such maize.

The most serious health concern related to GM maize is the claim it causes cancer in mammalian species (Séralini et al., 2012). However, that claim has been discredited (Blair and Regenstein, 2015). The report, which was published in the journal Food and Chemical Toxicology resulted in a considerable amount of controversy in the scientific community and in the media which publicized the findings worldwide.

Specifically, the paper reported that male and female laboratory rats fed diets containing Roundup Ready (GM) maize or the herbicide Roundup in drinking water for a prolonged period (2 years) had a higher percentage of tumors and kidney and liver damage than normal controls and died at a higher rate (particularly females) than rats fed a control diet. The GM maize used in the study was authorized for food and feed use in the EU.

The data showed that male and female rats in all treatment groups had higher mortality than the control group but not in a dose-related pattern typically found with toxic agents. For example, males fed the diets containing the highest level of GM grain from crops sprayed with Roundup showed the lowest mortality, similar to that of the controls.

Publication of the report resulted in a large number of letters to the journal in question. A common criticism was that the study had a poor design that did not permit a proper statistical analysis, an inadequate total number of animals, an inadequate number of control animals, a poor choice of animal, and an inadequate description of the dietary regimen. The strain of rat used is known to be susceptible to cancer when aged (incidence 70%−95.8% during a lifetime of 89−105 weeks), and for ethical reasons are generally not employed in such studies. The company supplying the rats reported that the incidence of spontaneous tumors in the strain of rats used and receiving no special diet or treatment is identical with those reported by Séralini et al. (2012). The ethical supervision of the animals was criticized in that the prolonged duration of the trial caused unnecessary suffering for publicity purposes and was contrary to accepted guidelines in that a different set of protocols should have been used to investigate possible long-term effects. Another criticism was that the researchers displayed a bias against GM foods in the design and conduct of the study and that funding support had been received from an anti-GM agency (CRIIGEN: Committee for Research and Independent Information on Genetic Engineering), of which the lead researcher is the President, which many saw as a potential conflict of interest. Several letters requested a full disclosure of the data. The French Society of Toxicologic Pathology refused to support any of the scientific claims made or any relevance to human risk assessment.

As a result of the criticism the paper was withdrawn by the journal.

A logical interpretation of the Séralini et al. (2012) report is that the cancer incidence is likely to have been spontaneous and unrelated to treatment. The study was too small to differentiate the separate effects of strain of rat, aging, and dietary treatment, a point conceded by Séralini et al. (2013) in a rebuttal to the criticisms ("The variability in rates of mortality can indeed, if looked at in isolation, arise in principle by chance"). Additionally, the toxic effects claimed were not dose-related, unusual if the GM maize is indeed toxic.

The European Food Safety Authority (EFSA, 2012) issued an official response to the paper by Séralini et al. (2012) stating that it did not meet acceptable scientific standards and there was no need to reexamine previous safety evaluations of the GM maize in question. This followed separate and independent assessments carried out by EFSA and by six EU Member States (Belgium, Denmark, France, Germany, Italy, and the Netherlands).

Similar reviews and rejection of the claims made by Séralini et al. (2012) and a decision to make no change to the existing authorization for the use of glyphosate-tolerant maize and the herbicide glyphosate (Roundup) in food production were made by Health Canada and the CFIA, the German Federal Institute for Risk Assessment (BfR), Food Standards Australia New Zealand (FSANZ), and the French Agence nationale de sécurité sanitaire de l'alimentation de l'environnement et du travail (Anses). These agencies reviewed information submitted previously to the regulatory agencies as well as published scientific literature on Roundup Ready Maize and Roundup in addition to the Séralini et al. (2012) data.

It should be noted that Séralini and coworkers claimed in previous publications (Séralini et al., 2007; de Vendomois et al., 2009) that GM crops caused liver and kidney pathologies. However the claims have not been substantiated by regulatory agencies or other scientists (Blair and Regenstein, 2015). Thus, other than the Séralini (2012) study, all similar studies reported in peer-reviewed publications showed no safety issues. No other investigators appear to have replicated the findings reported by Séralini et al. (2012). In an interesting development, Séralini et al. (2014) republished the rejected paper in an open-access environmental journal.

Another paper claiming deleterious effects in pigs (and by implication, humans) as a result of consuming feed based on GM maize (a mixture of cultivars) and GM soybean meal was published in the *Journal of Organic Systems* by Carman et al. (2013). It stated that pigs given GM-based feed had more severely inflamed stomachs and that female pigs had enlarged uteri, compared with pigs fed a diet based on conventionally grown maize and soybean meal. No significant differences were found between pigs fed the GM and non-GM diets for feed intake, weight gain, mortality, or blood biochemistry parameters. Although was no difference in overall mortality between the two groups (13% and 14% for the non-GM and GM-fed groups, respectively), it was unacceptably high by industry standards. Also a high percentage of all pigs were found at slaughter to show signs of pneumonia (57% and 60%, respectively). These findings call into question the overall management and welfare conditions under which the pigs were raised. Other shortcomings in the design were pointed out by other researchers, resulting in the findings being dismissed as failing to meet acceptable standards. Since the lead researcher was an Australian and the GM diet was derived from plant cultivars approved for food use in Australia and New Zealand (and other countries), FSANZ (2013) issued a report on the study. In summary the report stated:

Overall, the data presented in the paper are not convincing of adverse effects due to the GM diet and provide no grounds for revising FSANZ's conclusions about the safety of previously approved glyphosate-tolerant and insect-protected GM corn lines and glyphosate-tolerant GM soy lines.

Several cultivars of GM rice have been approved internationally, but no large-scale commercial production of GM rice is taking place in any country. Other GM lines are being developed, with the aim of enhancing the nutritional value of rice since this grain is known to contain insufficient amounts of iron and vitamin A for populations using rice as a staple. GM rice (Golden Rice) with an enhanced content of beta-carotene, a precursor of vitamin A in the diet, is one of these and has been approved for food use in the United States, Australia, New Zealand, and Canada. It also has an enhanced content of iron, of potential importance since the World Health Organization has stated that iron deficiency affects 30% of the world's population. It is called Golden Rice due to its yellow color.

Oilseed crops

Approved GM oilseed crops include soybeans, canola, and cotton, which are major sources of oil and protein for human and animal feeding. Soybeans are the most important of these crops since both the beans and extracted oil are used as human food. Only the oil from canola and cottonseed are used as human food, the fat-extracted meals being used as animal feed: thus the fraction consumed by humans is devoid of any modified DNA. Results of scientific investigations confirm the approval granted to GM cultivars by regulatory authorities, and a few contrary findings published by some investigators (e.g., Carman et al., cited above) have not been accepted as credible by the scientific community.

The safety of glyphosate-tolerant soybeans has been demonstrated in several other studies, using a variety of techniques. For instance (Brake and Evenson, 2004) reported no negative effects on fetal, postnatal, pubertal, or adult testicular development in mice and no differences in litter size or body weight when fed a diet containing glyphosate-tolerant soy in place of conventional soy. Zhu et al. (2004) conducted a nutritional and safety assessment of soy protein from glyphosate-tolerant or conventional soybeans using rats. No adverse effects of GM soybean meal were observed even at a dietary level as high as 900 g/kg, based on growth and mortality rates, gross necropsy findings, hematological and urinalysis values, and clinical serum parameters. In a similar study, Sakamoto et al. (2008) reported that the inclusion of GM soybeans in the diet of rats at a level of 300 g/kg for 104 weeks had no adverse effects on body weight gain, feed intake, gross necropsy findings, hematological and serum biochemical parameters, and organ weights. Pathological examination showed no increase in incidence or in any specific type of nonneoplastic or neoplastic lesions in either sex fed the diet containing GM soybeans.

The main concerns about potentially adverse effects of GM protein foods on health are allergenicity and toxicity, soybean and peanut proteins being known to be allergenic in some human subjects. The potential for allergenicity in a protein can generally be predicted from a comparison of the amino acid sequences to those in databases of known allergenic sequences, but possible allergenicity still needs to be tested and proven to be absent prior to official approval of the product. This has been done with both GM soybeans and canola.

Allergenicity and toxicity

Batista et al. (2005) tested the potential allergenicity of protein extracts prepared from GM maize (insect and/or herbicide-tolerant) and soybeans (glyphosate-tolerant Roundup Ready) and from non-GM control samples in two sensitive groups: children with food and inhalant allergies and individuals with asthma rhinitis. No adverse reactions were observed, and no individuals tested showed any detectable antibodies against the pure modified proteins.

The allergenicity and immuno-reactive components of conventional and GM (glyphosate-tolerant) soybeans were compared in allergic adults who had been sensitized to soybeans (Kim et al., 2006). To evaluate the effects of digestive enzymes and heat treatment, the soybean extracts were heated or preincubated with or without simulated gastric and intestinal fluids. Sensitization rates to non-GM and GM soybean were found to be identical (3.8% of allergic adults), and levels of circulating antibodies specific for the two extracts were comparable.

Gizzarelli et al. (2006) tested the potential allergenicity of GM and conventional soybeans in mice given protein extracts by gastric lavage and found that levels of specific antibodies produced in spleen cell cultures and cytokine production were comparable.

Delaney et al. (2008) showed that the amino acid sequences of the protein in glyphosate-tolerant GM soybeans did not demonstrate any similarities to known allergenic or toxic proteins. Their study also showed that the GM protein was rapidly degraded in simulated gastric fluid containing pepsin and in simulated intestinal fluid containing pancreatin and was completely inactivated at temperatures above 56°C.

These data indicate that the allergenicity of conventional and approved GM cultivars of soybeans for humans is similar.

Fate of GM proteins in the gastrointestinal tract and absorption into bodily tissues

A main factor determining whether a protein food has toxic properties is its fate in the gastrointestinal tract. A possible result of the ingestion of a GM protein is the transfer of transgenic protein fragments to intestinal microorganisms or animal and human cells. This aspect has been investigated in a substantial number of studies.

Harrison et al. (1996) used mice to measure the in vitro digestion of the proteins expressed in GM soybeans (glyphosate-tolerant) and reported a rapid breakdown by proteolytic enzymes. No deleterious effects were recorded when a single dose of the GM protein was administered to mice by gavage at a concentration of up to 572 mg/ kg body weight, based on visual observation, food intake and body weight gain, and gross necropsy findings. The concentration of 572 mg/kg body weight was calculated to exceed 1000-fold the anticipated consumption level by humans of food products potentially containing the GM protein. Using a similar approach, Delaney et al. (2008) assessed the acute toxicity of the modified protein in glyphosate-tolerant soybeans by oral administration of the purified protein to mice via oral gavage. All mice survived the duration of the study, and no clinical signs of systemic toxicity were observed in any of the treatment groups given up to 2000 mg/kg of the modified protein or doses of 10, 100, or 1000 mg/kg/day.

A 90-day toxicity study was conducted by Papineni et al. (2017) using rats to evaluate the safety of herbicide-tolerant soybeans compared to a related non-GM soybean and three commercially available non-GM soybeans. Rats were given diets formulated with either 100 or 200 g/kg soybean meal and 10 or 20 g/kg soybean hulls for 90 days. Animals were evaluated by clinical observation, ophthalmic examination, body weights/body weight gains, feed consumption, hematology, prothrombin time, urinalysis, clinical chemistry, organ weights, and gross and histopathologic examinations. No treatment-related effects were found.

The findings on safety can be explained by consideration of the fate of the DNA from the GM protein in the gastrointestinal tract of humans and farm stock and whether it is digested differently than regular DNA from conventional food and feed. Results indicate that DNA (and RNA) in conventional food is degraded by pancreatic enzymes, and that GM foods are digested by animals in the same way as conventional foods (Blair and Regenstein, 2015). For instance, Aumaitre et al. (2002) reported the results of studies on the feeding of GM maize, canola, and soybean meal to farm animals, showing substantial equivalence of these cultivars with non-GM cultivars in terms of dietary composition and effects on productivity, body and meat composition, meat flavor, milk composition, and nitrogen and ruminal metabolism. DNA from the modified proteins in the GM feedstuffs was detected in the diets but not in the gut, feces, or milk of dairy cows; muscle, liver, kidneys, or spleen of broilers; eggs or excreta of laying hens, or in the liver, kidneys, or spleen of fattening bulls. In addition the published findings show no reports in the scientific peer-reviewed literature demonstrating that an active gene has been transferred from GM plants into animal or human tissues (Blair and Regenstein, 2015).

One of the few studies *involving* human subjects showed that GM protein did not survive passage through the intact gastrointestinal tract of human subjects fed GM soybeans (Netherwood et al., 2004). The data were obtained from human ileostomic patients (individuals in which the terminal ileum section of the gut is resected and digesta are diverted to a colostomy bag) and from volunteers with intact gastrointestinal systems. DNA from the modified protein was detected in the digesta at the terminal end of the ileum, the maximum amount being 3.7% in one of the patients. Results with 12 human volunteers who had intact gastrointestinal systems and were fed a diet containing GM soybeans showed that 90%−98% of an indigestible marker was recovered in the feces but no DNA from the modified protein was detected. It was therefore concluded that a small amount of DNA from GM soy can survive passage through the small intestine of ileostomists, but it is completely degraded in the large intestine.

Beagle et al. (2006) studied the digestive fate in growing pigs of a GM maize cultivar modified to improve protein utilization. The cultivar had not been released for commercial use. DNA from the transgenic protein was detected in 71.4% of stomach and 1.8% of the ileal ingesta samples but was not detected in the large intestine, white blood cells, plasma, liver, or muscle. These data indicated that intestinal degradation of the modified protein began in the stomach was completed mainly in the small intestine and was complete by the time the ingesta had reached the large intestine. These findings support the above data obtained in humans.

On the other hand, the results of some studies suggest that DNA fragments (naturally occurring and transgenic) in the feed do survive to the terminal gut of ruminants and that some uptake into gut epithelial tissues does occur (Sharma et al., 2006). However the researchers concluded that there was no evidence to suggest that transgenic DNA is processed differently in the gut than natural-occurring DNA present in the feed (Sharma et al., 2004).

Sharma et al. (2004) reported that conventional and GM (glyphosate-tolerant) canola were substantially equivalent in terms of degradation of DNA during incubation in rumen fluid. Harrison et al. (1996) confirmed these findings, reporting a statistically significant reduction in the amount of GM canola protein as the digesta passed from the rumen to the small intestine, colon, and feces. These and similar findings by other researchers indicate that plant DNA in the ruminant gut is found only in intact plant cells and that once the DNA is released during fermentation in the rumen environment, it is degraded almost immediately. Plant debris was evident throughout an incubation period of meals and diets for 48 h, but the GM gene fragments were not detectable beyond 4 or 8 h—consistent with the previous study indicating that the DNA in disrupted plant cells is rapidly degraded by nucleases present in ruminal contents (Alexander et al., 2002).

Alexander et al. (2006) measured the concentration of transgenic DNA in digesta, feces, and blood collected from sheep fitted with ruminal and duodenal cannulae and fed forage-based or concentrate-based diets containing GM (glyphosate-tolerant) canola meal. No fragments of transgenic DNA were detected in these fluids, blood, liver, and kidney or in microbial DNA. In addition they reported that the fragments of transgenic DNA found in supernatant fractions from rumen fluid and duodenal fluids and varying in size were not amplifiable. These data can be interpreted as showing that transgenic DNA is completely degraded as it passes through the intestine of sheep.

Work with pigs (Jennings et al., 2003) showed that neither small fragments of transgenic DNA nor immune-reactive fragments of transgenic protein were detectable in loin muscle samples of pigs fed a diet containing glyphosate-tolerant soybean meal. Walsh et al. (2011) tested the presence of transgenic DNA and protein in the tissues of pigs fed a diet containing herbicide-tolerant or the non-GM parent-line maize for 31 days. They reported that detection of the transgene gene and protein was limited to the gastrointestinal digesta, and that antibodies to the transgene were not detected in plasma, kidney, liver, spleen, muscle, heart, or blood.

Ash et al. (2003) investigated the extent of deposition of genetically modified protein from glyphosate-tolerant soybeans in tissues and eggs of laying hens. The GM soybeans, soybean meal, and complete diets were found to contain transgenic proteins. However, whole eggs, egg albumen, liver, and excreta were all negative for residues of transgenic protein, indicating complete digestion of the GM soy. Research by Deauville and Maddison (2005) showed that transgenic DNA could be detected in gizzard digesta in poultry but not in intestinal digesta 96 h following the ingestion of diets containing a source of GM maize and/or soybean meal. Except for a single detection of lectin (nontransgenic single copy gene) in the extracted DNA from one bursa tissue sample, there was no positive detection of any naturally occurring or transgenic single copy genes in either blood, breast meat, liver, gizzard, heart, spleen, kidney, or bursa. A naturally occurring gene present in the feed (rubisco, the gene controlling photosynthesis in plants) was detected in 23% of tissues and in low numbers in blood.

Rossi et al. (2005) found that endogenous DNA was progressively degraded as the digesta moved through the digestive tract of meat chickens. A fragment of transgenic gene was detected only in the crop and gizzard of birds fed a diet containing insect-resistant maize. No significant difference in DNA detection was observed between birds fed the GM and an isogenic (non-GM) maize, indicating that the DNA derived from GM feed undergoes the same fate as from conventional feed. Tony et al. (2003) reported similar findings, results showing that an insect-resistant GM maize cultivar was digested in the same way as a conventional cultivar and that transgenic DNA was degraded in different parts of the gut in the same way as the DNA of the control maize cultivar. No residues of transgenic protein were found in blood or in pectoral or thigh muscle, liver, spleen, kidney, heart muscle, bursa, or thymus gland.

Work with fish has produced findings similar to those described above and has provided further information on possible uptake of transgenic material from the gut into animal tissues. For instance, Sanden et al. (2004) investigated the survival of fragments of GM feedstuffs (herbicide-tolerant maize and phosphate-tolerant soybean flour) in the gut of Atlantic salmon. Residues of the transgenic protein were found in the diet containing GM soy, but only a small DNA fragment could be isolated from the contents of the stomach, pyloric region, midintestine, and distal intestine. No DNA fragments from GM or conventional soy were detected in liver, muscle, or brain tissues. A subsequent investigation (Sanden et al., 2006) showed the presence of dietary DNA from GM soybean meal in some epithelial cells in the salmon intestine and in the cellular vacuolar system. Other work with fish suggests that uptake of residues of GM feedstuffs does not appear to be different from the uptake of non-GM residues. In a study involving zebra fish, dietary DNA fragments from the naturally occurring rubisco gene and from insect-resistant GM maize were detected in several organs, but DNA fragments from GM soybean meal were not detected (Sissener et al., 2011). An investigation involving diets containing GM soybean meal found fragments of the transgenic protein in a few muscle samples of fish after continuous feeding but none were detected 2 days after changing to a non-GM diet (Suharman et al., 2009). Similar research by Ran et al. (2009) reported transgenic DNA soy fragments in heart, liver, stomach, intestine brain, brachia, spleen, and muscle of tissue of tilapia after 4 weeks of a GM diet but did not report any data on residues of non-GM DNA. These findings indicate that dietary DNA fragments, both from GM and non-GM feedstuffs, can be absorbed from the fish intestine and can be detected in internal organs. However, the fragments appear to be below a size able to code for functional proteins.

The available research findings indicate that the transgenic proteins in GM feedstuffs are substantially degraded by feed processing and by passage through the digestive tract of humans, cattle, sheep, pigs, poultry, and fish. There is no evidence to suggest that transgenic DNA is digested in the gut differently from naturally occurring DNA in the food or feed. Little or no GM residues are absorbed, although some investigations have reported the presence of residues of both GM and non-GM proteins in certain organs of some species of fish. The GM residues do not appear to be absorbed preferentially, and there is no evidence to suggest that the absorbed DNA can be incorporated and expressed in the genotype of humans or animals. They are, therefore, not a safety concern; although further work is recommended. No GM residues have been reported in meat, milk, or eggs, suggesting that fish may differ from other species in their utilization of plant-derived diets, possibly because of their different digestive system.

Further data on this topic were reported by Nicolia et al. (2014), who showed that the transgenic DNA is diluted greatly by the total of ingested DNA, that dietary DNA is largely degraded by cooking, and that ingestion of transgenic DNA does not pose a higher risk than ingestion of any other type of DNA. This study confirmed that some feed-ingested DNA fragments (naturally occurring and transgenic) do survive to the terminal gut and that uptake into epithelial tissues does occur. However, there was no evidence to suggest that transgenic DNA is processed in the gut in a manner different from non-GM feed-ingested DNA. Also, there are no reports available in the scientific peer-reviewed literature demonstrating that an active gene has transferred from GM plants into animal or human tissues (Hohlweg and Doerfler, 2001; Thomson, 2001; Van den Eede et al., 2004).

Several recent comprehensive reviews from various authors summarize the results of feeding food-producing animals with the current generation of GM crops (Deb et al., 2013; Flachowsky, 2013; Tufarelli et al., 2015; Van Eenennaam and Young, 2014). The studies have involved sheep, goats, pigs, chickens, quail, cattle, water buffalo, rabbits, and fish fed different GM crop varieties, the results consistently revealed that the performance and health of GM-fed animals were comparable with those fed near isogenic non-GM lines and commercial varieties.

Chemical residues

The available data indicate that cereal grains contain chemical and pesticide residues but show that the amounts are too small to be of concern in relation to human health. Many of the residues found are at the limit of detection. In spite of these findings the possibility of chemical residues in food may be of greater concern to many consumers than the possibility that the food being consumed is derived from GM crops. Therefore, the significance of possible glyphosate residues in grains and oilseeds is an important consideration. It is useful, therefore, to summarize the available evidence relating to humans and animals.

Glyphosate is one of the least toxic pesticides to animals (Duke and Powles, 2008; Kniss, 2017). According to these researchers, glyphosate is less acutely toxic than common chemicals such as sodium chloride or aspirin, with an LD_{50} for rats of over 5 g per kg compared to sodium chloride at 3000 mg/kg (rat) and aspirin at 200 mg/kg. It is not characterized as a carcinogen or a reproductive toxin, and has relatively low chronic toxicity. No toxic effects were observed in a chronic feeding study with dogs fed up to 500 mg/kg body weight/day, the highest dose tested (US Environmental Protection Agency, 1992).

Williams et al. (2000) reviewed the data related to the safety of the herbicide Roundup and its active ingredient, glyphosate, for humans. It included assessments of aminomethylphosphonic acid (AMPA, the breakdown product of glyphosate), Roundup formulations, and the predominant surfactant polyethoxylated tallow amine (POEA) used internationally in Roundup formulations. The studies reviewed included those conducted for regulatory purposes as well as published research reports. These reviewers found that the oral absorption of glyphosate and AMPA is low, and that both materials are eliminated via the urine essentially unmetabolized. The reported evidence also showed that neither glyphosate nor AMPA bio-accumulates in any animal tissue. Acute risks were assessed by comparison of oral LD_{50} values with estimated maximum acute human exposure. Based on the available evidence, the authors concluded that, under present and expected conditions of use, Roundup herbicide does not pose a health risk to humans. Results of a large study conducted in the USA (Agricultural Health Study) confirm these assessments, concluding "no consistent pattern of positive associations indicating a causal relationship between total cancer (in adults or children) or any site-specific cancer and exposure to glyphosate" (De Roos et al. 2005; Mink et al., 2012). A similar conclusion was reached in relation to glyphosate exposure and a range of non-cancer conditions (Mink et al., 2011).

The rat study conducted by Séralini et al. (2012), which was outlined above, included groups provided with drinking water containing glyphosate. The treatments were: (1) regular water, (2) water containing 50 ng/L of glyphosate (described as the contamination level of some regular tap waters), (3) water containing 400 mg/kg glyphosate (described as the US maximum residue level (MRL) of glyphosate and present in some GM feed), and (4) water containing 2.25 g/L glyphosate (described as half of the minimal agricultural working dilution). All four groups were fed a control diet containing conventional maize. The results showed that total deaths (or removals due to morbidity) over a 600-day test period were, respectively; 5/20, 8/20, 9/20, and 5/20. Although these data indicated no clear evidence of a linear effect (which would be expected if glyphosate was toxic at the levels used), Séralini et al. (2012) reported pathological changes in the livers of rats given the glyphosate-supplemented water. The data to support on this conclusion do not allow an accurate assessment of liver damage and appear to again show a nonlinear effect. For instance in males the incidence of nonregressive tumors was lowest in treatment 2 and highest in treatment 4. The significance of possible glyphosate contamination of soyabean products is similar to that of maize crops, the currently available data suggesting no proven negative effects on the health of animal or human consumers. Several studies claim to have demonstrated harmful effects in animals fed GM feed. For instance Vecchio et al. (2004) reported that Sertoli cells in the testes of the mice fed a diet containing GM (glyphosate-tolerant) soybean meal showed enlarged vesicles of the smooth endoplasmic reticulum at 2 and 5 but not at 8 months of age. This result does not appear to have been replicated in any other independent studies. The authors speculated that the effects reported might have been due to the presence of glyphosate residues in the diet containing GM soybean meal, although no analytical data on glyphosate residues were presented.

Sanchez and Parrott (2017) in their review of studies usually cited as evidence of adverse effects of GM food/feed pointed out that the report by Vecchio et al. (2004) shows methodological flaws that invalidate any conclusions of adverse effects.

EFSA (2018) evaluated data published subsequent to its previous assessments of the health risks to humans from exposure levels to glyphosate residues in food and concluded that current exposure levels to glyphosate residues do not pose a risk to human health or to the health of cattle, sheep, pigs, horses, or poultry. A similar finding was reported by the FDA (2018).

Microorganisms

Several GM microorganisms have been approved for food use, the yeast *Saccharomyces cerevisiae* being the first GM organism to be approved for use in food production. GM yeasts are an important source of enzymes used in food production (e.g., cheese-making) and in improving the quality of beer and wine. GM bacteria are used in the production of enzymes such as milk-clotting enzymes for cheese production and food/feed additives such as aspartame and L-lysine. An important feature relating to the safety of these approved GM microorganisms is that they have been modified by utilizing genetic material from within the host species and from microorganisms with GRAS (Generally Regarded As Safe) status (in Europe QPS—Qualified Presumption of Safety).

The safety of the approved GM microorganisms as components of food and livestock feed is attested to by the fact that no authenticated reports of allergenicity or toxicity have been published in any peer-reviewed journals.

GM animals

A GM salmon was approved for commercial food production by Health Canada in 2013. The modification involved the introduction of a growth hormone gene from Chinook salmon into the genome of Atlantic salmon, resulting in faster growth and a reduction in the time to reach market size. Approval was based on assessment of safety, toxicity and allergenicity, and nutritional quality in comparison with conventional salmon. Approval was also provided by the CFIA and by Fisheries and Oceans Canada and Environment Canada who concluded that the GM salmon was not harmful to the environment when produced in containment facilities that prevented their escape or reproduction in the wild. The FDA approved the sale of the GM salmon in the United States in 2015.

Scientists in other countries have conducted similar research on GM fish, e.g., Cuban scientists who developed a faster-growing strain of GM tilapia, *Oreochromis hornorum* L. (Guillén et al., 1999). The fish were shown to be acceptable for food use, following clinical and pathological testing. Also no effects were detected in healthy human volunteers after the consumption of the GM tilapia for 5 days, based on examination of blood hemoglobin, total serum proteins, glucose, creatinine, cholesterol, leukocytes, and erythrocyte levels. One explanation for these findings in the human volunteers is that fish growth hormone is not bioactive in primates (Dunham, 2004) and furthermore would be degraded by cooking and during digestion in the human gut.

Production of GM fish is also an area of active research in China.

Foods derived from animals fed diets containing GM feedstuffs

Most of the GM food crops are fed to farm stock. It is important, therefore, to ensure that the milk, meat, and eggs produced are safe for consumers. A large number of studies has been conducted on these issues, including studies required by regulatory agencies.

Blair and Regenstein (2015) reviewed the available evidence related to the inclusion of approved GM feed ingredients in the diet of food-producing animals and concluded that the nutritional composition, nutritive value, and safety of these food and feed sources were essentially equivalent to their related non-GM counterparts. They also concluded that meat, milk, and eggs produced by farm stock fed diets containing approved GM ingredients are as wholesome, safe, and nutritious as similar foods produced by stock fed diets based on conventional feed ingredients. Reports published subsequent to the Blair and Regenstein (2015) review are in agreement with these conclusions (Tufarelli et al., 2015; Korwin-Kossakowska et al., 2016; Panchin and Tuzhikov, 2017; de Vos and Swanenburg, 2018).

Several studies have examined the possibility that functional transgenes from GM feedstuffs might be present in milk, meat, and eggs. While DNA in biologically active genes and proteins is commonly present in food and feed, it is known to be degraded rapidly during digestion. Also it has been shown that the cooking and processing of GM crops into human food and livestock feed disrupts the cellular structure and breaks up the DNA sequences (Blair and Regenstein, 2015), reducing the possibility of absorption of active DNA sequences into the edible tissue from these animals.

However, fragments of both types of DNA have been shown to be absorbed in the gut, though not on a consistent basis, and uptake of DNA fragments from the intestinal tract can be regarded as a normal physiological process. Importantly there are no reports available in the scientific peer-reviewed literature demonstrating that an active gene can be transferred from GM plants into animal or human tissues (Hohlweg and Doerfler, 2001; Thomson, 2001; Van den Eede et al., 2004; Korwin-Kossakowska et al., 2016; Van Eenannaam and Young, 2017). Also the available data do not provide evidence for the transfer of transgenic DNA from ingesta to the gut microorganisms.

One effect of these findings is that a valid and reliable assay to establish whether or not food-producing animals have been fed GM feed is very difficult (or impossible) to develop.

Consensus on safety

There is broad scientific consensus that all approved foods and feeds been derived from GM crops being marketed currently are safe to eat. This conclusion is based on the findings of independent scientists, regulatory agencies, and scientific agencies in many countries. In its assessment, the American Association for the Advancement of Science (AAAS, 2012) found that the World Health Organization, the American Medical Association, the US National Academy of Sciences, the European Joint Research Centre, the British Royal Society, and every other respected organization that has examined the evidence has come to the same conclusion: consuming foods containing ingredients derived from GM crops is no riskier than consuming the same foods containing ingredients from crop plants modified by conventional plant improvement techniques. Other reviews have reached similar conclusions (US National Academies (NRC, NAS, NAM) 2016. Genetically Engineered Crops: Experiences and Prospects. The National Academies of Sciences, Engineering, and Medicine, Washington, DC 20001; European Commission, 2008; Batista and Oliviera, 2009; Domingo and Bordonaba, 2011; Snell et al., 2012; ChileBio, 2013; Nicolia et al., 2014; Blair and Regenstein, 2015; Korwin-Kossakowska et al., 2016; Panchin and Tuzhikov, 2017; Sanchez and Parrot, 2017; de Vos and Swanenburg, 2018).

A consistent finding in these reviews is that much, or all, of the transgenic DNA is degraded in the gastrointestinal tract of the human or animal consumer and that none is absorbed into the tissues. Although some consumers have concerns about the safety of GM foods, this can be attributed largely to the fact that they have not been made aware of the extensive database of favorable findings. In some cases consumers prefer not to know about this extensive database or choose to ignore it.

In a recent review, Van Eenennaam and Young (2014) assessed the scientific literature on performance and health of animals consuming feed containing GM ingredients and composition of products derived from them, since on a global basis, food-producing animals consume 70%—90% of the biomass of GM crops. Data on livestock productivity and health were collated from publicly available sources from 1983, before the introduction of GM crops in 1996, through 2011, a period with high usage levels of GM feedstuffs. These datasets, representing over 100 billion animals following the introduction of GM crops, did not show any unfavorable trends of concern in livestock health and productivity. Also, the researchers found that no study has shown any differences in the nutritional profile of animal products derived from GM-fed animals.

In 2016, the US National Academies of Sciences, Engineering, and Medicine released a report concluding that biotech crops are no different from conventionally bred crops in terms of risks to human health and the environment. This was followed by the declaration of more than 100 Nobel Laureates, together with other scientists, calling upon biotech critics to cease and desist opposition to GM crops (specifically Golden Rice), and for governments around the world to reject campaigns against biotech crops.

In spite of these findings and recommendations, not all countries and regions have adopted biotechnology to improve the quality and yield of food crops, in particular Europe. According to recent assessments by leading European scientists, this can be attributed to a current policy which discriminates against the cultivation of GM crops (e.g., Masip et al., 2013), based on a stated uncertainty of the technology and the public attitude to GM foods. This policy has been criticized as a trade barrier to the importation of cereal grains and grain products from countries using GM technology, resulting in the United States bringing a case to the World Trade Organization (WTO) against the EU's failure to implement a timely, science-based approval system for food and feed products enhanced through biotechnology. Several other countries, including Argentina, Australia, Canada, Chile, Colombia, El Salvador, Honduras, Mexico, New Zealand, Peru, and Uruguay joined the United States in the complaint because they also wished to ensure that science-based determinations are applied to regulatory decisions. In 2006 the WTO ruled that the EU had failed to meet its WTO obligations of implementing a timely, science-based system for the approval of biotech-enhanced agricultural products. As a result, the European Community in 2006 announced its intention to implement the ruling. In spite of this declaration some critics point out that Europe has still to adopt rational, science-based principles for the harmonization of agricultural policies (e.g., Masip et al. (2013)).

An important assessment of EU policy was issued by EASAC, the European Academies Science Advisory Council (2013). This body was formed by the national science academies of the EU member states to enable them to collaborate in providing advice to European policy-makers. Their assessment stated: *"The scientific literature shows no compelling evidence to associate such crops, now cultivated worldwide for more than 15 years, with risks to the environment or with safety hazards for food."* They also pointed out several other authoritative reports confirming the safety of approved GM food products. For instance, a comprehensive assessment by the Swiss National Science Foundation (2012) of over 2000 studies found that no health or environmental risks related to GM technology had been identified.

The EASAC report also emphasized that any regulatory system had to be evidence-based. The report found "an inconsistent and inefficient connection" between the recommendations of EFSA and political action for final expeditious approval of GM cultivars. The regulatory system in the EU focuses on the technology used in the development of GM crops, whereas countries like Canada regulate new crop cultivars on the basis of the traits expressed and not on the basis of the method used to introduce the traits, whether achieved using conventional breeding, mutagenesis, or GM technology. The US policy is similar to that in Canada in that it is focused on the product of genetic modification techniques, not the process itself; that regulation is based on verifiable scientific risks; also that GM products are on a continuum with existing products, so that existing regulations are sufficient to assess the products. This approach acknowledges the fact that it is the product, and not the process, that warrants regulation because it is the presence of novel traits in a new crop that potentially pose an environmental or health risk, and not how the traits were specifically introduced. Regulations for biotechnology-derived crops should therefore be focused on those cultivars that possess traits sufficiently different from the same or similar species as to require an assessment of risk.

Some observers regard the US policy in this regard as lax and that the precautionary approach adopted in Europe is more appropriate in spite of the scientific evidence (e.g., Bühl et al., 2016). However it is useful to point out that the response to a major food-related problem (bovine spongiform encephalopathy [BSE] commonly known as mad cow disease, affecting cattle and capable of being passed to humans that had eaten infected meat) over 2 decades ago was handled very effectively in the USA (and in Canada), resulting in far fewer deaths in livestock and humans than in some European countries and testifying to the effectiveness of the US food regulations.

Special labeling of GM products is a controversial topic, and EASAC found the policy to be scientifically indefensible for products that are substantially the same as those of non-GM origin. The EASAC study received backing from the national academies of all EU member states, plus Norway and Switzerland. The report is therefore a major contribution to this debate on GM foods as it reflects the view of Europe's most eminent scientists. The European Union's chief scientific advisor Anne Glover fully supported the report published by EASAC (http://www.euractiv. com/science-policymaking/chief-eu-scientist-backs-damning-news-530693).

This background helps to explain the restrictive approach taken on GM products in the EU. This policy is demonstrated in trade issues and in the labeling policy adopted in the EU, which conveys a negative image of the quality of GM foods to consumers.

Consumers in several countries would like to have information about the GM status on the food label, but given the current climate it is likely that a mandatory labeling requirement for GM foods will have the effect of deterring consumers from purchasing these foods, either from a lack of knowledge or from prejudice. As a result the United States adopted a voluntary policy of labeling of GM foods, and Canada has adopted a policy of requiring no special labeling of GM foods.

The whole issue of what foods should be excluded and included in any mandatory label of GM foods needs to precede any discussion on labeling.

The American Association for the Advancement of Science (AAAS, 2012) stated that: "*it is the long-standing policy of the Food and Drug Administration (FDA) that special labeling of a food is required if the absence of the information provided poses a special health or environmental risk. The FDA does not require labeling of a food based on the specific genetic modification procedure used in the development of its input crops. Legally mandating such a label can only serve to mislead and falsely alarm consumers.*"

The US Council for Agricultural Science and Technology (CAST, 2014) commissioned a study on the topic. According to their assessment, people have the right to know what is in their food and its nutrient content, but the right to know what is in food is different from the right to know how it was produced. Furthermore, this uniquely singles out GM technology—not other production methods and processes—for such a right-to-know claim. There is no science-based reason to single out GM foods and feeds for mandatory process-based labeling.

One unfortunate effect of mandatory requirement for the special labeling of GM foods without scientific justification in developed countries is that countries that do not yet have the benefit of advanced food safety regulations are liable to adopt the same requirement, alarming their consumers unnecessarily about on the safety of GM foods and possibly impairing their nutritional well-being.

As reported by Blair and Regenstein (2015), the Catholic Pontifical Academy of Sciences and 33 outside experts made a passionate endorsement in 2009 of GMOs for global food security and development. Their report (Meldolesi, 2011) stated that *"there is a moral imperative"* to make the benefits of genetic engineering technology *"available on a larger scale to poor and vulnerable populations who want them,"* urging opponents to consider the harm that withholding this technology will inflict on those who need it most. *'Technology, in this sense, is a response to God's command to till and to keep the land (cf. Gen 2:15) that he has entrusted to humanity, and it must serve to reinforce the covenant between human beings and the environment, a covenant that should mirror God's creative love."* The Danish Council on Ethics (2019) made a similar plea. Both Jews and Muslims through their formal processes of food certification for compliance with their food laws (kosher and halal, respectively) have accepted microbial and plant-based GM products.

GM crops are being grown by Amish farmers in the United States, a group that follows a very traditional lifestyle.

Health benefits of GM crops

Although the main focus in assessing the relationship between GM crops and human health is safety, it is important to point out that the introduction of GM crops has had demonstrable human health benefits. These benefits can be attributed to reductions in chemical use, increased crop yields and improved farm profits (Klümper and Qaim, 2014). Grain quality has also been improved and, importantly, dangerous mould contamination decreased as a result of prevention of insect damage to crops.

As outlined by Smyth (2019) small landholder farmers in developing countries gain most of the human health benefits because they generally lack the mechanized systems of pesticide application and the necessary protective clothing used in developed countries. These benefits can be categorized as follows.

Reductions in pesticide poisonings

Most or all of the fieldwork (seeding, weeding, spraying and harvesting) is done by hand on the typically small farms in developing countries. Pesticide applications, especially on crops such as cotton and brinjal (eggplant, *Solanum melongena*), require numerous applications throughout the course of the growing season to ensure that insect damage is minimized. This can result in skin absorption of chemical residues by the farmers and pesticide poisoning. The introduction of GM crops, particularly Bt cotton, has resulted in significant reductions in farmer pesticide poisoning cases in China, India, Pakistan and South Africa due to fewer applications and reduced levels of insecticide exposure (Bennett et al., 2003; Hossain et al., 2004; Kouser and Qaim, 2011, 2013; Zhang et al. 2016; Zilberman et al., 2018; Smyth, 2019). It is clear from these data that glyphosate is a safer herbicide than alternative pesticides (as explained earlier in this chapter) and requires a lower application rate.

Reductions in farmer suicide

India has a high rate of reported suicides and researchers have examined the relationship between farmer suicide and the adoption of GM cotton in that country. The findings of Gruère and Sengupta (2011) indicate a plateauing of the suicide rate after the commercialization of Bt cotton, followed by a reduction and a plateauing. The reduction has been explained by the facts that while farmers growing Bt cotton have annual costs higher than non-GM farmers, the costs of pesticides are reduced and yields are improved. Thus net farmer returns are on average 58.2% higher (Klümper and Qaim, 2014), the improvement in financial well-being promoting better mental health and resulting in the reduction in suicides. Three clear conclusions emerge from the Gruère and Sengupta (2011) data: (1) there is no observed correspondence (or causality) between the national Bt cotton adoption rate and farmer suicides, contradicting a claim by opponents of GM technology that Bt cultivation is responsible for the farmer suicides; (2) the annual growth in suicides actually diminished after the introduction of Bt cotton; and (3) the largest increase in adoption happened during years with reduced suicides.

Any interpretation of the situation that adoption of Bt cotton in India has had a beneficial effect in reducing farmer suicides is contested by other researchers with some suggesting that the high costs of GM crops are a cause of suicides. However there is support for the Gruère and Sengupta (2011) conclusions. Plewis (2014) examined the data under the aegis of the UK Royal Statistical Society and found that pattern of changes in suicide rates over the previous 15 years was consistent with a beneficial effect of Bt cotton, though not in every cotton-growing state in India. This is an important but controversial issue that merits further research to determine quantitatively the relationship between Bt cotton adoption and suicide rate in Indian farmers. Importantly the results to date contradict the claim by opponents of GM technology that Bt cotton cultivation is directly responsible for the farmer suicides (Smyth, 2019).

Lowering cancer incidences

The development of insect-resistant crop varieties has begun to have a noticeable potential to improve human health through a reduction in cancer rates (Smyth, 2019). Prior to the commercialization of Bt crops (maize in particular), insect damage to the harvested crop increased the potential for the development of products harmful to health due to mould contamination. A study of 21 years of maize production found that Bt maize contained lower concentrations of mycotoxins (29%), fumonisins (31%) and thricotecens (37%) (Pellegrino et al., 2018). Mycotoxins are both toxic and carcinogenic to humans and animals and are of most concern in developing countries (WHO, 2018) related to factors such as climate, lack of food choices and food regulations. Fumonisins have been linked to higher rates of neural tube defects in consumers of high maize-based diets (Missmer et al., 2006).

Nutritional benefits

GM crops have made significant contributions (Smyth 2019) to address the United Nations Sustainable Development Goals, in particular goals (1) reducing poverty and (2) reducing hunger and improving food security. Bio-enhanced GM crops for human consumption have been developed, with increased micronutrient content (Hefferon, 2014), and are likely to become of particular importance in developing countries (Smyth, 2019). Nutritionally enhanced foods improve nutrient intake in consumers, preventing and/or helping to reduce mortality from cancer, diabetes, cardiovascular disease, and hypertension, as well as providing significant childhood health improvements such as reducing blindness due to the lack of vitamin A availability. In many developing countries, plant-based food accounts for one hundred per cent of an individual's nutrient intake, emphasizing the importance of nutritionally enhanced crops.

Addressing consumer concerns

It is clear from all surveys and reports in the popular media that there is a substantial amount of distrust among consumers about the quality and safety of GM foods, although there is no foundation for this concern in the scientific evidence.

As the journal *Nature Biotechnology* (Anon, 2013) asked in an editorial "Three decades after transgenes were first introduced into plants, why do so many consumers remain so negative about genetically modified (GM) food?" "*It does not matter that no adverse health effects have been recorded from eating them. Nor does it matter that august agencies, such as the World Health Organization, the US National Academy of Sciences, the European Commission or the American Medical Association, have come out with ringing endorsements of their safety. The fact is, negative attitudes remain entrenched and widespread. And changing them will require a concerted and long-term effort to develop GM foods that clearly provide convincing benefits to consumers—something that seed companies have conspicuously failed to do over the past decade.*"

In its analysis, the editorial outlined various factors that have contributed to the situation. One is that reports claiming negative effects on health are seized upon by anti-GM activists "*no matter how flimsy the evidence or flawed the study design*" and "*All too often, an uncritical and sensationalist media leaps upon negative findings, continuing the cycle of scares, urban myths, and downright mistruths about GM food, all of which serve to stoke consumer paranoia.*"

The editorial found also that the public mistrusts most mainstream sources of data on GM foods, including large corporations, regulators, governments, and even scientists. In addition, European regulators have deepened the existing prejudices "*by creating a regulatory system that singles out GM products as sufficiently threatening to merit special attention.*"

A recent survey in the United States (IFIC, 2018) found that 36% of respondents knew very little or nothing at all about bioengineered or genetically modified foods, the same number as those who knew at least a fair amount. Despite the low level of knowledge, 47% said they avoid GMO foods at least part of the time. The vast majority (85%) of those who avoid GMOs did so out of human health concerns. Fernbach et al. (2019) obtained similar findings in a survey of consumers in the

USA, France and Germany, extreme opponents knowing the least about GM foods but thinking they knew the most.

Addressing this issue by ensuring that consumers are better informed on the established facts relating to GM foods should therefore be considered a priority. However, a major challenge will be determining and applying the most effective method of doing so while warning notices still appear on the labels of GM foods, indicating that politicians also need to become better informed about GM foods.

It is likely that consumers, particularly young people, are now more receptive to news about GM foods than previously. More balanced reports on food quality are being published in the popular media, written by better-educated journalists. This may explain why a recent survey conducted by the New Scientist (Lawton, 2018) in the United Kingdom on public attitudes to science, technology, medicine, and environment found that the UK public is well-informed and supportive of current developments in science and technology. The survey was conducted in August 2018 with a representative sample of 2026 UK adults, not all of whom were readers of the *New Scientist* magazine. Results showed that the issues of most importance were genetic engineering, artificial intelligence, cancer, and climate change, since they were regarded as most likely to have an impact on society and human life. In addition, the survey showed that majority (69%) were in favor of genetically modified (GM) crops, stating that they could help feed the world. A large percentage (80%) also believed that genetic engineering could help cure or eradicate diseases. Social media were perceived by survey respondents negatively, largely because of fake news, trolls, and peer pressure on young people. One surprising finding of the survey was that politicians were regarded as ignoring public hopes and fears, reinforcing the suggestion above that politicians need to become better informed on current issues in science and technology particularly in relation to GM foods.

In a welcome initiative in Africa, the Uganda Biosciences Information Center is conducting a series of teachers' training workshops in 2018 to create and increase countrywide appreciation of integration of biosciences in the country's formal education system. Developing a better appreciation of the benefits of biotechnology in young people is an objective that should be adopted universally.

Conclusions

Biotechnology continues to play a very important role in the production of new cultivars of crops, and this was recognized in the award of the 2013 World Food Prize to a team of scientists who had made outstanding contributions to this science. A necessary component of this development in crop production is the need to ensure that the GM cultivars are as safe and nutritious for food and feed use as their conventional counterparts. There is broad scientific consensus that all approved foods and feeds that have been derived from GM crops being marketed currently are safe to eat, and consumers need to be convinced of these findings. Consumers in several countries would like to have information about the GM status on the food label, but it is clear that a mandatory labeling requirement for GM foods has the effect of deterring consumers from purchasing these foods, either from a lack of knowledge or from prejudice. The whole issue of what foods should be excluded and included in any mandatory label on GM foods needs to precede any discussion on labeling. Ethical concerns about GM foods might best be addressed by religious leaders.

References

AAAS, 2012. Statement by the American Association for the Advancement of Science Board of Directors on Labeling of Genetically Modified Foods. http://www.aaas.org/news/releases/2012/media/AAAS_GM_statement.pdf.

Alexander, T.W., Sharma, R., Okine, E.,K., Dixon, W.T., Forster, R.J., Stanford, K., McAllister, T.A., 2002. Impact of feed processing and mixed ruminal culture on the fate of recombinant EPSP synthase and endogenous canola plant DNA. FEMS Microbiology Letters 214, 263−269.

Alexander, T.W., Reuter, T., Okine, E., Sharma, R., McAllister, T.A., 2006. Conventional and real-time polymerase chain reaction assessment of the fate of transgenic DNA in sheep fed Roundup Ready rapeseed meal. British Journal of Nutrition 96, 997−1005.

Anon, 2013. Editorial. Contrary to popular belief: three decades after transgenes were first introduced into plants, why do so many consumers remain so negative about genetically modified (GM) food? Nature Biotechnology 31, 767.

Aumaitre, A., Aulrich, K., Chesson, A.C., Flachowsky, G., Piva, G., 2002. New feeds from genetically modified plants: substantial equivalence, nutritional equivalence, digestibility, and safety for animals and the food chain. Livestock Production Science 4, 223−238.

Ash, J., Novak, C., Scheideler, S.E., 2003. The fate of genetically modified protein from roundup ready soybeans in laying hens. Journal of Applied Poultry Research 12, 242−245.

Batista, R., Oliveira, M.M., 2009. Facts and fiction of genetically engineered food. Trends in Biotechnology 27, 277−286.

Batista, R., Nunes, B., Carmo, M., Cardoso, C., José, H.S., de Almeida, A.B., Manique, A., Bento, L., Ricardo, C.P., Oliveira, M.M., 2005. Lack of detectable allergenicity of transgenic maize and soya samples. Journal of Allergy and Clinical Immunology 116, 403−410.

Beagle, J.M., Apgar, G.A., Jones, K.L., Griswold, K.E., Radcliffe, J.S., Qiu, X., Lightfoot, D.A., Iqbal, M.J., 2006. The digestive fate of *Escherichia coli* glutamate dehydrogenase deoxyribonucleic acid from transgenic corn in diets fed to weanling pigs. Journal of Animal Science 84, 597−607.

Bennett, R., Buthelezi, T.J., Ismael, Y., Morse, S., 2003. Bt cotton, pesticides labour and health: a case study of smallholder farmers in the Makhathini Flats Republic of South Africa. Outlook on Agriculture 32, 123−128.

Blair, R., Regenstein, J.M., 2015. Genetic Modification and Food Quality: A Down to Earth Analysis. Wiley-Blackwell, Oxford, UK, 276 pp.

Brake, D.G., Evenson, D.P., 2004. A generational study of glyphosate-tolerant soybeans on mouse fetal, postnatal, pubertal and adult testicular development. Food and Chemical Toxicology 42, 29−36.

Bühl, L., Malarciuc, C., Völlmecke, A., 2016. Transatlantic Differences in GMO Regulation: A Case Study Approach. http://www.openjournals.maastrichtuniversity.nl/Marble/article/download/285/232.

Carman, J.A., Vlieger, H.R., Ver Steeg, L.J., Sneller, V.E., Robinson, G.W., Clinch-Jones, C.A., Haynes, J.I., Edwards, J.W., 2013. A long-term toxicology study on pigs fed a combined genetically modified (GM) soy and GM maize diet. Journal of Organic Systems 8, 38–54.

CAST, 2014. The Potential Impacts of Mandatory Labeling for Genetically Engineered Food in the United States. Issue Paper Number 54, April 2014. Council for Agricultural Science and Technology, Ames, Iowa.

Chen, Y., Hwang, W., Fang, T.J., Cheng, Y., Lin, J., 2011. The impact of transgenic papaya (TPY10-4) fruit supplementation on immune responses in ovalbumin-sensitised mice. Journal of the Science of Food and Agriculture 91, 539–546.

ChileBio, 2013. 610 Scientific Articles Confirm Safety of Food and Feeds Derived From Genetically Modified Crops. http://www.isaaa.org/kc/cropbiotechupdate/article/default.asp?ID=11295.

Danish Council on Ethics, 2019. GMO and Ethics in a new era. http://www.etiskraad.dk/~/media/Etisk-Raad/en/Publications/DCE_Statement_on_GMO_and_ethics_in_a_new_era_2019.pdf?la=da.

De Roos, A.J., Blair, A., Rusiecki, J.A., Hoppin, J.A., Svec, M., Dosemeci, M., Sandler, D.P., Alavanja, M.C., 2005. Cancer incidence among glyphosate-exposed pesticide applicators in the Agricultural Health Study. Environmental Health Perspectives 113, 49–54.

de Vendomois, J.S., Roullier, F., Cellier, D., Séralini, G.-E., 2009. A comparison of the effects of three GM corn varieties on mammalian health. International Journal of Biological Sciences 5, 706–726.

de Vos, C.J., Swanenburg, M., 2018. Health effects of feeding genetically modified (GM) crops to livestock animals: a review. Food and Chemical Toxicology 117, 3–12.

Deaville, E.R., Maddison, B.C., 2005. Detection of transgenic and endogenous plant DNA fragments in the blood, tissues, and digesta of broilers. Journal of Agricultural and Food Chemistry 53, 10268–10275.

Deb, R., Sajjanar, B., Devi, K., Reddy, K., Prasad, R., Kumar, S., Sharma, A., 2013. Feeding animals with GM crops: boon or bane? Indian Journal of Biotechnology 12, 311–322.

Delaney, B., Zhang, J., Carlson, G., Schmidt, J., Stagg, B., Comstock, B., Babb, A., Finlay, C., Cressman, R.F., Ladics, G., Cogburn, A., Siehl, D., Bardina, L., Sampson, H., Han, Y., 2008. A gene-shuffled glyphosate acetyltransferase protein from Bacillus licheniformis (GAT4601) shows no evidence of allergenicity or toxicity. Toxicological Sciences 102, 425–432.

Domingo, J.L., Bordonaba, J.G., 2011. A literature review on the safety assessment of genetically modified plants. Environment International 37, 734–742.

Duke, S.O., Powles, S.B., 2008. Glyphosate: a once-in-a-century herbicide. Pest Management Science 64, 319–325.

Dunham, R.A., 2004. Aquaculture and Fisheries Biotechnology Genetic Approaches. CAB International, Wallingford, UK.

EFSA, 2012. Review of the Séralini et al. (2012) publication on a 2-year rodent feeding study with glyphosate formulations and GM maize NK603 as published online on 19 September 2012 in Food and Chemical Toxicology. EFSA Journal 10, 2910.

EFSA, 2018. Review of the existing maximum residue levels for glyphosate according to article 12 of Regulation (EC) No 396/2005. EFSA Journal 16, 5263.

European Commission, 2008. Scientific and technical contribution to the development of an overall health strategy in the area of GMOs. In: Report EUR 23542 EN, Joint Research Centre − Institute for Health and Consumer Protection. Office for Official Publications of the European Communities, Luxembourg, 56 pp, Scientific and Technical Research series - ISSN 1018-5593.

Ewen, S.W., Pusztai, A., 1999. Effect of diets containing genetically modified potatoes expressing *Galanthus nivalis* lectin on rat small intestine. Lancet 354, 1353−1354.

FDA, 2018. Glyphosate Residues in Foods. https://www.fda.gov/Food/FoodborneIllness Contaminants/Pesticides/ucm618247.htm.

Fermín, G., Keith, R.C., Suzuki, J.Y., Ferreira, S.A., Gaskill, D.A., Pitz, K.Y., Manshardt, R.M., Gonsalves, D., Tripathi, S., 2011. Allergenicity assessment of the papaya ringspot virus coat protein expressed in transgenic rainbow papaya. Journal of Agricultural and Food Chemistry 59, 10006−10012.

Fernbach, P.M., Light, N., Scott, S.E., Inbar, Y., Rozin, P., 2019. Extreme opponents of genetically modified foods know the least but think they know the most. Nature Human Behaviour 3, 251−256.

Flachowsky, G., 2013. Feeding studies with first generation GM plants (input traits) with food-producing animals. In: Flachowsky, G. (Ed.), Animal Nutrition with Transgenic Plants. CAB International Biotechnology Series. CABI, Oxford, UK, pp. 72−93.

FSANZ, 2013. Response to a feeding study in pigs by Carman et al. Food Standards Australia New Zealand FSANZ Canberra. Australia, and Wellington, New Zealand. www. foodstandards.gov.au/consumer/gmfood/Pages/Response-to-dr-Carman%27s-study.aspx.

Gizzarelli, F., Corinti, S., Barletta, B., Iacovacci, P., Brunetto, B., Butteroni, C., Afferni, C., Onori, R., Miraglia, M., Panzini, G., Di Felice, G., Tinghino, R., 2006. Evaluation of allergenicity of genetically modified soybean protein extract in a murine model of oral allergen-specific sensitization. Clinical and Experimental Allergy 36, 238−248.

Gruère, G., Sengupta, D., 2011. Bt cotton and farmer suicides in India: an evidence-based assessment. Journal of Development Studies 47, 316−337.

Guillén, I., Berlanga, J., Valenzuela, C.M., Morales, A., Toledo, J., Estrada, M.P., Puentes, P., Hayes, O., de la Fuente, J., 1999. Safety evaluation of transgenic tilapia with accelerated growth. Marine Biotechnology 1, 2−14.

Harrison, L.A., Bailey, M.R., Naylor, M.W., et al., 1996. The expressed protein in glyphosate tolerant soybean, 5-enolpyruvylshikimate-3-phosphate synthase from Agrobacterium sp. strain CP4, is rapidly digested in vitro and is not toxic to acutely gavaged mice. Journal of Nutrition 126, 728−740.

Hefferon, K.L., 2014. Nutritionally enhanced food crops; progress and perspectives. International Journal of Molecular Sciences 16, 3895−3914.

Hohlweg, U., Doerfler, W., 2001. On the fate of plant or other foreign genes upon the uptake in food or after intramuscular injection in mice. Molecular Genetics and Genomics 265, 225−233.

Hossain, F., Pray, C., Lu, Y., Huang, J., Fan, C., Hu, R., 2004. Genetically modified cotton and farmers' health in China. International Journal of Occupational and Environmental Health 10, 296−303.

IFIC, 2018. IFIC Foundation Survey. Research With Consumers to Test Perceptions and Reactions to Various Stimuli and Visuals Related to Bioengineered Foods (Washington, DC).

Jennings, J.C., Kolwyck, D.C., Kays, S.B., Whetsell, A.J., Surber, J.B., Cromwell, G.L., Lirette, R.P., Glenn, K.C., 2003. Determining whether transgenic and endogenous plant

DNA and transgenic protein are detectable in muscle from swine fed Roundup Ready soybean meal. Journal of Animal Science 81, 1447−1455.

Joint FAO/IAEA Programme, 2014. Mutant Variety Database. http://mvgs.iaea.org/AboutMutantVarities.aspx.

Kim, S.H., Kim, H.M., Ye, Y.M., Kim, S.H., Nahm, D.H., Park, H.S., Ryu, S.R., Lee, B.O., 2006. Evaluating the allergic risk of genetically modified soybean. Yonsei Medical Journal 47, 505−512.

Klümper, W., Qaim, M., 2014. A meta-analysis of the impacts of genetically modified crops. Plos One 9, e111629.

Kniss, A.R., 2017. Long-term trends in the intensity and relative toxicity of herbicide use. Nature Communications 8, 14865.

Korwin-Kossakowska, K., Sartowska, G., Tomczyk, B., Prusak, B., Sender, G., 2016. Health status and potential uptake of transgenic DNA by Japanese quail fed diets containing genetically modified plant ingredients over 10 generations. British Poultry Science 57, 415−423.

Kouser, S., Qaim, M., 2011. Impact of Bt cotton on pesticide poisoning in smallholder agriculture: a panel data analysis. Ecological Economics 70, 2105−2113.

Kouser, S., Qaim, M., 2013. Valuing financial, health, and environmental benefits of Bt cotton in Pakistan. Ecological Economics 44, 323−335.

Lawton, G., 2018. Revealed: What the UK Public Really Thinks about the Future of Science. www.newscientist.com/article/2179920-revealed-what-the-uk-public-really-thinks-about-the-future-of-science/.

Lin, H., Yen, G., Huang, T., Chan, L., Cheng, Y., Wu, J., Yeh, S., Wang, S., Yang, L., 2013. Toxicity assessment of transgenic papaya ringspot virus of 823-2210 line papaya fruits. Journal of Agricultural and Food Chemistry 61, 1585−1596.

Masip, G., Sabalza, M., Perez-Massot, E., Banakar, R., Cebrian, D., Twyman, R.M., Capell, T., Albajes, R., Christou, P., 2013. Paradoxical EU agricultural policies on genetically engineered crops. Trends in Plant Science 18, 312−324.

Meldolesi, A., 2011. Vatican panel backs GMOs. Nature Biotechnology 29, 11.

Mink, P.J., Mandel, J.S., Lundin, J.I., Sceurman, B.K., 2011. Epidemiologic studies of glyphosate and non-cancer health outcomes: a review. Regulatory Toxicology and Pharmacology 61, 172−184.

Mink, P.J., Mandel, J.S., Sceurman, B.K., Lundin, J.I., 2012. Epidemiologic studies of glyphosate and cancer: a review. Regulatory Toxicology and Pharmacology 63, 440−452.

Missmer, S.A., Suarez, L., Felkner, M., Wang, E., Merrill Jr., A.H., Rothman, K.J., Hendricks, K.A., 2006. Exposure to fumonisins and the occurrence of neural tube defects along the Texas-Mexico border. Environmental Health Perspectives 114, 237−241.

Netherwood, T., Martín-Orúe, S.M., O'Donnell, A.G., Gockling, S., Graham, J., Mathers, J.C., Gilbert, H.J., 2004. Assessing the survival of transgenic plant DNA in the human gastrointestinal tract. Nature Biotechnology 22, 204−209.

Nicolia, A., Manzo, A., Veronesi, F., Rosellini, D., 2014. An overview of the last 10 years of genetically engineered crop safety research. Critical Reviews in Biotechnology 34, 77−88.

Panchin, A.Y., Tuzhikov, A.I., 2017. Published GMO studies find no evidence of harm when corrected for multiple comparisons. Critical Reviews in Biotechnology 37, 213−217.

Papineni, S., Murray, J.A., Ricardo, E., Dunville, C.M., Sura, R.K., Thomas, J., 2017. Evaluation of the safety of a genetically modified DAS-444Ø6-6 soybean meal and hulls in a 90-day dietary toxicity study in rats. Food and Chemical Toxicology 109, 245−252.

Pellegrino, E., Bedini, S., Nuti, M., Ercoli, L., 2018. Impact of genetically engineered maize on agronomic, environmental and toxicological traits: a meta-analysis of 21 years of field data. Nature Scientific Reports 8, 1−12.

Powell, M., Wheatley, A., Omoruyi, F., Asemota, H., Williams, N.P., Tennant, P.F., 2008. Effects of subchronic exposure to transgenic papayas (*Carica papaya L.*) on liver and kidney enzymes and lipid parameters in rats. Journal of the Science of Food and Agriculture 88, 2638−2647.

Ran, T., Mei, L., Wang, L., Aihua, L., Ru, H., Jie, S., 2009. Detection of transgenic DNA in tilapias (*Oreochromis niloticus*, GIFT strain) fed genetically modified soybeans (Roundup Ready). Aquaculture Research 40, 1350−1357.

Rossi, F., Morlacchini, M., Fusconi, G., Pietri, A., Mazza, R., Piva, G., 2005. Effect of Bt corn on broiler growth performance and fate of feed-derived DNA in the digestive tract. Poultry Science 84, 1022−1030.

Royal Society UK, 1999. Review of data on possible toxicity of GM potatoes. Annual Review of Plant Biology 59, 771−812.

Sakamoto, Y., Tada, Y., Fukumori, N., Tayama, K., Ando, H., Takahashi, H., Kubo, Y., Nagasawa, A., Yano, N., Yuzawa, K., Ogata, A., 2008. A 104-week feeding study of genetically modified soybeans in F344 rats. Shokuhin Eiseigaku Zasshi (Journal of the Food Hygienic Society of Japan) 49, 272−282.

Sanchez, M.A., Parrott, W.A., 2017. Characterization of scientific studies usually cited as evidence of adverse effects of GM food/feed. Plant Biotechnology Journal 5, 1227−1234.

Sanden, M., Bruce, I.J., Rahman, M.A., Hemre, G.I., 2004. The fate of transgenic sequences present in genetically modified plant products in fish feed, investigating the survival of GM soybean DNA fragments during feeding trials in Atlantic salmon, *Salmo salar* L. Aquaculture 237, 391−405.

Sanden, M., Krogdahl, A., Bakke-Mckellep, A.M., Buddington, R.K., Hemre, G.I., 2006. Growth performance and organ development in Atlantic salmon, *Salmo salar L. parr* fed genetically modified (GM) soybean and maize. Aquaculture Nutrition 12, 1−14.

Séralini, G.-E., Cellier, D., de Vendômois, J.S., 2007. New analysis of a rat feeding study with a genetically modified maize reveals signs of hepatorenal toxicity. Archives of Environmental Contamination and Toxicology 52, 596−602.

Séralini, G.-E., Clair, E., Mesnage, R., Gress, S., Defarge, N., Malatesta, M., Hennequin, D., de Vendômois, J.S., 2012. Long term toxicity of a Roundup herbicide and a Roundup-tolerant genetically modified maize. Food and Chemical Toxicology 50, 4221−4231 (paper retracted).

Séralini, G.-E., Mesnage, R., Defarge, N., Gress, S., Hennequin, D., Clair, E., Malatesta, M., de Vendômois, J.S., 2013. Answers to critics: why there is a long term toxicity due to NK603 Roundup-tolerant genetically modified maize and to a Roundup herbicide. Food and Chemical Toxicology 53, 476−483.

Séralini, G.E., Clair, E., Mesnage, R., Gress, S., Defarge, N., Malatesta, M., Hennequin, D., de Vendômois, J.S., 2014. Republished study: long-term toxicity of a Roundup herbicide and a Roundup-tolerant genetically modified maize. Environmental Sciences Europe 26, 14.

Sharma, R., Alexander, T.W., John, S.J., Forster, R.J., 2004. Relative stability of transgene DNA fragments from GM rapeseed in mixed ruminal cultures. British Journal of Nutrition 91, 673−681.

Sharma, R., Damgaard, D., Alexander, T.W., Dugan, M.E.R., Aalhus, J.L., Stanford, K., McAllister, T.A., 2006. Detection of transgenic and endogenous plant DNA in digesta and tissues of sheep and pigs fed Roundup Ready canola meal. Journal of Agricultural and Food Chemistry 54, 1699–1709.

Sissener, N.H., Sanden, M., Krogdahl, Å., Bakke, A.-M., Johannessen, L.E., Hemre, G.-I., 2011. Genetically modified plants as fish feed ingredients. Canadian Journal of Fisheries and Aquatic Sciences 68, 563–574.

Snell, C., Bernheim, A., Bergé, J., Kuntz, M., Pascale, G., Paris, A., Ricroch, A.E., 2012. Assessment of the health impact of GM plant diets in long-term and multigenerational animal feeding trials: a literature review. Food and Chemical Toxicology 50, 1134–1148.

Suharman, I., Satoh, S., Haga, Y., Takeuchi, T., Endo, M., Hirono, I., Aoki, T., 2009. Utilization of genetically modified soybean meal in Nile tilapia *Oreochromis niloticus* diets. Fisheries Science 75, 967–973.

Thomson, J., 2001. Horizontal transfer of DNA from GM crops to bacteria and to mammalian cells. Journal of Food Science 66, 188–193.

Tony, M.A., Butschke, A., Broll, H., Grohmann, L., Zagon, J., Halle, I., Dänicke, S., Schauzu, M., Hafez, H.M., Flachowsky, G., 2003. Safety assessment of Bt 176 maize in broiler nutrition: degradation of maize-DNA and its metabolic fate. Archiv fur Tierernahrung 57, 235–252.

Tufarelli, V., Selvaggi, M., Dario, C., Laudadio, V., 2015. Genetically modified feeds in poultry diet: safety, performance, and product quality. Critical Reviews in Food Science and Nutrition 55, 562–569.

US Environmental Protection Agency, 1992. Pesticide tolerance for glyphosate. Federal Register 57, 8739–8740.

Van den Eede, G., Aarts, H., Buhk, H.J., Corthier, G., Flint, H.J., Hammes, W., Jacobsen, B., Midtvedt, T., Van der Vossen, J., Von Wright, A., Wackernagel, W., Wilcks, A., 2004. The relevance of gene transfer to the safety of food and feed derived from genetically modified (GM) plants. Food and Chemical Toxicology 42, 1127–1156.

Van Eenennaam, A.L., Young, A.E., 2014. Prevalence and impacts of genetically engineered feedstuffs on livestock populations. Journal of Animal Science 92, 4255–4278.

Van Eenennaam, A.L., Young, A.E., 2017. Detection of dietary DNA, protein, and glyphosate in meat, milk, and eggs. Journal of Animal Science 95, 3247–3269.

Vecchio, L., Cisterna, B., Malatesta, M., Martin, T.E., Biggiogera, M., 2004. Ultrastructural analysis of testes from mice fed on genetically modified soybean. European Journal of Histochemistry 48, 449–453.

Walsh, M.C., Buzoianu, S.G., Gardiner, G.E., Rea, M.C., Gelencsér, E., Jánosi, A., Epstein, M.M., Ross, R.P., Lawlor, P.G., 2011. Fate of transgenic DNA from orally administered Bt. Mon810 maize and effects on immune response and growth in pigs. PLoS One 6, e27177.

Wikipedia, 2013. Mutation Breeding. http://en.wikipedia.org/wiki/Mutation_breeding.

Williams, G.M., Kroes, R., Munro, I.C., 2000. Safety evaluation and risk assessment of the herbicide Roundup and its active ingredient, glyphosate, for humans. Regulatory Toxicology and Pharmacology 31, 117–165.

World Health Organization (WHO), 2018. Mycotoxins. http://www.who.int/news-room/factsheets/detail/mycotoxins.

Zhang, C., Hu, R., Huang, J., Huang, X., Shi, G., Li, Y., Yin, Y., Chen, Z., 2016. Health effects of agricultural pesticide use in China: implications for the development of GM crops. Nature Science Reports 6, 1–8.

Zhu, Y., Li, D., Wang, F., Yin, J., Hong, J., 2004. Nutritional assessment and fate of DNA of soybean meal from roundup ready or conventional soybeans using rats. Archives of Animal Nutrition 58, 295–310.

Further reading

EFSA, 2007. Statement on the Fate of Recombinant DNA or Proteins in Meat, Milk and Eggs From Animals Fed With GM Feed. Available at. http://www.efsa.europa.eu/en/efsajournal/doc/744.pdf.

FSANZ, 2012. Response to Séralini Paper. Food Standards Australia New Zealand FSANZ Canberra,. Australia, and Wellington, New Zealand. www.foodstandards.gov.au/consumer/gmfood/seralini/pages/default.aspx.

Omobowale, E.B., Singer, P.A., Daar, A.S., 2009. The three main monotheistic religions and gm food technology: an overview of perspectives. BMC International Health and Human Rights 9, 18–35.

Swiss Academies, 2013. Gentechnisch veranderte Nutzpflanzen – und ihre Bedeutung Fur eine nachhaltige Landwirtschaft in der Schweiz. Swiss Academies of Arts and Sciences. http://www.akademien-schweiz.ch/index/Publikationen/Berichte.html.

Case studies

Genetically modified (GM) food in South Africa

6.1

Jan-Hendrik Groenewald, BSc, BSc(Hons), MSc, PhD

Executive Manager-Biosafety South Africa, Somerset West, Western Cape, South Africa

Contextualizing the two-decades-old debate on GM foods

Generally speaking, members of the public and scientists have very different perceptions regarding the utility, safety, and desirability of genetic modification (GM) technology and the genetically modified organisms (GMOs) that result from it. In fact, in the United States, the science-related issue with the greatest difference in opinion between the public and scientists (37 vs. 88%) is that of the safety of GM foods (Funk and Rainie, 2015). This divide and resulting publicly accessible debate is almost exclusively focused on GM foods/crops, while GM-based medicines and industrial applications of GM technology are rarely discussed or considered to be controversial. The reasons for this state of affairs are varied, complex, interdependent, and context specific, but three, broad thematic contributing factors have crystallized over the past 2 decades since GM crops were first commercialized:

1. *The specialized nature of GM-related topics*: The specialized nature of genetics, GM technology, risk analysis, etc. places these subjects well outside the frame of reference of the general public. In addition, the average person's limited exposure to GMOs, including exposure to the direct benefits they offer, has also limited the value of heuristic decision-making. As a consequence, much uncertainty exists and many have no other option than to base their personal opinion and risk-benefit judgments on the limited, oversimplified and often intentionally inaccurately framed information, which is publicly accessible.

2. *Inaccurate risk-benefit perceptions*: Internationally, the predominant GM crops are commodity products, e.g., maize, soybeans, and cotton, with GM traits that improve their agricultural input characteristics, e.g., insect resistance, and herbicide tolerance. The direct benefits associated with such GM traits, e.g., reduced agricultural input costs and higher yields, are therefore experienced by the farmers, rather than the consumer who ends up buying a final product, which is mostly indistinguishable from the conventional one. In addition, consumers are exposed to claims of increased risks via the public debate on GMOs— personal risk-benefit perceptions regarding GM foods are therefore strongly

prejudiced. Two different experiences gained since GM products were first commercialized support this strong link between positive risk-benefit perceptions and the acceptance of GM products. Firstly, farmers from around the world have enthusiastically accepted GM crops and those who do not yet have access to them, continue to petition their availability. Secondly, GM-based medicines, where the benefits to the individual patient are clear and direct, are accepted without apparent objection.

3. *Food's social context*: Food is not a purely functional object but also represents a magnitude of societal, cultural, and emotional values. Many of the criticisms leveled against GM food relate to these broader social issues, rather than any of the inherent characteristics of the crops or derived foods themselves. The association of many of the currently available GM crops with multinational companies, intellectual property, industrial-scale farming, a commodity nature, etc. has seemingly placed GM crops in conflict with some of these evolving societal values.

In combination, these factors have resulted in the GM debate evolving into a value-based, rather than a purely fact-based discussion. The use of GM technology, particularly in food crops, has therefore become controversial, not because of any tangible, well-definable, or quantifiable inherent characteristics of GMOs, but rather because it represents a watershed between different value systems—ostensibly placing "technological advancement" and a "nature ideology" in direct conflict. Exacerbated by the fact that it is a technology that is applied to living organisms, i.e., nature itself. GMOs have therefore developed into one of the quintessential examples dividing these apparently contrasting value systems.

In addition, identity-protective cognition theory suggests that science-based arguments alone will not bring an end to such value-based debates, because facts alone do not change value perceptions (Kahan, 2010). People's value systems divert them from using their reasoning to identify and recognize what the facts are and instead redirect them to conform to beliefs that predominate their value system (Kahan, 2017). This value-based, cognitive bias is the reason why data are always disputed and areas of uncertainty ever expanded in scope and detail. In fact, one of the most noticeable characteristics of the anti-GMO narrative over the past 2 decades is that the arguments against the use of GM technology have evolved continually to exploit new areas of apparent uncertainty, in support of personal value systems, when preceding doubts have been addressed successfully through research.

Distinguishing between "science" and "value" conversations is critically important to make sense of the "GMO debate". Although a final decision regarding "acceptance" will always remain a personal choice, influenced by values, emotion, and dogma, these should be kept out of science-based discussions of GMOs, as not to dilute fact and/or unduly impact access for those with different, personal value choices.

Opposition based on emotion and dogma contradicted by data must be stopped. How many poor people in the world must die before we consider this a crime against humanity?

From: Open letter to Greenpeace, the UN and Governments around the world signed by 107 Nobel Laureates in medicine, chemistry, physics and economics, June 2016.

Genetically modified organism science
Genetics and genetic modification

Genetic modification relates to the deliberate design, editing, and/or assembly of genetic sequences using recombinant DNA technologies and is aimed at changing the genetic characteristics of a living organism. GM technology is not constrained by sexual reproduction and allows researchers to transfer a specific genetic sequence (a particular gene or genetic trait) to any another organism to generate novel individuals, i.e., GMOs, with novel trait combinations. In other words, a GMO is a living organism identical to its conventional counterpart except for the addition of one or two extra genetic traits, e.g., insect resistance and herbicide tolerance, which were transferred to the organism using GM techniques.

Although GM technology is relatively young ($\sim$40 years) and for the first time allows the routine transfer of genetic material between unrelated species, the exact same underlying genetic principles still apply to GM genes and GMOs. GM genes do not behave differently or are not "unique" or "unnatural" as a matter of principle. GM technology is only the directed application of what has been learned from nature (and happens in nature; Kyndt et al., 2015) and is a natural continuation of age old genetic design technologies such as selective breeding, hybrid development, polyploidy, mutation, breeding, etc. GM genes can, however, change the phenotypic traits of the resulting GMO in a novel way and are for this reason subject to regulation, which requires confirmation that the new GM trait(s) does not introduce any biosafety (food/feed/health or environmental safety) concerns, before the GMO can be commercialized.

Why do we want to use GM technology?

GM technology is a very powerful tool with which the genetic traits of organisms can be changed in very particular and useful ways. It is:

- **specific**, allows the addition/removal/change of a particular gene(s),
- **accurate**, only the targeted genes are impacted at the level of intervention, and
- **unrestrictive** in terms of transferring genetic trait between organisms.

It can therefore be used as a powerful research tool to elucidate biological research questions or as an innovation tool with which to develop novel, useful biotech products.

When these GM products are developed within a framework that ensures their sustainability, they can effectively address social, environmental, and technical challenges associated with biological systems in, for example, the health, agriculture, and manufacturing sectors. The unique potential benefits of GM technology are especially important within the context of responsible economic and social development, accessible healthcare, sustainable agriculture aimed at feeding a growing world population using limited natural resources, and climate change.

Genetically modified organism regulation and sustainable use in South Africa

Why are genetically modified organisms regulated?

GMOs are potentially novel, living organisms with a genetic trait that may not have been associated with the particular organism previously, and this new trait may impact the way the organism interacts with its environment—e.g., grow, propagate, or ability to act as a food source for other organisms. A GMO's potential impact on human/animal health and the environment therefore has to be assessed scientifically to ensure it is safe before it is released and consumed.

The assessment and management of these potential risks are the reason for and objective of all GMO regulations, in the same way road safety regulations, for example, govern the risks associated with driving a vehicle on a public road. However, keeping the analogy in mind, it is critically important that regulatory requirements remain proportional to the possible risks they govern, to ensure they do not unintentionally inhibit appropriate application and the loss of all associated benefits.

How are genetically modified organisms regulated in South Africa?

Although some binding international agreements regarding GMOs are in place, e.g., the Cartagena Protocol on Biosafety and the CODEX Alimentarius, it is important to realise that GMOs are primarily governed based on national legislation. Every country or territory therefore has the right and ability to decide exactly how they would like to use and regulate GMOs. The "regulatory unit" (the entity that receives approval) of all GMO regulatory systems around the world is the "GM event"—a genetically unique GM *individual*. In the case of GM crops, this individual is subsequently used in breeding programs to propagate the GM trait in its progeny to yield the various varieties farmers plant. Every GM event must be approved by every national regulatory authority where it may be imported or cultivated. Typically, the GMO events that have been commercialized in South Africa have therefore been subjected to the regulatory requirements and scrutiny of various other countries as well.

All activities with GMOs in South Africa are primarily regulated under the GMO Act (Act 15 of 1997). This includes research and development, import/export, production, consumption, and other uses of GMOs and their products. The GMO Act establishes minimum standards to ensure the food/feed (health) and environmental safety, as well as the socioeconomic viability of all activities involving GMOs (see the "GMO sustainability" section below for more details on these parameters).

It further establishes the necessary operational procedures and infrastructure required for the regulation of GMOs:

- The Registrar, seated within the Department of Agriculture, Forestry and Fisheries (DAFF), is responsible for administrating the Act.
- Inspectors are responsible for ensuring permit conditions are adhered to.
- The Advisory Committee (AC) is a panel of independent scientists that does a science-based evaluation of all applications.
- The Executive Council (EC) is the decision-making body and consists of 10 members representing seven different state agencies, i.e., DAFF, as well as the departments of Health (DoH), Science and Technology (DST), Environmental Affairs (DEA), Trade and Industry (dti), Labour (DoL), and Water Affairs and Sanitation (DWS).

Decisions by the EC are based on the information in the permit application, the AC's science-based recommendations, and the public's inputs and are interpreted within government's policy framework. A unanimous resolution is required for a permit to be issued, ensuring all possible perspectives from this widely representative body are critically considered.

Additional regulations, specifically pertaining to GMOs, are also contained under legislation of the DoH, e.g., food safety and labeling requirements, DEA, e.g., postrelease monitoring and triggers for environmental impact assessments (EIAs) and dti, e.g., labeling (Fig. 6.1.1).

The top five facts about South Africa's regulatory framework for genetically modified organisms

1. The goal of the GMO Act (1997) as defined in its preamble is "*to provide for measures to promote the responsible development, production, use and application of GMOs,*" emphasizing the balanced and accountable approach of the regulatory framework. Although risk management is the primary focus of the Act, it does so within a context of recognizing the benefits associated with biotechnological innovation.
2. South Africa's regulatory framework for GMOs was one of the earliest established anywhere in the world (initiated in the late 1970s by local scientists), which allowed South Africa to be an early adopter of GM technology—resulting in South Africa now having one of the most experienced, robust, and respected regulatory systems in the world. To date, the system has processed more than 5400 individual permit applications.
3. It is widely representative and a well-balanced system, allowing direct policy interpretations from various government departments and public inputs, while maintaining a solid science basis. Examples of policy interpretations, based on

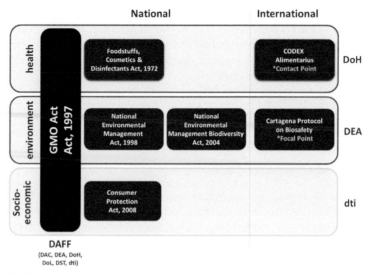

FIGURE 6.1.1

South Africa's regulatory framework for GMOs. National acts and international agreements directly pertaining to the regulation of GMOs, the associated government departments, and the scope of the respective legislation are indicated. *DAFF*, Department of Agriculture, Forestry and Fisheries; *DEA*, Department of Environmental Affairs; *DoH*, Department of Health; *DoL*, Department of Labour; *DST*, Department of Health Science and Technology; *dti*, Department of Trade and Industry; *GMO*, genetically modified organism.

socioeconomic impact assessments, which have been enforced over the years include safeguarding South Africa's international markets, ensuring competition within the relevant sectors and retaining minimum levels of choice for the end user. This close collaboration and wide consultation of experts underlay the fact that no confirmed negative impacts have been reported for the commercialized GMOs in the country.

4. Public participation in regulatory decision-making is a legislated prerequisite for confined use, commodity clearance and general release permit applications. Government has also invested substantially over the past 2 decades in communication and engagement programs to inform the public about biotechnology and GMOs. First in the form of the Public Understanding of Biotechnology (PUB) Program within the South African Agency for Science and Technology Advancement (SAASTA) and subsequently via the biosafety communication and engagement program of the national biosafety service platform, Biosafety South Africa.

5. The regulatory system continues to improve and evolve as required. For example, the GMO Act was amended in 2006 to include the requirements of the Cartagena Protocol on Biosafety, to which South Africa acceded in 2003. In addition,

various guideline documents have been developed over the years to help ensure quality and compliance and to inform the public on the workings of the regulatory system. Guideline updates have been included over the years to keep them aligned with international best practice and to accommodate issues such as the management of stacked traits, new breeding techniques, low-level presents, etc.

Genetically modified organism sustainability
Sustainability as the minimum standard for genetically modified organism use

Broadly defined, "*being sustainable*" is the minimum requirement a GMO should adhere to before it will be considered for commercial release in South Africa. GMO sustainability can be divided into its biosafety components, i.e., food/feed (health) and environmental safety, and its viability components, i.e., sociopolitical (governance) and technoeconomic feasibility (Fig. 6.1.2).

Before continuing to discuss the sustainability of GMOs, it is critically important to appreciate the fact that these details can only be sensibly and accurately considered at the hand of a specific, individual GM product. A GM tomato containing an insecticidal protein is very different from a GM sugarcane containing a gene that makes it tolerant to a certain herbicide, when considering the respective sustainability components, e.g., food safety, environmental interactions, and potential socioeconomic benefits. Broad, generalized statements regarding the safety, utility, value, effectivity, or any other attributes of "GMOs" or "GM products" as a broad, undifferentiated group can therefore never be accurate as they fall prey to the *generalization fallacy*. Sweeping statements like "*GMOs are unsafe*" or "*GMOs increase pesticide use*" are therefore inaccurate, in the same way a statement such as "*Birds are blue*" is, as they lack context and do not recognize the possible vast differences between diverse entities, constituents, requirements, contexts, applications, etc.

The food and feed safety (health) aspects of a GMO are evaluated in terms of the organism that has been transformed (the host), the organism from which the transgene was obtained (the donor), the specific genes or genetic sequences that were used for transformation, and the final GMO event/individual. Among others, food/feed properties such as toxicity, allergenicity, and nutritional value are analyzed and evaluated. Because food safety data are transferable, these are often shared between regulatory authorities around the world.

Environmental risk assessments for GMOs consider all possible interactions between the specific GMO and its receiving environment, including aspects such as gene flow, nontarget impacts, resistance development, persistence, and associated treatments such as herbicide use.

Sociopolitical and technoeconomic assessments consider wide-ranging issues such as the existence and requirements of the national biosafety regulatory framework and its competent authority, the economic viability of the product, stakeholder,

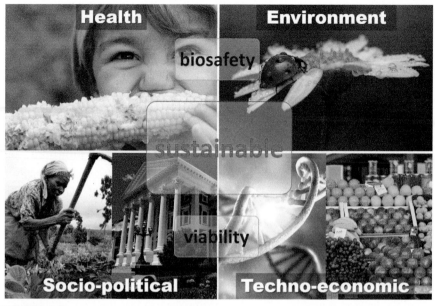

FIGURE 6.1.2

Defining GMO sustainability. To be sustainable, a GMO needs to adhere to minimum health, environmental, sociopolitical, and technoeconomic standards. *GMO*, genetically modified organism.

and consumer preferences, possible market impacts, diversity and choice in the market, etc.

Risk in context

A quick search of the internet may leave one convinced that GMOs and in particular GM crops and foods are hazardous, harmful, risky, and/or unsafe. To understand how the potential risks associated with GMOs are assessed and managed and to be able to better judge these claims for oneself, a better understanding of the vocabulary and context of risk analysis is required. Understanding the meaning of the terms most often used in GMO risk analysis is important, not only because it helps to define the context of the discipline but also because it can assist individuals in doing their own basic risks assessments.

- Hazard—is any potential source of harm (the possibility to cause harm).
- Harm—is an adverse outcome or impact.
- Risk—is the probability of a harm occurring under defined circumstances.
- Safety—is the condition of not being exposed to or being protected from harm.

Hazards are fairly easy to identify because many examples are part of our daily lives, e.g., a bottle of bleach under the sink. Similarly, it is easy to come up with examples of possible harms associated with a particular hazard, e.g., bleach poisoning. In contrast, it is more difficult to explain and understand the concept of risk because it is not something concrete, but rather a probability or chance of something happening. Risk is the "probability link" between hazard and harm, considering *both* the mechanisms of exposure and the extend of the harm:

$$\text{hazard} \xrightarrow{\text{exposure}} \text{harm}$$

In other words, risk defines the chance that a hazard (bleach) will result in a harm (poisoning) and implies exposure (access to and ingestion of the bleach) and a harmful result (poisoning/illness).

In formal, science-based risk assessments, the extent of a risk is estimated (or characterized) by considering both the likelihood and consequence of a harm occurring

$$\text{risk} = \text{likelihood} \times \text{consequence}$$

Reducing either of these, e.g., locking the cupboard in which the bleach is stored or only storing bleach at highly diluted concentrations, will therefore reduce the risk of bleach poisoning. Note that although both these risk management interventions have reduced the risk of bleach poising, none of them has changed the chemical structure or hazardous nature of bleach per se.

Finally, everything we do involves some level of risk and NO activity is absolutely safe. Moreover, our *perceptions* regarding specific risks are influenced by a wide array of personal factors such as familiarity (either technical knowledge or personal experience), biases, dread (or absence thereof), experienced benefits, etc., resulting in risk perceptions that are very different from the actual, technical risk. For example, millions of people get into their cars and drive on public roads every day without really contemplating the risks associated with it. We generally perceive the associated risks to be acceptable because we are familiar with them and the context in which they occur, realise, based on experience, that we can manage them well, and the risks are clearly outweighed by the benefits of high mobility. When discussing risk one should therefore always remember that:

- there is no such thing as zero risk or absolute safety,
- risk should be assessed in the relevant context,
- risks can be managed, and
- experienced benefits counteract the associated risk perceptions.

Risk analysis as basis for sound decision-making

Sustainability as a minimum standard for the use of technology is a widely agreeable goal, but is it possible to accurately assess and obtain this for a GMO?

The answer is, YES, by subjecting potential GM products to a scientific risk analysis.

Risk analysis is by no means new or unique to GMOs, but GMO-specific risk analysis frameworks have evolved into sophisticated, robust, and powerful design and decision-making tools over the past 30 years (Johnson et al., 2007; Wolt et al., 2010). Risk analysis is in principle the contextualized, iterative integration of risk assessment, risk management, and risk communication. Although slightly different frameworks may be used by different risk assessors and although the details may vary between an environmental risk assessment and a food safety assessment, the same broad risk analysis principles are shared among the various assessments and act as the critically important science basis for all these assessments (Fig. 6.1.3).

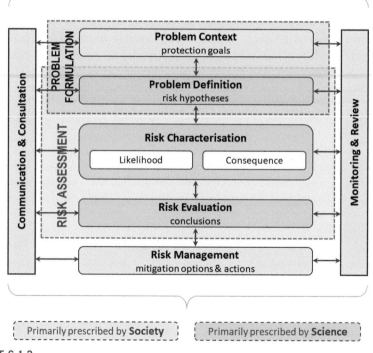

FIGURE 6.1.3

GMO risk analysis framework. *GMO,* genetically modified organism.

Adapted from Johnson, K.L., Raybould, A.J., Hudson, M.D., Poppy, G.M., 2007. How does scientific risk assessment of GM crops fit within the wider risk analysis? Trends in Plant Science 12(1), 1—5 & Wolt, J.D., Keese, P., Raybould, A., Fitzpatrick, J.W., Burachik, M., Gray, A., Olin, S.S., Schiemann, J., Sears, M., Wu, F., 2010. Problem formulation in the environmental risk assessment for genetically modified plants. Transgenic Research 19, 425—436.

The most important principles and steps of risk analysis can be summarized as follows:

- It is not a science- or scientist-only activity. Several of the activities are aimed at or fully integrated with society and/or societal values, in fact, some of the most important inputs into the process, such as the identification of protection goals, are based on societal values, not the scientific method (refer to the yellow blocks in Fig. 6.1.3).
- Generally speaking, the first step of risk analysis is to consider the context, both in terms of those tangible parameters that directly relate to the specific GMO, e.g., the host and donor organisms and receiving environment, as well as the more generic and intangible parameters such as values, e.g., what constitutes a harm, and protection goals.
- The second step, problem formulation, basically entails asking the question "*What can go wrong within the specific context?*". This is asked from all the different perspectives, which together constitute sustainability, i.e., possible health, environmental, and socioeconomic impacts, and then evaluated in terms of possible scientific risk hypotheses. To be able to develop meaningful hypotheses a clear pathway to harm must exist.
- If any of these hypotheses are found to be plausible, the next step is to characterize the associated risk in terms of the likelihood that harm may occur and the consequence thereof. If the risk is ascertained to be unacceptably high, the product will be discarded, or, if possible, risk mitigation strategies may be incorporated into its design or use to reduce the risk to acceptable levels.
- Only when the risks associated with a *specific* GMO is found to be acceptable, will it be released for commercial use, but even then, it will still be subject to postrelease monitoring. Monitoring data are fed back into the risk analysis process to continuously verify if the original risk analysis conclusions remain accurate.
- The steps of risk analysis are therefore not strictly sequential, but rather iterative, meaning that information obtained from a risk assessment can be used to inform risk management decisions and vice versa. Similarly, data generated from risk communication activities, e.g., public engagement, are used to define the outcomes of the risk analysis process.

Local and international experience with genetically modified organism use

When discussing the sustainable or safe use of GMOs in the South African context, i.e., judging the performance of "GMOs" based on historic data, it is important to remember the following:

- GM-based medicines, generally referred to as recombinant DNA (rDNA) medicines, have also long been commercialized, but are seldom discussed or criticized (refer to "Contextualizing the two-decades-old debate on GM foods").

Public debates on "GMO use in South Africa" therefore predominantly relates to GM crops or GM foods.

- In terms of GM crops, only a few, specific GMOs, i.e., maize, cotton, and soy, each having either one or a combination of only two GM traits, i.e., insect resistance and herbicide tolerance, are relevant, as only these have been commercialized in South Africa. To be clear, no other GM crops, fruits, or vegetables are currently available on the South African market.
- One should distinguish between "a theoretical" and "the relevant" GMO discussion, i.e., the discussion should be limited to what is applicable—the few approved GMOs within the South African context. For example, in theory pollen-mediated gene flow, often, disparagingly referred to as "genetic contamination," is indeed possible and for that reason always forms part of GMO risk analysis, but within the specific context of an approved GMO within a particular environment, such broad assertions may be irrelevant at best and malevolent at worst.

The local perspective

South Africa approved its first GM crop, insect resistant cotton, in 1998. Since then, GM crops were widely adopted by farmers because of the value they derive from the GM traits. Currently approximately 85% of the maize, 95% of the soy, and 100% of the cotton planted in South Africa contain GM traits (ISAAA, 2017). To date, the estimated economic gains for South Africa since 1998 are ~US$ 2.1 billion; at ~US$ 237 million per annum (Brookes and Barfoot, 2017). Although the benefits may not be as apparent for the end consumer, studies have shown that GM adoption has stabilized the growth rate in maize prices, thereby reducing price risks (Abidoye and Mabaya, 2014). However, these authors continue to emphasize that direct benefits, derived from commodities such as maize, by the end consumer, are influenced much more by the off-farm part of the food system, unrelated to the fact that they are GM or not.

Seminal research regarding the possible socioeconomic benefits of GM crops for South African smallholder and subsistence farmers has been done over the past decade by Dr Marnus Gouse and coworkers of the University of Pretoria. They found that although South Africa's smallholder farmers do derive direct economic benefits from certain GM crops, they generally rate the social benefits associated with these crops in their particular context, as more important. These benefits include time and drudgery savings due to the reduced labor requirements and the elimination of the challenges associated with the application of chemical insecticides—which of course also has a safety benefit. An insect-resistant grain stored in informal systems also has lower levels of fungal/mycotoxin contamination due to the lower levels of insect damage (Gouse et al, 2004, 2005a, b, 2006, 2016; Gouse, 2012; Pray et al., 2013).

No confirmed food/feed or environmental safety issues have been raised during the 2 past decades regarding the approved GMO crops (or medicines) in South

Africa (Gouws and Groenewald, 2012). Similarly, no environmental issues have been identified (Van den Berg and Van Wyk, 2007; Van Wyk et al., 2008). Although insect resistance has developed against the first generation of Bt maize (Van Rensburg, 2007), this does not represent an environmental impact, and the potential economic impacts have been mitigated through appropriate risk management practices, including refugia compliance management and the introduction of stacked Bt genes.

The international perspective

A recent review by the US National Academies of Sciences, Engineering, and Medicine, which represents the current seminal work on this topic, is presented as the international consensus. It is entitled *"Genetically Engineered Crops: Experiences and Prospects"* and is available at http://www.nap.edu/23395:

- More than 20 scientists worked for longer than 2 years and considered more than 900 different publications and studies on GMOs, spanning more than 20 years, and read more than 700 submissions by the public to come to the conclusion that *"**no substantiated evidence that foods from GM crops were less safe than foods from non-GM crops could be found.**"*
- The use of insect-resistant or herbicide-resistant crops did not reduce the overall diversity of plant and insect life on farms, in fact, sometimes insect-resistant crops resulted in increased insect diversity, the study found.
- The available evidence indicates that GM soybean, cotton, and maize have generally had favorable economic outcomes for producers who have adopted these crops, but outcomes have varied depending on pest abundance, farming practices, and agricultural infrastructure. Although GM crops have provided economic benefits to many small-scale farmers in the early years of adoption, enduring and widespread gains will depend on such farmers receiving institutional support, such as access to credit, affordable inputs such as fertilizer, extension services, and access to profitable local and global markets for the crops.

Conclusion

GM technology is a powerful tool that has already made significant positive contributions to agricultural and industrial practice, productivity, and sustainability, as well as human healthcare around the world. It is indeed possible to develop and use GMOs sustainably, and risk analysis is an appropriate, robust, and effective design and decision-making tool to help ensure this within an appropriate sustainability framework; a framework that should also carefully consider the issues related to the social license required for the successful deployment of GM products.

South Africa has a well-established, representative, robust, and competent regulatory framework for GMOs, which has enabled it to be an early adopter of GM technology and has therefore greatly benefited from its implementation in terms of (1) human healthcare and food production, (2) the protection and justifiable, sustainable use of our environmental resources, and (3) enabling socioeconomic development and growth.

References

Abidoye, B.O., Mabaya, E., 2014. Adoption of genetically modified crops in South Africa: effects on wholesale maize prices. Agrekon 53 (1), 104−123.

Brookes, G., Barfoot, P., 2017. Farm income and production impacts of using GM crop technology 1996−2015. GM Crops and Food 8 (3), 156−193.

Funk, C., Rainie, L., 2015. Public and Scientists' Views on Science and Society. Pew Research Center Study on Science Literacy, Undertaken in Cooperation with the American Association for the Advancement of Science (AAAS). http://www.pewinternet.org/2015/01/29/public-and-scientists-views-on-science-and-society/.

Gouse, M., Pray, C.E., Schimmelpfennig, D., 2004. The distribution of benefits from Bt cotton adoption in South Africa. AgBioForum 7 (4), 187−194.

Gouse, M., Kirsten, J., Shankar, B., Thirtle, C., 2005a. Bt cotton in KwaZulu natal: technological triumph but institutional failure? Agbiotechnet 7 (1), 1−7.

Gouse, M., Pray, C.E., Kirsten, J., Schimmelpfennig, D., 2005b. A GM subsistence crop in Africa: the case of Bt white maize in South Africa. The International Journal of Biotechnology 7 (1/2/3), 84−94.

Gouse, M., Piesse, J., Thirtle, C., 2006. Output and labour effects of GM maize and minimum tillage in a communal area of KwaZulu-Natal. Journal of Development Perspectives 2 (2), 71−86.

Gouse, M., 2012. GM maize as subsistence crop: the South African smallholder experience. AgBioForum 15 (2), 163−174.

Gouse, M., Sengupta, D., Zambrano, P., Falck Zeped, J., 2016. Genetically modified maize: less drudgery for her, more maize for him? Evidence from smallholder maize farmers in South Africa. World Development 83, 27−38.

Gouws, L.M., Groenewald, J.H., 2012. How safe are South Africa's GM foods? South African Food Science and Technology Magazine 2, 21−23.

ISAAA, 2017. Global Status of Commercialized Biotech/GM Crops in 2017: Biotech Crop Adoption Surges as Economic Benefits Accumulate in 22 Years. ISAAA Brief No. 53. ISAAA, Ithaca, New York.

Johnson, K.L., Raybould, A.J., Hudson, M.D., Poppy, G.M., 2007. How does scientific risk assessment of GM crops fit within the wider risk analysis? Trends in Plant Science 12 (1), 1−5.

Kahan, D.M., 2010. Fixing the communications failure. Nature 463 (7279), 296−297.

Kahan, D.M., 2017. Misconceptions, Misinformation, and the Logic of Identity-Protective Cognition. Cultural Cognition Project Working Paper Series No. 164; Yale Law School, Public Law Research Paper No. 605; Yale Law & Economics Research Paper No. 575. https://ssrn.com/abstract=2973067.

Kyndt, T., Quispe, D., Zhai, H., Jarret, R., Ghislain, M., Liu, Q., Gheysen, G., Kreuze, J.F., 2015. The genome of cultivated sweet potato contains Agrobacterium T-DNAs with expressed genes: an example of a naturally transgenic food crop. Proceedings of the National Academy of Sciences 112 (18), 5844–5849.

Pray, C., Rheeder, J.P., Gouse, M., Volkwyn, Y., Van der Westhuizen, L., Shephard, G.S., 2013. Bt maize and fumonisin reduction in South Africa: potential health impacts. In: Falck-Zepeda, J., Gruere, G., Sithole-Niang, I. (Eds.), Genetically Modified Crops in Africa: Economic and Policy Lessons from Countries South of the Sahara. International Food Policy Research Institute (IFPRI), Washington DC, USA.

Van den Berg, J., Van Wyk, A., 2007. The effect of Bt maize on Sesamia calamistis in South Africa. Entomologia Experimentalis et Applicata 122, 45–51.

Van Rensburg, J.B.J., 2007. First report of field resistance by the stem borer, Busseola fusca, (Fuller) to Bt-transgenic maize. Plant and Soil 24, 5.

Van Wyk, A., Van den Berg, Van Hamburg, H., 2008. Diversity and comparative phenology of Lepidoptera on Bt and non-Bt maize in South Africa. International Journal of Pest Management 54, 77–87.

Wolt, J.D., Keese, P., Raybould, A., Fitzpatrick, J.W., Burachik, M., Gray, A., Olin, S.S., Schiemann, J., Sears, M., Wu, F., 2010. Problem formulation in the environmental risk assessment for genetically modified plants. Transgenic Research 19, 425–436.

Further reading

Andreotti, G., et al., 2018. Glyphosate use and cancer incidence in the agricultural health study. Journal of the National Cancer Institute 110 (5) (in press).

Burger, A., Groenewald, J.-H., 2009. Maize and *Bacillus thuringiensis* cry protein allergenicity. In: Biosafety South Africa Policy Brief. www.biosafety.org.za.

EFSA, 2015. Conclusion on the peer review of the pesticide risk assessment of the active substance glyphosate. EFSA Journal 13 (11), 4302.

FAO, WHO, 2016. Joint FAO/WHO Meeting on Pesticide Residues – Summary Report. http://www.who.int/foodsafety/areas_work/chemical-risks/jmpr/en/.

IARC Preamble, 2006. IARC Monographs on the Evaluation of Carcinogenic Risks to Humans – Preamble. http://monographs.iarc.fr/ENG/Preamble/index.php.

Mashele, N., Auerbach, R.M.B., 2016. Evaluating crop yields, crop quality and soil fertility from organic and conventional farming systems in South Africa's southern Cape. South African Journal of Geology 119.1, 25–32.

National Academies of Sciences, Engineering, and Medicine, 2016. Genetically Engineered Crops: Experiences and Prospects. The National Academies Press, Washington, DC. https://doi.org/10.17226/23395.

Nature (2017). doi:10.1038/nature.2017.23044 http://www.nature.com/news/european-union-nations-vote-to-keep-using-controversial-weedkiller-glyphosate-1.23044.

Reuters, 2017. In Glyphosate Review, WHO Cancer Agency Edited Out "Non-Carcinogenic" Findings. https://www.reuters.com/investigates/special-report/who-iarc-glyphosate/.

The Lancet Oncology, 2016. When is a carcinogen not a carcinogen? Editorial The Lancet Oncology 17.

Genetically modified bananas for communities of the great lakes region of Africa

6.2

Namanya Priver, PhD, Tindamanyire Jimmy, PhD, Buah Stephen, PhD, Namaganda Josephine, PhD, Kubiriba Jerome, PhD, Tushemereirwe Wilberforce, PhD

National Agricultural Research Laboratories-Kawanda, National Agricultural Research Organisation, Kampala, Uganda

Introduction

Over 50 million people in the East and Central African region including Uganda, Tanzania, Rwanda, Burundi, DR Congo, and Kenya depend on the East African Highland banana (EAHB, AAA-EA, Musa spp.), a unique type of cooking bananas, as a staple food and for income. East and Central Africa are considered a secondary center of diversity for the EAHBs, also called Matooke. Annual regional production is worth US$ 4.3 billion, which is about 5% of the East and Central African (ECA) region's gross domestic product (FAOSTAT, 2014). Banana has the unique advantage of producing acceptable yields amid erratic rainfall, coupled with an all-year-round fruiting characteristic. It is therefore, not surprising, that there is relatively less poverty and food insecurity incidences among the banana-dependent communities. The banana's extensive root system and leaf canopy have environmental benefits in terms of reduced soil erosion and stabilizing agroecologies (Karamura et al., 2016). Furthermore, the banana forest—like plantations capture significant amounts of carbon dioxide from the atmosphere, which is quickly recycled into soil organic matter (Kamusingize et al., 2017).

The average yield of the banana crop on-farm is estimated at 10 ton/ha/year in Uganda, yet the crop's potential is over 60—70 ton/ha/year; while the commercial systems of India and Ecuador are reported to produce bananas up to 120 ton/ha/year. This yield gap is attributable to a complex of biotic constraints such as banana bacterial wilt (also called banana *Xanthomonas* wilt, BXW), weevils, fusarium wilt, nematodes, black Sigatoka; and abiotic stresses (nutrient deficiencies and moisture/

drought stress) (Wairegi et al., 2010). There have been attempts to increase production by increasing the land area under banana cultivation over the past 50 years in order to meet the escalating food demands from a high population growth rate of about 9.1 million people per year (AfrDB, 2012). However, this is not sustainable since the available arable land area is limited. Uganda's National Banana Research team with its global network of research for development continuously generates and deploys technologies that aim at adequately addressing the above problems to increase production per unit area per unit labor force. The yield losses from some of the most important biotic and abiotic constraints of banana are summarized in Table 6.2.1.

The key pests and diseases can be feasibly managed using sanitation practices and clean planting materials. However, sanitation practices are labor intensive and therefore not sustainable. For instance cultural control for the destructive BXW has very high implementation costs arising from the need for whole communities to act in order to manage the disease. This involves engaging not only many farmers but also their supportive and massive administrative and political machinery (Kubiriba and Tushemereirwe, 2014). As is the case for all crops, the most effective way of addressing the problems is through use of host plant resistance. Using conventional breeding to develop the resistant bananas is the preferred approach in Uganda. However, most preferred varieties are sterile and so cannot be improved through conventional breeding. Furthermore, the few that have minimal fertility have to date yielded hybrids that are less acceptable to consumers than the land races largely because the resistance is obtained from inedible wild sources. The only option available to address these challenges is to use genetic engineering to insert the lacking traits.

Using biotechnology for development of banana with pest and disease resistance

Banana researchers have made great strides in crop improvement through conventional breeding leading to the release of high-yielding banana hybrids. However, consumer acceptability is vital for products with resistance to major pests and diseases such as weevils, nematodes, banana bacterial wilt (BXW)m and *Fusarium*

Table 6.2.1 Yield Loss due to abiotic and biotic constraints of banana.

Constraint	Yield loss (%)	Source
Black Sigatoka	30–50	Tushemereirwe et al. (2003)
Banana *Xanthomonas* Wilt (BXW)	80–100	Kubiriba et al. (2014)
Banana weevil	60	Okech et al. (2004)
Fusarium wilt	60%–100%	Kangire, 1998.
Soil Nutrient deficiency (K and N)	28–68	Nyombi et al. (2010)
Drought stress	20–65	van Asten et al. (2011)

oxysporum cubense (FOC). For example, the FHIA banana hybrids—developed by Fundación Hondureña de Investigación Agrícola (FHIA) of Honduras, with resistance to FOC, have had acceptability limitations in East and Central Africa due to changes in the preferred taste for a dessert banana (Karamura et al., 2016). For a more complex disease, because of its rapid spreading and very destructive nature, banana bacterial wilt has no known source of resistance in the *Musa* germplasm.

Recently, the banana researchers started to employ biotechnology approaches to complement conventional breeding thereby offering opportunities to introgress genes that are outside the Musa species domain for improved banana products. For example, out of successful efforts of conventional breeding, National Agricultural Research Organisation (NARO) developed and released a number of EAHB hybrids, primarily resistant to black Sigatoka, including KABANA 6H and KABANA 7H, released in 2010 and 2011 and NAROBAN banana Hybrids 1, 2, 3, and 4 released in 2017 (Nowakunda et al., 2015; Tumuhimbise et al., 2017). Because of this NARO does not use biotechnology tools to develop resistance to black Sigatoka in bananas. However, in order to develop varieties with multiple resistance, biotechnology approaches are being explored to add traits such as bacterial wilt resistance into officially released elite conventional EAHB hybrids.

Using biotechnology to address human nutritional deficiencies

Vitamin A deficiency (VAD) and iron-deficiency anemia (IDA) are major global public health problems. In Uganda, VAD is estimated at 33% among children less than 5 years and 35% among reproductive women (UDHS, 2011). Options for addressing micronutrient deficiencies including supplements and food fortification have not been able to reach some poor community members who rely on staple starch foods like bananas and those who do not visit health facilities where the supplements are supplied. There are some banana varieties with high levels of provitamin A (pVA) such as Fe'i bananas that exist in Micronesia (Englberger et al., 2006). However, these Fe'i bananas do not have the acceptable taste attributes to consider for direct adoption for Eastern and Central African banana consumers. GM bananas enhanced with pVA are considered among the sustainable options for addressing VAD in hard to reach banana-dependent communities. When adopted, it is expected that pVA-enhanced GM bananas will significantly contribute to reducing the number of people with VAD in Uganda.

In order to harness the potential of biotechnology for enhancement of pVA, a banana-derived gene, phytoene synthase (PSY2a), was isolated from Fe'i cultivar ASUPINA bananas (Mlalazi et al., 2012). The proof-of-concept studies were first conducted in Cavedish bananas in Australia (Paul et al., 2018, 2017). pVA—rich EAHBs have been developed using the banana PSY2a genes and are in confined field trials in Uganda. Phytoene synthase is the enzyme that catalyzes the first committed step or the turning point in the biochemical process in plants that leads to the formation of pVA carotenoids.

The genetically modified development pipeline

The process of producing GM bananas involves several stages starting from establishing the first building blocks of life which are banana cells, growing them into a fully grown plant (Namanya et al., 2014), Fig. 6.2.1. The cells are the units of the plant that have the natural ability to receive genetic material and reproduce it. Similarly, there is a naturally occurring soil bacterium *Agrobacterium tumefaciens*, which interacts with plants and has the ability to transfer its genetic material. Scientists have studied the gene transfer system of *Agrobacterium* so that the disease-causing genes have been removed and replaced with "preferred" genes leaving its transfer system intact (Gelvin, 2003). Under optimum conditions, the bacterium is conditioned to transfer the "preferred good attributes" (such as pVA-enhancing genes, disease-resistance genes) when brought in contact with the plant cells. The good attributes are then introduced into any plant cell utilizing the natural ability of a "tricked/disarmed" *Agrobacterium* to transfer its genes into plant cells. The process of introducing such attributes into plant cells is what is referred to as genetic engineering. Plants regenerated from such banana cells are genetically modified (GM). Therefore genetic engineering utilizes natural systems of plant–bacteria interaction, whereby GM banana plants are developed from single cells of known banana varieties and not injected with chemicals as perceived by some stakeholders.

GM banana plants go through various stages of rigorous screening to select those that will have taken up the good trait into the DNA in the nucleus of the cell before taking them to subsequent stages of development. Through the plant development cycle, the DNA of the transformed individual banana plant is screened using PCR (polymerase chain reaction)—a molecular method that confirms that the plants have taken up the introduced genetic material. In order to check the function of

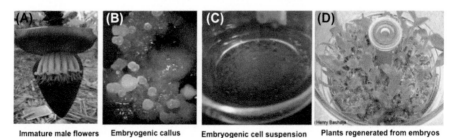

| Immature male flowers | Embryogenic callus | Embryogenic cell suspension | Plants regenerated from embryos |

FIGURE 6.2.1

Banana cells suspensions are developed from meristematic tissues in immature male flowers of a choice cultivar. (A) Immature male flower, (B) Embryogenic callus, (C) Embryogenic cell suspension, (D) Plants regenerated from embryos.

the incorporated trait, the GM plants that consistently test positive for the trait are weaned, potted into soil, and subjected to specific stresses under screenhouse conditions (providing a netted shield, decreased humidity, natural lighting, and room temperature for the potted plants). For example, GM banana plants transformed with bacterial wilt resistance genes are inoculated with the bacteria in the screenhouse to select resistant lines (Fig. 6.2.2).

Selected GM banana lines from the screenhouse are progressed to confined fields and further subjected to specific stresses under natural field conditions to select resilient lines. An example for selection of GM bananas under confined field conditions has been demonstrated for resistance to banana bacterial wilt disease (Tripathi et al., 2014). GM bananas that have pVA-enhancing genes incorporated are only evaluated under field conditions where the fruit is assessed after harvest. In addition to the disease resistance or enhanced pVA content, GM bananas are selected for normal growth characteristics including their ability to produce suckers, plant height, flowering time, maturity period, and fruit characteristics to ascertain conformity to the original identity of the variety, with no difference from the untransformed variety. Yield data are collected to ensure that there is no yield penalty associated with the desired attribute.

Once the selected lines have the attribute (gene) of interest that is functional, with normal growth and yield, the selected GM lines go through advanced molecular checks to ascertain that the genetic makeup of the new variety has not changed except for the intended improvement. This includes gene function, interaction with the existing genetic composition of the plant, and ensuring that the attribute of interest is properly incorporated in the banana genome such that no undesirable gene products are created.

Bananas grow in different agroecological conditions. Therefore, GM bananas need to be selected for adoption in different agroecologies of banana-growing communities of varying social economic setups. Consequently, the performance of the selected GM banana lead lines is further assessed in multilocation-confined field trials (MLTs) in different agroecologies to ascertain stability of the trait and their

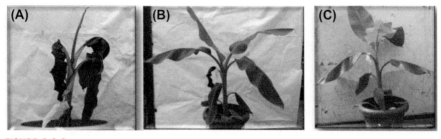

FIGURE 6.2.2

Selection of bacterial wilt resistant lines in potted GM bananas in screenhouse. (A) Susceptible nontransgenic control, (B) Only the infected leaf of GM banana wilts, (C) No wilting in infected GM banana plant.

performance, food safety, and nutritional integrity. All the data collected from the beginning up to field selection stage contribute to a dossier for release of GM banana product by the national regulator as guided by the national laws.

Genes and their safety

The choices made from inception of GM development cycle take into consideration the concerns about the safety of GM bananas under development. Initially, the choice of attributes (genes) incorporated into the banana is carefully sourced from edible plants or naturally occurring organisms that already interact with plants. For example, the genes that were constitutively expressed to confer resistance to banana bacterial wilt disease, *HRAP* (hypersensitive response-assisting protein) or *PFLP* (plant ferredoxin–like protein), originated from sweet pepper (Capsicum annuum) (Chen et al., 2000). Similarly, the genes for enhancement of pVA in banana were sourced from another type of banana variety, Asupina (Fe'i), an edible banana found in the Pacific Islands (Mlalazi et al., 2012). There is therefore a long history of safe use for the HRAP, PFLP, and pVA proteins incorporated into banana. Furthermore, for many generations in the history of mankind, pVA carotenoids have been safely consumed from a wide range of vegetables and fruits by humans and animals.

The strategy for safety assessment of GM bananas follows provisions of internationally recognized principles and practises such as those provided for through Allergen Online and Codex Alimentarius. The first level of safety considers that the choice of gene has no potential to cause allergens. Bioinformatic searches for the HRAP and PFLP proteins against the Allergen Online database (http:www.allergenonline.org/databasefasta.shtml) did not show any significant alignments with any allergens. The HRAP and PFLP protein had less than 35% cross-reactivity below the threshold recommended by Codex Alimentarius, above which the gene would have been rejected. Before release, strategies are already in place to pretest GM banana food products for allergenicity and toxicity, following FAO/WHO's Codex Alimentarius standards relating to foods, food production, and food safety.

Biodiversity and environmental safety

There is a perception that farmers will loose their traditional banana varieties when superior GM crops are introduced. On the contrary, GM bananas will add to the diversity of varieties in cultivation. For example, banana bacterial wilt decimates all banana cultivars in cultivation. In specific cases where there is no known resistance to such biotic stresses, GM has the potential to introduce improved varieties with desired resistance. Therefore, introducing genes for resistance into such cultivars would preserve them. However, with or without biotechnology, biodiversity continues to be lost due to climate stresses and known and unknown outbreaks of pests and diseases. Unlike conventionally bred hybrids where many characteristics of the variety change, picking some from the male parent and others from the female parent during the conventional development process, the change in the GM banana is only specific to the target attribute, thereby preserving all other characteristics for the target variety. This provides an advantage to cultivar preservation. For example, in the pVA-biofortified GM Nakitembe (AAA-EA), the banana product remains an EAHB cultivar Nakitembe in all characteristics except for enhanced pVA levels.

No unintended effects on nontarget organisms

Scientists are aware of potential introgression of the introduced genetic material into naturally occurring flora and fauna, either through cross-pollination or lateral gene flow. In the case of banana, all cultivated EAHB are naturally sterile. They do not cross-pollinate by themselves, even assisted seed production during hybrid development is difficult and consequently they reproduce vegetatively. Therefore there are no biosafety concerns of gene flow from any of the GM banana cultivars to wild species or other traditional banana varieties.

Furthermore, studies have been conducted to determine the effect of GM bananas on nontarget microorganisms in the soil and plant environment. Nimusiima et al. (2015) studied the effect of transgenes for BXW resistance, HRAP, and PFLP, in confined field trials of transgenic bananas 3 years after establishment. Transgenic and nontransgenic lines and their associated microbiome were investigated by molecular fingerprinting. There were no significant differences found in the profiles of the bacterial communities associated with transgenic and nontransgenic banana plants. In a separate confined field trial conducted at NARO (National Agricultural Research Organisation) for transgenic banana plants transformed with genes conferring nematode resistance, faunal analysis was conducted after 3 years. Again, these studies showed no significant differences in nematode diversity for nontarget nematode species including the bacterial, fungal, and carnivorous feeders, between plots of transgenic and nontransgenic banana plants (Fig. 6.2.3, NARO-ABSPII end of project report, 2016—unpublished).

The choice of genes incorporated into banana varieties for traits such as enhancement of pVA or resistance to BXW was derived from plant species with a long history of safe use. In future, when varieties with resistance to pest and diseases have been deployed into cultivation, they will require minimal or no use of pesticides, an invaluable addition to environmental safety. There are reports showing that use of biotechnology crops has reduced carbon footprints of active ingredients of chemicals. An example report by Brookes and Barfoot (2017) shows reduction in pesticide use and environmental impact quotient, a measure of pesticide effect on the environment, by 17.6% and 18.5% in 2014 and 2015 translating into 6.4% and 6.1% pesticide saving, respectively. Such contributions to the environment must be recognized while taking keen consideration for regulatory regimes that harness strict adherence to safety.

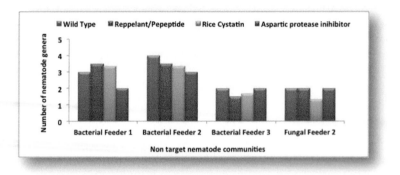

FIGURE 6.2.3

Shows nontarget nematode communities identified from a confined field trial for nematode resistance under plots cultivated with transgenic banana plants.

Economics and trade implications

Just like most countries in the world, biotechnology and its products are not without controversy in Uganda. Some stakeholders share concerns that introducing GM crops could disrupt Uganda's trade with the EU markets who have a stand against GM crops. Although global trade in agricultural commodities especially to the EU constitutes a significant 24% share of Uganda's GDP (gross domestic product), a negligible amount of bananas are exported from Uganda. Currently Ugandan scientists are focusing on applying modern technologies primarily to meet the domestic needs first, especially the food security of an increasing population. Besides, the skepticism toward production and use of GM crops in EU has been gradually changing. For example, EU annually imports 32M tonnes of soybean of which 90% is GM, 2.5 Mton maize (25% is GM), and 2 Mton (20% is GM) of rapeseed (USDA-GAIN, 2016). By 2016, some of the EU countries such as Portugal, Spain, Czech Republic, and Slovakia had increased their acreage of biotechnology crops (James, 2016). While the short-term targets are for local needs, the prediction for the future global markets is positive.

GM bananas are expected to have significant social economic and health benefits on communities translating to national and regional impacts. Studies by Ainembabazi et al. (2015) show that 65% of the farmers (Fig. 6.2.4) were ready to adopt GM banana with BXW resistance immediately. The expected rate of adoption was up to 74% farmers covering 40% acreage allocated to banana production with a yield gain of 54% per ha. Overall, it was estimated that Ugandan farmers would, over 25 years, earn up to $953m worth of bananas at present value. In earlier related studies, Kikulwe et al. (2013) predicted willingness among banana end users to adopt GM banana resistant to the fungal disease black Sigatoka after assessing potential benefits, costs, consumer perceptions, and related policy implications.

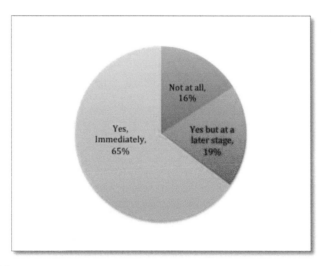

FIGURE 6.2.4

Farmers response and willingness to adopt genetically modified banana with BXW resistance in Uganda.

Source: Ainembabazi, J.H., Tripathi, L., Rusike, J., Abdoulaye, T., Manyong, V., 2015. Ex-ante economic impact assessment of genetically modified banana resistant to Xanthomonas wilt *in the great lakes region of Africa. PLoS One 10, e0138998. https://doi.org/10.1371/journal.pone.0138998.*

Partnerships, ownership, patents, and access

The GM development cycle may be viewed as a six-step process from discovery of genes to release of a product. Ugandan scientists have for the last 15 years acquired capacity and expertise to develop products for the Ugandan consumers covering all aspects of the GM product development cycle from tissue and cell culture, genetic engineering, laboratory and field testing, and recent regulatory trials (Fig. 6.2.5, Table 6.2.2). The regulatory system and policy framework has grown and evolved along with the science and will finally bring the GM banana products through to release. In the process, National Agricultural Research Organisation (NARO) has established strong national and international partnerships in training, technology access, as well as technical backstopping with institutions such as the Queensland University of Technology (QUT)—Australia, Cornell University—USA, Makerere University—Uganda, University of Pretoria—South Africa, AATF—Kenya, IITA—Nigeria, University of Ghent—Belgium, University of Leeds—UK.

However, the NARO drives the agenda for GM research on banana in Uganda. Technical partnerships are governed by agreements that ensure the developed products addressing public needs as public goods. For example, genes incorporated into GM bananas for development of pVA enhancement were accessed directly from Queensland University of Technology, Australia, who are technology partners under the Grand Challenges in Global Health Initiative. The intellectual property for the

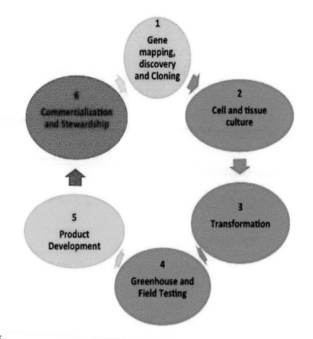

FIGURE 6.2.5

Shows the pipeline for GM development from gene discovery through to commercialization.

Table 6.2.2 Skills developed at Masters and Doctoral level for GM banana development.

Number of scientists	Skills acquired	Level of deployment
7	Gene isolation and bioinformatics	Medium
5	Cell culture and tissue culture	High
16	Genetic engineering	High
2	Biosafety, food standards, and regulation	Medium

pVA-enhanced banana is governed by the global access agreements whereby products are developed for charitable markets without encumbrances (Gates Foundation, n.d). As a result, GM bananas developed with enhanced pVA will be accessed and owned by small holding farmers. Upon release, farmers will be able to access initial planting materials from NARO and Ugandan private tissue culture laboratories. Consequently the recipient farmers have full control of the banana seed system requiring no on-going costs to access new planting material, no restrictions to sharing suckers or replanting them, because farmers can reproduce their own suckers since the banana is clonally propagated.

Regulatory aspects

The regulatory framework for GM research in Uganda is gradually evolving with the progressing research for different products. While the National Banana Research Program has released conventionally bred banana varieties in the past, there are no GM bananas on-farmers fields yet. All GM bananas are still going through the selection process in experimental-confined field trials restricted on research stations only and none on farmers' fields. The confined field experiments were approved by National Biosafety Committee (NBC) comprised of independent representative experts who evaluate, guide, and approve the research applications under the biosafety framework and mandate of the Uganda National Council for Science and Technology (UNCST) as the overall regulator of all science and technology research in Uganda (UNCST statute 1990). All banana GM research is regulated by NBC-UNCST in accordance with national and international biosafety practices and considerations.

Conclusion

Millions of people in East and Central Africa still eke their livelihoods out of bananas. The problems that affect banana production are still largely unresolved by available management approaches including conventional breeding. Biotechnology, therefore, as a complementary tool, has potential to provide the products that will address food production and nutrition constraints. Most of the concerns toward genetic engineering technology whether regulatory or safety are addressed along the development cycle, and the benefits of biotech crops in terms of financial, environmental, and humanitarian gain are phenomenal. The future of GM products in Uganda is very bright with up to 65% Ugandan farmers ready to accept GM bananas immediately. The number of people willing to embrace the technology with a positive attitude is increasing, the stakeholders' trust in the regulatory regime to address their fears is high, and the process of building functional structures for implementing the necessary policies has finally and gradually gained momentum. And it is becoming increasingly clear that the challenges of increasing food production and nutrition will be meaningfully addressed if all options available to scientists are harnessed.

Acknowledgments

The authors acknowledge Uganda Government, the United States Agency for International Development (USAID) through the ABSPII (Agricultural Biotechnology Support Project) for financial support. We acknowledge technical collaboration with Queensland University of Technology (QUT), Australia, in training, technology, and product development for pVA-enhanced bananas. We acknowledge International Institute of Tropical Agriculture (IITA) as technical partners in development of BXW resistance. We also acknowledge Academia Sinica, Taiwan, for the genes for BXW resistance and African Agricultural Technology Foundation (AATF) for their role in accessing technologies for BXW resistance from Academia Sinica.

References

African Development Report, 2012. Towards Green Growth in Africa. African Development Bank (AfDB) Group, ISBN 978-9938-882-00-1.

Ainembabazi, J.H., Tripathi, L., Rusike, J., Abdoulaye, T., Manyong, V., 2015. Ex-ante economic impact assessment of genetically modified banana resistant to *Xanthomonas wilt* in the great lakes region of Africa. PLoS One 10, e0138998. https://doi.org/10.1371/journal.pone.0138998.

van Asten, P.J., Fermont, A.M., Taulya, G., 2011. Drought is a major yield loss factor for rainfed East African highland banana. Agricultural Water Management 98 (4), 541−552.

Brookes, G., Barfoot, P., 2017. Environmental impacts of genetically modified (GM) crop use 1996−2015: impacts on pesticide use and carbon emissions. GM Crops and Food 8, 117−147. https://doi.org/10.1080/21645698.2017.1309490.

Chen, C., Lin, H., Ger, M., Chow, D., Feng, T., 2000. cDNA cloning and characterization of a plant protein that may be associated with the harpinPSS-mediated hypersensitive response. Plant Molecular Biology 43, 429−438. https://doi.org/10.1023/A:1006448611432.

Englberger, L., Schierle, J., Aalbersberg, W., Hofmann, P., Humphries, J., Huang, A., Lorens, A., Levendusky, A., Daniells, J., Marks, G.C., Fitzgerald, M.H., 2006. Carotenoid and vitamin content of Karat and other Micronesian banana cultivars. International Journal of Food Sciences and Nutrition 57, 399−418. https://doi.org/10.1080/09637480600872010.

FAO, 2014. Statistical Yearbook. http://www.fao.org/3/a-i3590e.pdf.

Gelvin, S.B., 2003. Agrobacterium-mediated plant transformation: the biology behind the "Gene-Jockeying" tool. Microbiology and Molecular Biology Reviews 67, 16−37. https://doi.org/10.1128/MMBR.67.1.16-37.2003.

Gates Foundation, n.d. Global Acess [WWW Document]. The Role of IP in Global Access. URL (http://globalaccess.gatesfoundation.org/).

James, C., 2016. Global Status of Commercialized Biotech/GM Crops (No. Brief, 52), ISAAA Briefs. ISAAA.

Kamusingize, D., Mwanjalolo Majaliwa, J., Komutunga, E., Tumwebaze, S., Nowakunda, K., Namanya, P., Kubiriba, J., 2017. Carbon sequestration potential of East African highland banana cultivars (*Musa* spp. AAA-EAHB) cv. Kibuzi, Nakitembe, Enyeru and Nakinyika in Uganda. Journal of Soil Science and Environmental Management 8, 44−51. https://doi.org/10.5897/JSSEM2016.0608.

Kangire, A., 1998. Fusarium wilt (Panama disease) of exotic bananas and wilt of East African highland bananas (Musa, AAA-EA) in Uganda. Thesis submitted for the degree of Doctor of Philosophy. Department of Agriculture, Reading University, p. 304.

Karamura, E.B., Tinzaara, W., Kikulwe, E., Ochola, D., Ocimati, W., Karamura, D., 2016. Introduced banana hybrids in Africa: seed systems, farmers' experiences and consumers' perspectives. Acta Horticulturae 239−244. https://doi.org/10.17660/ActaHortic.2016. 1114.33.

Kikulwe, E., Birol, E., Wesseler, J., Falck-Zepeda, J.B., 2013. Benefits, costs, and consumer perceptions of the potential introduction of a fungus-resistant banana in Uganda and policy implications. In: Genetically Modified Crops in Africa: Economic and Policy Lessons from Countries South of the Sahara. IFPRI, Washington, DC.

Kubiriba, J., Tushemereirwe, W., 2014. Approaches for the control of banana *Xanthomonas wilt* in East and central Africa. African Journal of Plant Science 8, 398−404. https://doi.org/10.5897/AJPS2013.1106.

Mlalazi, B., Welsch, R., Namanya, P., Khanna, H., Geijskes, R.J., Harrison, M.D., Harding, R., Dale, J.L., Bateson, M., 2012. Isolation and functional characterisation of banana phytoene synthase genes as potential cisgenes. Planta 236, 1585−1598. https://doi.org/10.1007/s00425-012-1717-8.

Namanya, P., Mutumba, G., Magambo, S.M., Tushemereirwe, W., 2014. Developing a cell suspension system for Musa-AAA-EA cv. 'Nakyetengu': a critical step for genetic improvement of Matooke East African Highland bananas. In Vitro Cellular and Developmental Biology − Plant 50, 442−450. https://doi.org/10.1007/s11627-014-9598-0.

Nimusiima, J., Köberl, M., Tumuhairwe, J.B., Kubiriba, J., Staver, C., Berg, G., 2015. Transgenic banana plants expressing *Xanthomonas wilt* resistance genes revealed a stable non-target bacterial colonization structure. Scientific Reports 5, 18078.

Nowakunda, K., Barekye, A., Ssali, R.T., Namaganda, J., Tushemereirwe, W.K., Nabulya, G., Erima, R., Akankwasa, K., Hilman, E., Batte, M., Karamura, D., 2015. 'Kiwangaazi' (syn 'KABANA 6H') black Sigatoka nematode and banana weevil tolerant 'Matooke' hybrid banana released in Uganda. HortScience 50, 621−623.

Nyombi, K., Van Asten, P.J., Corbeels, M., Taulya, G., Leffelaar, P.A., Giller, K.E., 2010. Mineral fertilizer response and nutrient use efficiencies of East African highland banana (Musa spp., AAA-EAHB, cv. Kisansa). Field Crops Research 117 (1), 38−50.

Okech, S.H., Van Asten, P.J.A., Gold, C.S., Ssali, H., 2004. Effects of potassium deficiency, drought and weevils on banana yield and economic performance in Mbarara, Uganda. Uganda Journal of Agricultural Sciences 9 (1), 511−519.

Paul, J.-Y., Harding, R., Tushemereirwe, W., Dale, J., 2018. Banana21: from gene discovery to deregulated golden bananas. Frontiers of Plant Science 9. https://doi.org/10.3389/fpls.2018.00558.

Paul, J.-Y., Khanna, H., Kleidon, J., Hoang, P., Geijskes, J., Daniells, J., Zaplin, E., Rosenberg, Y., James, A., Mlalazi, B., Deo, P., Arinaitwe, G., Namanya, P., Becker, D., Tindamanyire, J., Tushemereirwe, W., Harding, R., Dale, J., 2017. Golden bananas in the field: elevated fruit pro-vitamin A from the expression of a single banana transgene. Plant Biotechnology Journal 15, 520−532. https://doi.org/10.1111/pbi.12650.

Tripathi, L., Tripathi, J.N., Kiggundu, A., Korie, S., Shotkoski, F., Tushemereirwe, W.K., 2014. Field trial of *Xanthomonas wilt* disease-resistant bananas in East Africa. Nature Biotechnology 32, 868−870. https://doi.org/10.1038/nbt.3007.

Tumuhimbise, R., Barekye, A., Kubiriba, J., Tushemereirwe, W., Ssali, R.T., Akankwasa, K., Oyesigye, N., Arinaitwe, J., Arinaitwe, I., Kabita, N.,B., Wasswa, W., Buregyeya, H., Namanya, P., Talengera, D., Batte, M., Nyiine, M., Nabulya, G., Lugolobi, N., Namaganda, J., 2017. A Submission to the Variety Release Committee for the Release of Four Cooking Banana Varieties M19, M20, M25 and M27. NARL-NARO.

Tushemereirwe, W.K., Kashaija, I.N., Tinzaara, W., Nankinga, C., New, S., 2003. A Guide to Successful Banana Production in Uganda: Banana Production Manual. New.

UDHS, 2011. Uganda Demographic and Health Survey. Kampala Uganda 2011,. Uganda Bureau of Statistics (UBOS) and ICF International Inc.. Uganda Bureau of Statistics, Kampala.

USDA-GAIN, 2016. Agricultural Biotechnology Annual EU-28 (No. GAIN Report Number FR1624).

Wairegi, L.W.I., van Asten, P.J.A., Tenywa, M.M., Bekunda, M.A., 2010. Abiotic constraints override biotic constraints in East African highland banana systems. Field Crops Research 117, 146–153. https://doi.org/10.1016/j.fcr.2010.02.010.

Trends in genetically modified crops development in Nigeria: issues and challenges

6.3

David Adedayo Animasaun, PhD [1], **Musibau Adewuyi Azeez, PhD** [2],
Amos Oladimeji Adubi, MSc [2,3], **Felicia Adejoke Durodola, MSc** [2],
Joseph Akintade Morakinyo, PhD [1]

[1]*Department of Plant Biology, Faculty of Life Sciences, University of Ilorin, Ilorin, Kwara State, Nigeria;* [2]*Laboratory of Ecotoxicology, Genetics and Nanobiotechnology, Environmental Biology Unit, Department of Pure and Applied Biology, Ladoke Akintola University of Technology, Ogbomoso, Oyo State, Nigeria;* [3]*Department of Biology, School of Science, College of Education, Lanlate, Oyo State, Nigeria*

Introduction

Food is generally a complex biochemical material. It is anything eaten to satisfy appetite, meet physiological needs for growth, maintain all body metabolic processes, and supply energy to regulate body temperature and activity. *Food, from the professional point of view, is any substance, whether processed, semiprocessed, or raw, which is intended for human consumption, and includes drink and any other substance which has been used in the manufacture, preparation, or treatment of "food,"* but does not include cosmetics or tobacco or substances used only as drugs. Because foods differ markedly in the amount of the nutrients they contain, they are classified on the basis of their composition and the source from which they are derived (Fashakin, 2008). Food is a basic requirement of life and as human population increases with projection to reach 9 billion by 2050 (UN, 2017), there is a growing concern about food security for the world's teaming population. Annual decrease in arable land together with global climate changes and poor agricultural practices in underdeveloped and developing countries are factors that will determine global food security. In addition, farmers in the third world countries with larger proportion of the world population have limited access to water resources, finance, and technologies required to effectively drive food production. It is therefore obvious that conventional techniques of food production would be grossly insufficient in meeting the world food requirement in the nearest future (Blancfield et al., 2008;

Mottaleb and Mohanty, 2015), making biotechnology application in food production highly imperative.

Genetically modified foods (GMFs) generally refer to crop plants whose genomes have been altered by purpose using modern molecular techniques for human and animal consumption (Taire, 2003). The genome of a crop plant may be altered or modified for a number of reasons that include conferring of resistance to pest and diseases, drought tolerance, herbicide resistance, and improvement in nutritional qualities among others (Paine et al., 2005; Fedoroff et al., 2010; Tester and Langridge, 2010). Traditional methods of plant breeding to achieve a desired improvement in plants are known to be laborious and usually inaccurate, but with the advent of molecular techniques, i.e., genetic engineering, it is possible to create plants with desired traits within very short period, with precision and required great accuracy (Whitman, 2000).

Biotechnology, genetic engineering, and genetically modified foods

Genetic modification refers to a set of technologies employed to alter the genetic makeup of living organisms such as animals, plants, or bacteria (Neil et al., 2000). Biotechnology and genetic modification are commonly used interchangeably, but biotechnology is a more general term, which refers to using living organisms or their components such as enzymes, to make products that include wine, cheese, beer, and yogurt (NGIN, 2002; Olaniyan et al., 2007). In the past, traditional processes which utilize living organisms in their natural form has been used for food, drink, and dairy production, whereas the modern techniques of biotechnology involve a more advanced modification of the biological system or organism in production processes. This of course results in high production turn over, increase in array of products, and reduction of production costs. With the advent and popularization of the concept of genetic engineering in the 1970s, there were great interests in medical and agricultural biotechnology research driven by the new technologies with the possibility to manipulate organisms' genetic material and composition. Decades after, biotechnology finds applications in many different disciplines such as biochemistry, genetics, agriculture, and molecular biology among others. In the recent decades, several medical, textiles, biochemical, biofuel, and agricultural products have been produced through biotechnology (Adams et al., 2002; Jacobsen and Schouten, 2008; Nielsen, 2013).

Genetic engineering, otherwise known as genetic modification or transgenic method, involves direct manipulation of an organism's genetic material using biotechnological procedures. The procedure employs modern technologies to change and manipulate the genetic configuration and makeup of the cell or organisms. Genetic engineering sometimes requires transfer of gene(s) within (intraspecific) and across species boundaries (interspecific) in order to improve or produce a novel strain or varieties of an organism. The aim of genetic modification is "to isolate single genes of known functions from one organism and transfer copies to a new host (in this case plant or food crops) with a view to elicit desirable characteristics" (Jarvis and Hickford, 1999). This is achieved by isolation of the desirable DNA fragment or gene and making copies of it through recombinant DNA procedure by artificial synthesis of the fragment. With the help of a suitable vector, the cloned fragment is transferred to the host organism. The desire DNA fragment can be inserted randomly to a selected host or target to a specific segment of the host genome. Genetic engineering could be used to insert a gene of interest into a host or to "knock out" a deleterious gene from an organism. In addition, it could also be used to silent a gene whose presence is affecting or inhibiting (epistatic gene) the expression of another of interest or even break undesirable linkage block.

In contrast to conventional modification of organisms that requires long time of conventional breeding, genetic engineering provides platforms for combining genes from different varieties and even organisms through recombinant DNA technology to produce a novel organism. The organism that is produced through the process of genetic engineering is known as genetically modified (GM) or transgenic organism. The method of modification for GMOs varies from the traditional method in an important respect. Boyer et al. (1973) made the first successful attempt in microbial engineering by describing a method of producing protein from microorganism. This was subsequently followed in 1974, by the creation of first genetically modified or transgenic animal; a mouse carrying an inserted DNA fragment (Jaenisch and Mintz, 1974). Since then several genetically manipulated organisms have been produced even at commercial level (Katsumoto et al., 2007). The release of "Flavr Savr" a genetically modified tomato in 1994 marked the beginning of commercial engineered food (Maryanski, 1995). Although, the tomato was modified for longer shelf-life, other crops have been modified for increased pest and herbicide resistance.

Genetic modification or transgenic method has helped to overcome some limitations inherent in conventional plant breeding such as:

(1) lack of practical access to useful germplasm due to sexual incompatibility barriers or undesirable linkage block;
(2) concomitant time lags in incorporating useful genes into existing varieties; and
(3) lack of suitable conventional approaches to dealing with a particular agronomic problem or need such as incidences of pests and diseases (e.g., rice sheath blight, cassava mosaic virus, potato leaf roll virus black sigatoka in plantain) (Spillane, 1999).

Furthermore, genetic modification has also been found useful in a situation where options provided by conventional breeding are very limited especially in the areas like nuclear male sterility, improved heterosis breeding, reducing toxic compounds, herbicide tolerance, generating novel resistance genes, etc.

The knowledge of genetic modifications has greatly expanded the range of gene pools available and accessible for crop improvement purposes (Flavell, 1999).

Useful genes from microorganisms such as vaccine antigens (Arakawa et al., 1998; Mason et al., 1996) and aluminum tolerance genes (de la Fuente et al., 1997) can be transferred through genetic engineering to food plant. In addition, isolated plant genes especially those conferring resistance to pests and pathogens can also be transferred between sexually incompatible crop plant species (Whitham et al., 1996; Wilkinson et al., 1997: Molvig et al., 1997), thus overcoming interspecific and intergenetic barriers. However, modern biotechnologies have also played major roles in any conventional crop improvement approaches that are restricted to use of genetic variation accessible within the primary to secondary gene pools.

Mutation breeding

Mutation breeding is another method that can be used to produce GMFs. This method employs physical agents (ionizing and nonionizing radiations) or chemical mutagens to produce inheritable change in the genome of an organism. According to Kharkwal and Shu (2009), Forster and Shu (2012), the three types of mutagenesis in mutation breeding include:

(1) induced mutagenesis as a result of irradiation or treatment with chemical mutagens;
(2) site-directed mutagenesis involving creation of a mutation at a defined site in a DNA molecule; and
(3) insertion mutagenesis due to DNA insertion, either through genetic transformation and insertion of T-DNA or activation of transposable DNA.

The radiations that are used for the purpose of induced mutation include UV-rays, X-rays, gamma rays, and fast neutron bombardment, of which gamma irradiation is known to be most commonly used and effective in inducing a wide range of mutations (Bado et al., 2015). Gamma ray is an electromagnetic radiation with short wavelength that penetrates deeper into target tissue than other radiation (Mba et al., 2012) This radiation splits water to produce highly reactive hydroxyl radicals (http://microbiologyon-line.blogspot.com) that react with cellular components to produce DNA mutations. Unlike gamma radiation, fast neutron bombardment causes translocations, chromosome losses, and large deletions (Sikora et al., 2011), which may not produce the required desirable mutations in most cases.

The most commonly used plant material for induced mutation is seed. However, material such as whole plant is also used while multiple forms of plant propagules viz. bulbs, tubers, corms, and rhizomes have now become very useful and efficient materials (Wani et al., 2014). In the later, scientists take advantage of totipotency (ability of a single cell to regenerate a whole plant through different intermediate stages of cell divisions and differentiation) using single cells and other forms of in vitro—cultured plant tissues (Mba, 2013). The mutations of importance in crop improvement are those usually involving single bases, which may or may not affect protein synthesis.

Physical mutagens induce gross lesions such as chromosomal aberration or rearrangements, while chemical mutagens are preferably used to induce point mutations (Kharkwal and Shu, 2009). Physical mutagens have been associated with high degree of accuracy and sufficient reproducibility (especially in the case of gamma ray with its uniform penetrating power in the tissue), which are major advantage over chemical mutagens. Chemical mutagens produce effects that are generally considered milder on plant materials, they can be applied without complicated equipment or facilities as in the case of physical mutagens and the resulting mutations are primarily single nucleotide polymorphisms (SNPs). However, the ratio of mutational to undesirable modifications is generally higher for chemical mutagens than for physical mutagens (Oldach, 2011). In order to add new traits to an already high-quality genetic background, such as varieties or elite breeding lines, a very low final doses of mutagenic treatment has been proposed (Maluszynski et al., 2009).

Nigeria as a case study

Farmers in many parts of Africa, including Nigeria, simply lack access to modern technology, and without the development of locally adapted technologies, there is no viable alternative to traditional practices. These conditions led to the development of a system of International Agricultural Research Centres (IARCs) that were eventually organized under the rubric of the Consultative Group for International Agricultural Research (CGIAR). By the late 1960s, the International Centres appeared to be making significant progress. Improvements in crop productivity were most apparent in the two major cereal grains produced in developing countries, wheat and rice. In both crops, improvement was based on a new "plant type." Specifically, this plant type was shorter and earlier maturing, with less photoperiod sensitivity than traditional tropical and subtropical varieties. The development of these plant types was not in any sense "miraculous." However, these new plant types were popularized as miracles and represented as the foundation for a "Green Revolution" in developing countries particularly Nigeria.

Taken together, the past 4 decades have been an era of rapid productivity and production gains in agriculture. In spite of historically unprecedented population increases and in spite of limited natural resources per capita, food production has increased in the recent years. Agricultural sectors have been transformed, not by industrialization, but by crop genetic improvement. Unfortunately, there was a drift and a serious shift of fall in the food production per capita due to insurgence, terrorism, and tribal wars compounded by drought and flooding. Consequently, a large proportion of the population suffers hunger and malnutrition. Nigeria's population is growing exponentially much faster that the rate of food production. Low yield, poor agricultural inputs, and obsolete crop production and processing techniques are the major bane of food sufficient in the country. The cost of food, drink, and dairy items are on the increase, the real price of food is much more than its level

50 years ago. Although the modern day technologies offer arrays of food products, millions of people could not still afford quality food (Evenson and Gollin, 2003).

Status of the genetically modified foods in Nigeria

In Africa generally and in particular sub-Sahara Africa, one of the zones with worse cases of food inadequacy and malnutrition, the adoption of GMF is comparatively poor. Although, some African countries like Kenya, South Africa, and Egypt are gradually embracing GMF, little or no progress toward the adoption of such products could be seen in West Africa countries. Nigeria, as the most populated African country, faces challenges of insufficient food for the ever-growing population (UN, 2017). The country is in dire need of biotechnology application to boost food production and quality, yet little attention is given to harnessing the benefits of GMFs to salvage the situation. Just like in many other countries, there have been serious and fierce debates over the introduction of GMF into Nigeria. The generated debates centered on the possibility of the GMF introducing new risks to food security, environment, and public health such as polluting the environment and also threatening of the biodiversity (Kuzma and Haase, 2012). There is general concern on the consequences of genetically modified crops on health and the environment, which include pesticide resistance, implication of the crops for farmers, and the crops role in feeding the world (Newswire, 2013). All these have greatly hindered the adoption of GMFs in Nigeria and consequently affecting research endeavors by National Research Centres and Universities within the countries. However, there could be a positive outlook in the years ahead, as some farmers in Nigeria are considering growing of cotton (Bt cotton) and maize (Bt maize) crops that are genetically modified for biotic stress.

Precisely, in July 2018, Nigeria took a remarkable step toward the use of biotech crop by approving its first commercially available GMO crops, giving farmers access to engineered soybean seeds designed to resist local pests. With much enthusiasm, it was hope that the release of the seeds would soon lead the way to other GMO options. It was believed that the use of biotech crops would improve and increase productivity in the agricultural sector, to impact positively on the socioeconomic status of Nigerian farmers as well enhanced national economic prosperity. According to Gbarada (2017), this is with a view to attract foreign investment and generate earnings from the safe modern biotechnology sector. It is also hope that the production of GM crops will stimulate environmental stability, create jobs/wealth from the modern biotechnology-based activities, produce more raw materials for industrial growth especially in the country's textile sector, develop plants/organisms that can ameliorate the impact of climate change, and serve in pollution remediation and improve medical sector by using various organisms that are readily available in the country. In the spirit of diversification of the nation's economy base, Nigerian government is making efforts to encourage commercial production of Bt cotton to supply raw materials and resuscitate the ailing textile sector of the economy. To achieve and sustain the country's agro-industrial drive, government has fashioned out polices to promote relatively low-energy cost, loan facilities, and tax waiver to attract both local and foreign investors into the agricultural biotechnology sector including production of modified food.

With the influx of new modified and biotech crops into global market, it is obvious that GMF has come to stay. A new wave of acceptance is evolving in the African continent, and Nigeria is on the way from field trial experiment to granting environmental release approvals of GMF. More so, some other West African countries: Burkina Faso and Ghana are gradually embracing GMF (GM Crop List, 2017), East African Ethiopia is also advancing policies of GMF production (Gebretsadik and Kiflu, 2018) while South Africa, Egypt, and Sudan are already ahead into GMF production (Pretty, 2008).

In one of the Nigerian daily newspapers (Vanguard, 2019), it was reported that GM crops and seeds have been introduced to the country and among these are the release of genetically modified cowpea to farmers, two transgenic cotton hybrid varieties into the Nigerian market, and the granting of permits by the federal government for confined field trials on genetically modified maize, rice, cassava, sorghum, and cowpea to ascertain their ability to resist insect attack etc. In another development, Nigerian government through National Biosafety Management Agency approved its first genetically modified crop for use by the Nigerian farmers. The genetically modified cowpea was a product of 10 years of extensive research efforts by the Institute for Agricultural Research (IAR) at the Ahmadu Bello University, Zaria. This cowpea has been found to manifest resistance to *Maruca vitrata*, a pod borer insect that can reduce yields by as much as 80% and can also reduce insecticide applications from about eight to about two times, thereby raising yields up to 20% (Isaac and Conrow, 2019).

Furthermore, in January 2018, the Ministry of Agriculture announced the Government decision to commercialize genetically engineered cowpea and cotton. Both crops are products of genetic engineering and contain genes for pest resistance. This development was a follow up to the country Biosafety Bill in 2015, thus making it eligible to grow and utilize GMFs. To this end, the National Biotechnology Management Agency (NBMA, Abuja) was saddled with regulatory functions of genetic engineering procedure and products. Meanwhile, according to the regulatory body, Bt cotton, Bt maize, nitrogen use efficient, water use efficient, and salt tolerant (NEWEST) rice are among the GM crops at final stages of trials and safety regulation before release.

Furthermore, Ngandwe (2005) reported that parasite-resistant maize varieties that can tolerate heavy striga infestations without suffering crop losses was developed by the Nigerian laboratory of the International Institute for Tropical Agriculture (IITA). These maize varieties known as Sammaz 15 and 16 contain genes that diminish the growth of parasitic flowering plants such as striga were found to dramatically cut losses due to this root-infecting parasite during the 2 years of trial cultivation by farmers in Borno state in Northern Nigeria (SciDev net news, 2008). This led to the distribution of the new parasite-resistant maize seeds since December

2008 (Okigbo et al., 2011). In addition, National Biotechnology Development Agency (NABDA) claimed that herbicide tolerance soybean and virus resistance cassava fortified with iron and zinc micronutrients will soon be available for farmers and agri entrepreneurs. With this development, researchers are optimistic that the GM crops may be ready for commercialization in about 3 years, as the time requires completing all the necessary backcrosses to transfer the desired traits to Nigerian local varieties.

Nigeria started well in the 1970s when the breeding activities by its research institutes and universities began. This effort was initiated by the establishment of the first botanical station by the colonial government in 1893. According to the Food and Agriculture Organization, the mandate crops of major interest were maize, sorghum, cowpea, and groundnuts, and generally, the main task was line evaluation in a highly favorable environment (FAO, 2019). Today, a lot of institutes and universities are involved in plant breeding and biotechnology research (Table 6.3.1), and Nigerian National Agricultural Research (NAR) system was adjudged historically as the largest in Africa. Unfortunately, this story has changed since early 1980s when the system started experiencing serious setbacks associated with drastic reduction in funding, frequent changes in government policies, inability of the national research institutions to effectively focus limited resources on priority areas, and lack of mechanisms for effective collaborations among NAR institutes, universities, extension, and private sector.

Genetic modification of crops by induced mutation

China has been at the forefront of mutation breeding research leading all other countries of the world by releasing 810 mutant varieties belonging to 46 different species. The major commercial varieties among the mutant crops released are rice, wheat, maize, barley, millet, mulberry, rapeseed, soybean, pepper, cotton, tomato, and groundnut. They have either been released for commercial production or as donor parents in cross-breeding. The country that is next in rank is Japan with the release of 481 mutant varieties. Among the African countries, Côte d'Ivoire ranked the topmost by releasing 25 mutant varieties, followed by Egypt with 9 mutant varieties while Nigeria, Congo and Kenya released 3 mutant varieties each (Table 6.3.2). The three (3) mutant released from Nigeria were registered between 1980 and 1988, which suggests very low participation of the country in even mutation breeding as observed for genetically modified crops till date. Nevertheless, there exist some reports of isolated research efforts by some researchers in research institutes and universities across Nigeria, but such uncoordinated efforts are inadequate to yield expected results. There have been several individual efforts toward mutation breeding in Nigeria, but most reports are basically on the effects of physical or chemical mutagens on one crop plant or another (Adamu et al., 2004; Animasaun et al., 2014, 2016; Olasupo et al., 2016). There are little or no decisive reports on the use of induced mutation to develop new varieties of crops.

Table 6.3.1 Some notable research and education institutes in Nigeria with activities in plant breeding (FAO, 2019).

	Institution/University	Mandate crop	Plant breeding efforts
1	Institute for Agricultural Research of Northern Nigeria, Ahmadu Bello University, Zaria	Sorghum, cotton, cowpea, groundnuts, maize, and other farming systems requirements	Aspects of crop improvement, i.e., genetic improvement
2	National Horticultural Research Institutes (NIHORT)	Production, processing, storage and marketing of tropical fruits, vegetables, and ornamental plants.	Plant breeding and biotechnology, especially in two aspects; molecular characterization and tissue culture
3	Cocoa Research Institute of Nigeria (CRIN)	Cocoa	Genetic diversity studies of cocoa germplasm and tissue culture
4	Forestry Research Institute of Nigeria (FRIN)	Forestry and forests product utilization, training of technical and subtechnical personnel, wildlife, watershed management, and agroforestry	Research in forestry, its products
5	University of Ado Ekiti (UNAD)	Majorly maize and others, i.e., cassava, cowpea, *Telfeiria* (flouted gourd)	Plant breeding and biotechnology, i.e., majorly line evaluation, breeding for resistance to abiotic stresses, and quality traits in maize and cassava
6	Federal University of Agriculture, Abeokuta (FUNAB)	Majorly maize, cowpea, and melons	Plant breeding and biotechnology, especially in tissue culture and genetic engineering of cowpea. Individual researchers work on several other crop using molecular biology tools
7	University of Ibadan (UI)	Majorly Maize, cowpea, and cassava	Plant breeding and biotechnology majorly line evaluation
8	Obafemi Awolowo University	Mainly with maize, cowpea, kenaf, vegetables and fruits. All other crops except cassava	Plant breeding and biotechnology; areas such as molecular characterization, tissue culture, genetic engineering, gene isolation, and wild crosses are covered
9	National Root Crops Research Institute (NRCRI)	crops are cassava, yams, cocoyam, ginger, potato, sweet potato, sugar beet, and other minor root crops	Genetic improvement, farming systems, processing, utilization, and marketing of root and tuber crops. Plant breeding and biotechnology, cell and tissue culture, genetic engineering. Since inception, the institute has official released and registered 38 and 11 improved varieties of cassava and yam, respectively

Note: There are several other institutions both public and private where pockets of plant breeding and biotechnology research are conducted but are not accommodated here due to lack of adequate information.

Table 6.3.2 Officially released mutant varieties in the Food and Agriculture Organization (FAO)/International Atomic Energy Agency (IAEA) Mutant Varieties Database (IAEA, 2015).

Country	Registration	No. of released varieties	Country	Registration	No. of released varieties
Albania	1996	1	Korea	1970–2008	35
Algeria	1979	2	Malaysia	1993–2002	7
Argentina	1962–87	6	Mali	1998–2000	15
Australia	1967–2010	9	Mexico	0	5
Austria	1959–95	17	Moldova	2004–07	7
Bangladesh	1970–2010	44	Mongolia	1984–2004	4
Belgium	1967–87	22	Myanmar	1975–2004	8
Brazil	1974–2005	13	Netherlands	1954–88	176
Bulgaria	1972–2010	76	Nigeria	1980–88	3
Burkina Faso	1978–79	2	Norway	1978–88	2
Canada	1964–2000	40	Pakistan	1970–2009	53
Chile	1981–90	2	Peru	1995–2006	3
China	1957–2011	810	Philippines	1970–2009	15
Congo	1972	3	Poland	1977–95	31
Costa Rica	1975–96	4	Portugal	1983	1
Côte d'Ivoire	1976–87	25	Romania	1992	1
Cuba	1990–2007	12	Russia	1965–2011	216
Czech Republic	1965–96	18	Senegal	1968	2
Denmark	1977–90	21	Serbia	1974	1
Egypt	1980–2011	9	Slovakia	1964–95	19
Estonia	1981–95	5	Spain	2010	1
Finland	1960–81	11	Sri Lanka	1970–2010	4
France	1970–88	38	Sudan	2007	1

Country	Years	No.	Country	Years	No.
Germany	1950–2005	171	Sweden	1950–88	26
Ghana	1997	1	Switzerland	1985	1
Greece	1969–70	2	Syria	2000	1
Guyana	1980–83	26	Taiwan	1967–73	2
Hungary	1969–2001	10	Thailand	2006	20
India	1950–2010	330	Tunisia	1977–2007	1
Indonesia	1982–2011	29	Turkey	1994–2011	9
Iran	2004–08	4	Ukraine	1997–2007	10
Iraq	1992–95	23	United Kingdom	1966–90	34
Italy	1968–95	35	United States	1956–2006	139
Japan	1961–2008	481	Uzbekistan	1966–91	9
Kenya	1985–2001	3	Vietnam	1975–2011	55
Total					3222

Issues and challenges of GMFs in Nigeria
Economic and ethics

The genetic modification of foods makes excellent economic sense for the major agribusiness and food corporations and has been strongly backed by them. Some of the biggest names in the food business openly use genetically modified components, while others will not disclose whether they use them or not. Such companies include Arnotts, Cadburys, Coca-Cola, Coles and Woolworths' house brands, Golden Circle, and Nestlé (Haung et al., 2005; Schmidt, 2005). Already, Nigeria has drafted a biosafety law allowing the use of GMF technology, which the National legislature is yet to approve for a long time (Zhu et al., 2000), until recently.

At the moment, the country also does not have a solid policy on the importation of GMF, unlike some African nations such as Angola, Lesotho, and Zambia, which have banned the import of GMFs. People do not see the possibility of the GMF being the panacea in alleviating hunger or reducing poverty among the common people. There is widespread belief that the GMF companies are more interested in profits than attending to possible challenges and risks that may be associated with the products. This has raised serious ethical issues why crops should be genetically modified in the first place and the concept is of great concern to religious organizations. In their opinion, conventional techniques of food production if well managed are sufficient for food sufficiency. They argued that scientists are playing God by creating varieties and mutant products of plants and animals by altering their natural genetic makeup, an opinion still in resonance among many religion faithful.

Although, biotechnology could contribute significantly toward Nigeria's potential role in agricultural leadership in the sub-Saharan Africa, it is imperative to look into factors that contribute to getting this far and the forces that long opposed GMOs adoption in the country. So much controversy has been generated over the adoption of GMFs, so much that it calls for a serious appraisal. There is no doubt that there are benefits and adverse effects of GMFs but in a situation where people's perception of the adverse effects greatly outweigh the benefits may be suicidal. The genetic modification of plants for food production stems from the challenges facing agriculture. The technology came about as a means of combating the problem of food shortage and hunger in the world. The United States of America has been giving GMFs to developing countries like Nigeria to help alleviate the problem of hunger and poverty in the countries. However, anxieties have been raised over the genetic and health implications of consuming the GMFs.

The driving force for the intention to adopt GMFs in Nigeria might not be unconnected with the ambition of Nigerian government to diversify her economy from monoeconomy of heavy dependence on crude oil. In addition, there is also the fear of looming crises of food security as a result of astronomically increasing population, coupled with heavy dependence on foreign foods. A number of factors such as incidence of drought, inadequate water resources, and poor soils along with other economic and social pressures have been identified as major problems responsible for food insecurity in Nigeria. The opinion of some Nigerians was that the decision to adopt GMFs must have been borne not only out of overall implications of GM crops on human and environmental health but also to provide future direction in agriculture; the implications of private-sector led research, livelihood and development options, ethical issues, and right concerns (Scoones, 2005).

The development, assessment, and release of GMOs/GMFs are with huge initial cost. Investors who channeled large funds to the processes of genetically modified crops production will ensure a profitable return on their investment. Consequently, most of the developed biotech seeds and food are either registered or patented under various intellectual protection laws, thus making its infringement a serious concern. This limits the access of potential agribusiness individuals with less capital, thus the big investors could have the monopoly of production and price control to maximize the profit. Of course, less number of players and competitors will lead to economic exploitation and the products may be beyond the rich of common farmer or people. Some individuals fear that because most farmers lack the technologies and skill required for GMOs/GMFs production, the market will be dominated by foreign capitalists, which may be counterproductive for the nation's economy. Furthermore, the consumer advocate group expressed worry that patenting of the newly developed biotech products will raise the price of seeds so high that local farmers will not be able to afford the seeds, thus widening the gap between the wealthy and the poor.

Meanwhile, the concern envisage by the inability of the poor and local farmers to afford GM seeds produced by private seed companies may not be a serious deterrent to GM seeds adoption as more developing countries in the recent years are making significant progress toward introduction of biotech seeds into their agricultural sectors (Pretty, 2008; Gebretsadik and Kiflu, 2018). The basic aim of every investment is to make profit, and agribusiness is not an exception. If the GM seeds would raise the profit margin of the farmers, they may be well disposed to it. In India and China, farmers quickly adopted Bt. cotton because of its high yield, greater productivity, and reduced occupational hazard due to less exposure to pesticide as the modified cotton required little or no pesticide applications (Pray et al., 2003; Hossain et al., 2004). By this, the farmers see as leverage on the initial high cost of the GM seeds.

Health and environmental safety concerns

Despite burden of problems being faced by the country, many individuals and pressure groups are of the opinion that rushing to adopt GMFs in the country may not be the best option as there are still a lot of unanswered questions. There are fears about the possible environmental consequences of GMFs, its health implications and socioeconomics. Environmental consequences may be in form of gene flow through pollen flow between the GM crops and its wild relatives and possibility of adverse effects of GM crops on nontarget organisms. For instance, Bt. toxins kill many species of insect larvae indiscriminately including those of positive agricultural and economic importance.

Health implication of consuming GMFs may arise in form of development of new allergies as creation of GMF involves routine transfer into the food supply, protein from organisms (such as viruses) that have never been consumed in food. Socio-economy may spur from corporate control of GMOs market and all associated chemicals through buying up of seed companies, patenting seeds, and locking farmers into exclusive agreement that may result in agricultural biodiversity and unsustainable farming (Lopez et al., 2004).

Like many other countries, in Nigeria, there are groups, civil societies, and individuals that are totally anti-GMO, while a number of other are reserved about the use of biotech seeds. The critics tend to focus mainly on health concern and safety of the biotech products for humans, animals, and the environment. For instance, a civil organization, Health of the Mother Earth Foundation (HOMEF) argued that the risks associated with the GMOs, and GMFs have not been adequately identified, evaluated, and appraised before releasing the seeds. Despite the currently available scientific position and consensus proclamation that the biotech procedure and products pose no greater risk to human health than conventional foods, notwithstanding, the anti-GMO critics are instigating fear and threat of death in potential users of the biotech products, put pressure on the regulating agencies to abrogate activities on genetically modified crops. In fact, there were repeated tales (though unsubstantiated and from nonscientists) and claims that consumption of GMFs has resulted into death of many people in the internally displaced camps (Id Camps) in the crises ridden parts of the country.

Moreover, in the view of some other anti-GMFs groups, there may be no benefit to the consumers as the approved GMFs and those pending approval are either herbicide-tolerant or insect-resistant. They pose real problem to the environments and offer absolutely no benefits to the consumer as they are neither cheaper nor better quality than conventional food. There may be dependency on chemical pesticides as the crops actually encourage chemical use, thereby posing threat to our foods, drinking water, and wildlife. Other problems include, creation of "super weeds," antibiotic-resistance, and increase toxins in plants (Lopez et al., 2004). All these serve as a pointer to the fact that the long-term effect of GMFs on the human population and the ecosystem in general needs to be addressed and properly researched. This is with a view to unravel and prevent any possible risks that may be associated with the consumption of the GMFs.

The politics of GMOs/GMFs in Nigeria

Lack of well-established legislative framework on biotechnological applications in Nigeria has created loophole to be exploited both by the proponent and anti-GMFs groups. The critics argued that GMFs supplied by the United States in aids to crises ridden internally displaced camps (Id camps) are to promote and grow foreign seed companies and as part of a starvation campaign to portrait Africa as a hungry continent. According to a report (Isah, 2018), since the official release of GM seeds to farmers by the government, the anti-GMO group have been lobbying the legislator to repeal or create an Act of Parliament that disallows growing or importation of any form of GMF into the country. Since the adoption of the modified seeds, the legislative arm of government has been foot-dragging to provide legislative framework for further development of biotech products in Nigeria.

In a bid to remove the sentiment, various scientists, farmers association, and research organizations have been involved in sensitization, seminars, and talk shows to win the heart of prospective stakeholders and consumers of genetic engineering technology and to educate the people on the opportunities and capacity of genetic engineering technologies to improve the quality and quantity of agricultural output in Nigeria. The regulating agency, NABDA, through the National Orientation Agency (NOA) has often time iterated that biotech seeds are safe and that Nigeria should explore the technologies involved into the fullest.

Intervention and outlook

As a way of boosting food production, there is need to review all agricultural practices in the country as more in-depth studies are needed to improve on the age-long practices. In one of the studies on commercial rice-growing fields, researchers found that thousands of Chinese farmers using agroecologic techniques experienced yield increase of 89% while completely eliminating some of their most common pesticides (Zhu et al., 2000; Haung et al., 2005; Schmidt, 2005). If the Nigerian farmers are sufficiently mobilized, they have the capacity to grow food that will be more than enough to feed the population. Individuals could also be encouraged to engage in small-scale farming of native crops because it enhances food production. This is corroborated by United Nations (UN) figures; for instance, in Asia, figures for Syria showed farms between 1 and 2.5 acres being more than three times as productive as farms over 35 acres. A similar study in Nigeria shows the small farms being more than four times as productive. This is because small farms tend to produce several crops at once, thus reducing nutrient depletion. Small farm and garden owners can compost any waste generated, use the land and other resources effectively more than large-scale agribusiness.

Although Nigeria has joined the League of Nations for GMFs by officially releasing GM seeds for production, there are hurdles to be crossed for the products to be accepted by the people. According to a report by the Centre for Food Safety (James, 2005; FAOSTAT, 2006), Nigeria still accepts GMFs as food aids, and the only condition for the importation is that the GMF food aid be milled. Presently, there is no law governing the production of food products by companies using genetically modified ingredients. There are many challenges ahead for the government, especially in the areas of safety testing, regulation, and internal policy. Moreover, every citizen has a right to know what he is consuming. There is a need to enlighten the general public on what GMFs are, highlighting the advantages and disadvantages of accepting it as a source of food. It is our opinion that GMFs may not be the ultimate solution to hunger in a developing country like Nigeria.

Conclusion

Food is very important to all living soul, as whenever there is no food, there is no possibility of existence. The trend of GMFs in Nigeria has revealed that the research in GMFs is still at its infancy and efforts in conventional breeding also have not been fully exploited. Conventional breeding still holds a lot of promises for the country if only government can make the once robust National Agricultural Research system work again by providing adequate and sustainable funding for research and product development, maintain stable policies, make national research institutions to effectively focus limited resources on priority areas, and devise a mechanism that will enhance effective collaborations among National Agricultural Research Institutes (NARIs), universities, extension, and private sector. This is the only way by which the country can be rescued from looming food insecurity as a result of its growing population and at the same time, seen to be creating wealth and employment for teeming youth. However, if Nigeria as a country must adopt GMFs; it must be done with caution at least by starting aggressive research into less controversial mutation breeding (induced mutation) and aspects of biotechnology that are less risky. The debates on adoption of GMFs is going to continue for some time, it is likely going to be the last option as the trend has shown that the country and its people are not yet fully ready nor prepared to handle the probable fallouts as a result of its adoption.

References

Adams, J.M., Piovesan, G., Strauss, S., Brown, S., 2002. The case for genetic engineering of native and landscape trees against introduced pests and diseases. Conservation Biology 16, 874–879.

Adamu, A.K., Chung, S.S., Abubakar, S., 2004. The effect of ionizing radiation (Gamma rays) on tomato (s.n.). Nigerian Journal of Experimental Biology 5 (2), 185–193.

Animasaun, D.A., Oyedeji, S., Azeez, M.A., Onasanya, A.O., 2014. Alkylating efficiency of sodium azide on pod yield, nut size and nutrition composition of SAMNUT 10 and SAM-NUT 20 varieties of groundnut (*Arachis hypogea* L.). African Journal of Food, Agriculture, Nutrition and Development 14 (7), 9497–9510.

Animasaun, D.A., Mustapha, O.T., Oyedeji, S., Yusuf, K.A., 2016. Chemo-sensitivity and determination of optimum exposure time of nitrous acid for growth and yield of *Digitaria exilis* (Haller). Journal of Pharmacy and Applied Sciences 3 (2), 8–13.

Arakawa, T., Chong, D.K.X., Langridge, W.H.R., 1998. Efficacy of a food plant-based oral cholera toxin B subunit vaccine. Nature Biotechnology 16, 292–297.

Bado, S., Forster, B.P., Nielen, S., Ghanim, A., Lagoda, P.J.L., Till, B.J., Laimer, M., 2015. Plant mutation breeding: current progress and future assessment. Plant Breeding Reviews 39, 23–88.

Blancfield, J.R., Lund, D., Spiess, W., 2008. In: Report on the Food Security Forum. Held in Conjunction with the 14th World Congress of Food Science and Technology, Shanghai, China, 19–23 October 2008.

Boyer, H.W., Chow, L.T., Dugaiczyk, A., Hedgpeth, J., Goodman, H.M., 1973. DNA substrate site for the EcoRII restriction endonuclease and modification methylase. Nature New Biology 244 (132), 40−43.

de la Fuente, J.M., Ramirez-Rodriguez, V., Cabrera-Ponce, J.L., Herrera-Estrella, L., 1997. Aluminium tolerance in transgenic plants by alteration of citrate synthesis. Science 276, 1566−1568.

Evenson, R.E., Gollin, D., 2003. Crop Genetic Improvement in Developing Countries: Overview and Summary in Crop Variety Improvement and its Effect on Productivity. FAO Report 2003. Rome, Italy.

FAOSTAT, 2006. Soybeans, Rapeseed, Maize and Cotton Harvested Areas in 2005. FAO Report 2003. Rome, Italy.

FAO, 2019. Global Partnership Initiative for Plant Breeding Capacity Building. Available at: http://www.fao.org/in-action/plant-breeding/our-partners/africa/nigeria/en/.

Fashakin, J.B., 2008. Principles of Food Science and Technology. Akwe. National Open University of Nigeria, Nigeria.

Flavell, R.B., 1999. Agriculture: a path of experiment and change. Nature Biotechnology (Suppl. 17), BV7.

Fedoroff, N.V., Battisti, D.S., Beachy, R.N., Cooper, P.J.M., Fischhoff, D.A., et al., 2010. Radically rethinking agriculture for the 21st century. Science 327, 833−834, 9.

Forster, B.P., Shu, Q.Y., 2012. Plant mutagenesis in crop improvement: basic terms and applications. In: Shu, Q.Y., Forster, B.P., Nakagawa, H. (Eds.), Plant Mutation Breeding and Biotechnology. CABI, Wallingford, pp. 9−12.

Gbarada, O., 2017. Genetically modified food (GMOs) and its environmental conflict situation in Nigeria. American Journal of Environmental Policy and Management 3 (5), 31−38.

Gebretsadik, K., Kiflu, A., 2018. Challenges and opportunities of genetically modified crops production; future perspectives in Ethiopia: review. The Open Agriculture Journal 12, 240−250.

GM Crops List (2017). Available at: (http://www.isaaa.org/gmapprovaldatabase/cropslist/). (Accessed 18 February 2019).

Haung, J., Hu, R., Rozelle, S., Pray, C., 2005. Insect resistant GM rice in farmer's fields: assessing productivity and health effects in China. Science 308, 688−690.

Hossain, F., Pray, C.E., Lu, Y., Huang, J., Fan, C., Hu, R., 2004. Genetically modified cotton and farmers health in China. International Journal of Occupational and Environmental Health 10, 296−303.

IAEA, 2015. IAEA Mutant Database. International Atomic Energy Agency, Vienna. Available at: http://mvd.iaea.org/.

Isaac, N., Conrow, J., 2019. Nigeria Approves its First GMO Food Crop. https://allianceforscience.cornell.edu/blog/2019/01/nigeria-approves-first-gmo-food-crop.

Isah, A., 2018. Embracing Biotech Crops and Why Nigeria's GMO Fight is Far From Over. Genetic Literacy Project, 2018 Report.

Jacobsen, E., Schouten, H.J., 2008. Cisgenesis, a new tool for traditional plant breeding, should be exempted from the regulation on genetically modified organisms in a step-by-step approach. Potato Research 51, 75−88.

Jaenisch, R., Mintz, B., 1974. Infection of mouse blastocysts with SV40 DNA: normal development of the infected embryos and persistence of SV40-specific DNA sequences in the adult animals. Proceedings of the National Academy of Sciences of the United States of America 71, 375−380.

James, C., 2005. Global Status of Commercialized Biotech/GM Crops in 2005. ISAAA, Ithaca, NY, 2005. v. 2006.

Jarvis, S., Hickford, J., 1999. Gene Technology. NZ Institute for Crop and Food Research, Christchurch.

Katsumoto, Y., Fukuchi-Mizutani, M., Fukui, Y., Brugliera, F., Holton, T.A., Karan, M., Nakamura, N., Yonekura-Sakakibara, K., Togami, J., Pigeaire, A., Tao, G.Q., Nehra, N.S., Lu, C.Y., Dyson, B.K., Tsuda, S., Ashikari, T., Kusumi, T., Mason, J.G., Tanaka, Y., 2007. Engineering of the rose flavonoid biosynthetic pathway successfully generated blue-hued flowers accumulating delphinidin. Plant and Cell Physiology 48 (11), 1589—1600. https://doi.org/10.1093/pcp/pcm131.

Kharkwal, M.C., Shu, Q.Y., 2009. The role of induced mutations in world food security. In: Shu, Q.Y. (Ed.), Induced Plant Mutations in the Genomic Era. Food and Agriculture Organization of the United Nations, Rome, pp. 33—38.

Kuzma, J., Haase, R., 2012. Genetically modified foods: policy context and safety. Food Policy Research Centre: Policy Brief 31.

Lopez, J., Doherty, A., Sarno, N., Bohlen, L., 2004. Genetically modified crops. Friend of the Earth International 105, 12—13.

Maluszynski, M., Szarejko, I., Bhatia, C.R., et al., 2009. Methodologies for generating variability. In: Ceccarelli, S., Guimar, E.P., Weltzien, E. (Eds.), Plant Breeding and Farmer Participation. Food and Agriculture Organization (FAO), Rome. Available from: http://www.fao.org/docrep/012/i1070e/i1070e00.htm.

Maryanski, J.H., 1995. "FDA's policy for foods developed by biotechnology" genetically modified foods: safety issues. In: Engel, Takeoka, Teranishi (Eds.), American Chemical Society, Symposium Series, vol. 605, pp. 12—22 (2).

Mason, H., Ball, J., Shi, J., Jiang, X., Estes, M., Arntzen, C., 1996. Expression of Norwalk virus capsid protein in transgenic tobacco and potato, and its oral immunogenicity in mice. Proceedings of the National Academy of Sciences of the United States of America 93, 5335—5340.

Mba, C., Afza, R., Shu, Q.Y., 2012. Mutagenic radiations: X-rays, ionizing particles, and ultraviolet. In: Shu, Q.Y., Forster, B.P., Nakagawa, H. (Eds.), Plant Mutation Breeding and Biotechnology, Joint FAO/IAEA Division of Nuclear Techniques in Food and Agriculture International Atomic Energy Agency, Vienna, pp. 83—90.

Mba, C., 2013. Induced mutations unleash the potentials of plant genetic resources for food and agriculture. Agronomy 3 (1), 200—231.

Molvig, L., Tabe, L.M., Eggum, B.O., Moore, A.E., Craig, S., Spencer, D., Higgins, T.J., 1997. Enhanced methionine levels and increased nutritive value of transgenic lupins (*Lupinus augustifolius* L.) expressing a sunflower albumin gene. Proceedings of the National Academy of Sciences of the United States of America 94, 8393—8398.

Mottaleb, K.A., Mohanty, S., 2015. Farm size and profitability of rice farming under rising input costs. Journal of Land Use Science 10 (3), 243—255. https://doi.org/10.1080/1747423X.2014.9196188.

Neil, A.C., Lawrence, G.M., Reece, J.B., 2000. Biology: Concepts and Connections. Wesley Longman, New York.

Nielsen, J., 2013. Production of biopharmaceutical proteins by yeast: advances through metabolic engineering. Bioengineered 4 (4), 207—211. https://www.tandfonline.com/doi/abs/10.4161/bioe.22856.

Newswire, P.R., 2013. Genetically Modified Maize: 'Doctors' Chamber Warns of "Unpredictable Results" to Humans".

NGIN, 2002. USDA Report Exposes GM Crop Economics Myth. http://ngin.tripod.com/230802a.htm.

Ngandwe, T., May 13, 2005. Zambian builds high tech lab to detect GM food imports. SciDev Net News.

Okigbo, R.N., Iwube, J.C., Ramesh, P., 2011. An extensive review on genetically modified (GM) foods for sustainable development in Africa. E-Journal of Science and Technology 3 (6), 25–44.

Olaniyan, S.A., Bakare, A.A., Morenikeji, O.A., 2007. Genetically modified foods in Nigeria: a long-lasting solution to hunger? Estudos de Biologia 29 (67), 191–202.

Olasupo, F.O., Ilori, C.O., Forster, B.P., Bado, S., 2016. Mutagenic effects of gamma radiation on eight accessions of Cowpea (*Vigna unguiculata* (L.) Walp.). American Journal of Plant Sciences 7, 339–351.

Oldach, K.H., 2011. Mutagenesis. In: Pratap, A., Kumar, J. (Eds.), Biology and Breeding of Food Legumes. CABI, Wallingford, pp. 208–219.

Paine, J.A., Shipton, C.A., Chaggar, S., Howells, R.M., Kennedy, M.J., et al., 2005. Improving the nutritional value of Golden Rice through increased pro-vitamin A content. Nature Biotechnology 23, 482–487.

Pray, C.E., Huang, J., Ma, D., Qiao, F., 2003. Impact of Bt cotton in China. World Development 29, 813–825.3.

Pretty, J., 2008. Agricultural sustainability: concepts, principles and evidence. Philosophical Transactions of the Royal Society, London B: Biological Sciences 363 (1491), 447–465. https://doi.org/10.1098/rstb.2007.2163.

Schmidt, C.W., 2005. Genetically modified foods: breeding uncertainty. Environmental Health Perspectives 13, A527–A533.

SciDev net news, 2008. Genetically Modified Crop in Africa. https://editors.eol.org/eoearth/wiki/Genetically_modified_crops_in_Africa.

Scoones, I., 2005. Governing technology development: challenges for agricultural research in Africa. Institute of Development Studies Bulletin 36 (2), 109–114.

Sikora, P., Chawade, A., Larsson, M., Olsson, J., Olsson, O., 2011. Mutagenesis as a tool in plant genetics. Functional Genomics and Breeding. International Journal of Plant Genomics, The Journal is a Hindawi Publication, online Journal usually with no page range but an ID. The ID for the publication is Article ID 314829. https://doi.org/10.1155/2011/314829.

Spillane, C., 1999. Recent developments in Biotechnology as they relate to plant genetic resources for food and agriculture. Commission on Genetic Resources for Food and Agriculture. Background Study Paper No. 9, 18–34.

Taire, M., 2003. Genetically Modified Foods, Keeping the Peace in Liberia [Internet], 2003 [access2006 Dec 11]. Available from: http://www.checkbiotech.org.

Tester, M., Langridge, P., 2010. Breeding technologies to increase crop production in a changing world. Science 327, 818–822.

UN (United Nations, Department of Economic and Social Affairs), 2017. Population Division. World Population Prospects: The 2017 Revision, Key Findings and Advance Tables Working Paper No. ESA/P/WP/248.

Vanguard newspaper, 2019. Are Genetically Modified Food (GMO) Safe? Available on. https://www.vanguardngr.com/2019/01/are-genetically-modified-foodsgmos-safe/.

Wani, M.R., Kozgar, M.I., Tomlekova, N., et al., 2014. Mutation breeding: a novel technique for genetic improvement of pulse crops particularly Chickpea (*Cicer arietinum* L.). In:

Parvaiz, A., Wani, M.R., Azooz, M.M., Lam-son, P.T. (Eds.), Improvement of Crops in the Era of Climatic Changes. Springer, New York (NY), pp. 217–248.

Whitham, S., McCormick, S., Baker, B., 1996. The N gene of tobacco confers resistance to tobacco mosaic virus in transgenic tomato. Proceedings of the National Academy of Sciences of the United States of America 93, 8776–8781.

Whitman, D.B., 2000. Genetically modified foods: harmful or helpful? An Overview. CSA 1–13.

Wilkinson, J.Q., Lanahan, M.B., Clark, D.G., Bleecker, A.B., Chang, C., Meyerowitz, E.M., Klee, H.J., 1997. A dominant mutant receptor from Arabidopsis confers ethylene insensitivity in heterologous plants. Nature Biotechnology 15, 444–447.

Zhu, Y., Chen, H., Fan, J., Wang, Y., Li, Y., Chen, J., 2000. Genetic diversity and control in rice. Nature 406, 716–722.

GMOs in Argentina

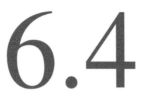

6.4

Moisés Burachik, PhD

Director, Regulatory Affairs, INDEAR, Rosario, Santa Fe Province, Argentina

Introduction

During the last two and half decades, the world has experienced great advances in the application of biotechnology to agricultural production and breeding practices. Argentina was an early adopter of these innovations: field tests of genetically modified (GM) crops (also called "transgenic") started in 1991, the first commercial product was released in 1996 and the number of commercial approvals to this date (November 2018) totals 52 (https://www.argentina.gob.ar/ogm-comerciales). This successful development was the result of several local factors, especially the setting up of a robust, science-based regulatory framework.

Although this process runs currently at a good pace, it had suffered in the past an interruption which sensibly impacted on the regulations: new labeling rules at the European Union (EU, an important market for Argentina's agricultural products) and the ensuing public debate over GM foods and crops forced the introduction of trade (i.e., nonscientific) issues in the approval process: approval of a product was granted if and when the EU market will also approve it (the so-called "mirror policy"). These difficulties, which resulted in a long (1998–2003) *de facto* moratorium of approvals at the EU, affected the regular processing of applications and negatively impacted the Argentine economy. At the time, this moratorium led Argentina, together with Canada and the United States (US), i.e., the "complaining parties," to engage in a trade dispute with the EU at the World Trade Organization (WTO). The complexity of the case demanded the WTO to establish a specific expert panel to address the issue (Burachik, 2013). A scientific exercise then ensued by which the panel asked questions to the parties, all of them reflecting the active debate already underway at the EU. As a result, regulatory scientists entered the interplay of arguments, scientific evidences, and rebuttals at stake in the debate. Because of the weight these arguments had not only in the EU versus Argentina trade dispute but also on the whole adoption process and worldwide acceptance of this new technology, they are also described here. Therefore, the structure of this chapter: the first part (I) will deal with the Argentine experience in the implementation of the genetically modified organisms (GMOs) and the second (II) develops

Genetically Modified and Irradiated Food. https://doi.org/10.1016/B978-0-12-817240-7.00009-7

some of the issues characterizing the GMO debate. At the end (III), I intend to draw some lessons learned in developing the above.

The Argentine case

The phase of adoption. Science-based regulatory framework

Argentina, an early adopter, is the third largest grower of transgenic crops in the world with 12% of the global biotech crop area (23.6 million hectares in 2017; ISAAA, 2017). Areas planted with transgenic crops were almost 100% for soybean (15 events) and cotton (4 events) and 96% for maize (29 events), performing as one of the highest adoption rates of innovations in Argentina's agriculture (ArgenBio, http://www.argenbio.org/index.php?action=cultivos&opt=5).

The early and subsequent fast development: (field tests started in 1991 and the first GM event was granted commercial approval in 1996) was the result of three major factors: the agronomic and scientific knowledge available from group of pioneering professionals, the immediate organization of an efficient, science-based regulatory framework (centered in advisory commissions with public and private membership), and the quick realization of the benefits of the technology by farmers. Research in molecular biology and genetics was (and continue to be) well advanced at the time, the prospective advantages were early perceived at the political decision level, and the regulatory commissions were able to integrate scientific basis with extensive field experience, leading to a proactive body of pragmatic biosafety rules. By setting conditions with the adequate level of precaution, confined trials allowed for 6 years (1991−96) of rich field experience.

An additional key factor in the introduction of transgenic crops in Argentina was the immediate adoption by the farmers of glyphosate-tolerant soybean (GTS), the first approved product (on March 25, 1996), which perfectly matched the zero-till practices already in use (Trigo et al., 2009). The further expansion of these two-coupled technologies has been one of the major technological events in the country's agricultural history, with an adoption rate of the GM crop even higher than in its original market in the United States (Trigo et al., 2009). Combining GTS with glyphosate use and zero-till practices resulted in a strong beneficial synergy: it introduced a sowing method which promoted conservation of soil structure, it facilitated the wheat−soybean double-cropping scheme, greatly simplified weed management with only one herbicide application almost at any time, versus several different at defined growth stages needed before, and reduced herbicides expenses by the soon expiry of Monsanto's glyphosate patent, which led to a price decline by the fierce competition from new manufacturers (Trigo et al., 2009).

When started, commercial approval of GM crops in Argentina required two independent, science-based risk assessments (RAs): the agroecosystem biosafety (by the National Advisory Commission on Agricultural Biotechnology, CONABIA) and the assessment of food/feed safety and nutritional equivalency with conventional counterparts (by the Technical Advisory Committee on the use of genetically modified organisms, within the National Service for Agri-food Health and Quality,

SENASA). Under this framework (Burachik, 2012), five GM crops were approved in the 1996—98 period. As the agriculture production of the country was strongly linked to exports of mainly soybean meal to the EU market, the timely European Commission (EC) decision (EC, 1996) approving GTS (on April 4, 1996) was a good news: it was expected that trade will grow and bring benefits to Argentina's economy. Moreover, based on strictly scientific criteria at the time prevailing at the EU, in the 1996—98 period, the EU granted approval to several transgenic crops, including insect-resistant maize MON810 (Monsanto) and Bt176 (Ciba—Geigy, also herbicide-tolerant), herbicide-tolerant maize T25 (AgrEvo), and oilseed rape Topas 19/2 (AgrEvo) (http://europa.eu/rapid/press-release_MEMO-04-102_en.htm?locale=en).

The trade-dependent phase. Not science-based requirements enter in the regulations

Unfortunately, this situation was soon to end: hostile criticism of the public toward GM foods was strongly promoted by opposing "nongovernmental organizations" (NGOs), fueled by a series of regulatory failures at the EU. Highly significant was the case of bovine spongiform encephalopathy, BSE, also known as "mad cow disease," which had nothing to do with GMOs. This incident reflected the failure of UK competent authorities to appropriately react to scientific advice warning about the disease. Food chain concerns were raised as early as 1988 (Holt and Phillips, 1988) and the belated recognition of the link with the human variant of Creutzfeldt—Jakob disease, vCJD in 1995, had the first-known victim in 1996. The context so created undermined the confidence of European consumers on the liability of regulatory officials to adequately protect the public's food safety. Realizing the power of food and environmental issues to generate strong emotions and drive political engagement led to partisanship exploitation (Kuntz, 2014) by several European Green Parties (https://europeangreens.eu/positions) resulting in new labeling rules submitted and approved in 1997 (European Parliament and the Council, 1997). Soon after, five EU Member States, acting as a "blocking minority," halted further approval of biotech products, and in 1998 the EU imposed a *de facto* moratorium until revised rules governing the approval, marketing, and labeling were implemented. New regulations for both food and feed were later approved (European Parliament and the Council, 2003a,b) requiring that any product with a GMO content of more than 0.9% be labeled. This moratorium was later challenged at the WTO by Argentina, Canada, and the United States in a remarkable dispute that ended ruling in favor of the complaining parties (Burachik, 2013).

It is interesting to place the above in the historical context, to see how development of agriculture biotechnology in Argentina, being dependent from the access to the EU market, was forced to make relevant regulatory changes, introducing not science-based requirements into the previous strictly scientific regulation. As Argentina's authorities were concerned by the possibility of shipments being rejected by European importers in the context of the *de facto* moratorium, a specific rule (Resolution N° 289/97; SAGPyA, 1997) was issued with a third decisive requirement for commercial approval: a confirmatory statement that commercial release will not cause negative impacts on trade. This nonscientific, overriding requirement affected the predictability for investment decisions on new product developments and resulted in socioeconomic and financial effects (see Smyth, 2017, on a discussion of these effects) which have never been estimated. A rough picture of these complex effects can be grasped from the yearly events approval rate within this critical period (Table 6.4.1).

Clearly, as shown in the Argentina case, opposition to GMOs may have profound institutional (regulations) and trade (asynchronic approvals) consequences. However, it may go still beyond and affect human welfare or even survival: in 2002, Zambia rejected a food aid donation of maize from the United States (Bohannon, 2002; Mwale, 2006, 2011) to feed 14 to 15 million hungry people because it was a transgenic maize. At the time, this GMO was already consumed in the United States, Argentina, Canada, Chile, Japan, Mexico, South Africa, and Uruguay, among other countries.

A University–Industry collaboration emerges

An interesting sign of the thrust of biotechnology in Argentina was the inception in 2003 of a university–industry collaboration between a research group belonging to the University of Litoral (Santa Fe Province) and headed by Dr. Raquel Lía Chan, with Bioceres, a seed producing company. Later, Bioceres created the Instituto de Agrobiotecnología Rosario (INDEAR), aimed at translating experimental findings on crops of agronomic interest from laboratory-level to the field. These efforts started with the laboratory-to-field development of two drought-tolerant GM crops, soybean and wheat, also expressing herbicide tolerance, based on the use of the sunflower transcription factor gene *HaHB4*, which had been discovered and characterized by Dr. Chan's academic group (Chan, 2009, 2014). Field trials with drought- and herbicide-tolerant soybean started in 2007 and obtained food safety clearance (SENASA, 2015) followed by similar science-based approval for the wheat event (SENASA, 2016).

However, both highly valuable GM products still wait for commercial release approval (as of November 2018) because the overriding condition of presumed negative market effects as explained above: the soybean waiting for China's approval (Ministerio de Agricultura and Ganadería y Pesca, MAGyP, 2015), and the wheat

Table 6.4.1 Approval rate of genetically modified (GM) events.

Period (Years)	1996–98	1999–2008	2009–18[a]
Rate (#events/year)	1.67	0.7	4.1
Characterization	Early adoption	EU "de facto" moratorium	EU approvals resumed

[a] *2018 counted as 0.83 year.*

Source: https://www.argentina.gob.ar/ogm-comerciales.

event, at least for Brazil's (Minagri, 2017), in both cases relevant markets for Argentina exports of these crops. It is expected that these delays will eventually subside allowing the placing on the market of these agricultural innovations. A further GM soybean, adding tolerance to a second herbicide to the drought-tolerant trait, is also subjected at the same approval condition (MPYT, 2018).

Other milestones in the achievements of INDEAR-Bioceres include commercial approval of GM safflower expressing chymosin (MAGyP, 2017, Minagri, 2017) and herbicide-tolerant alfalfa with low lignin content (Minagri, 2018).

Revisiting the regulatory framework

After two and a half decades of successful work of both the regulatory procedures and the development of agricultural biotechnology in Argentina, a group of academic, government, and industry scientists convened under the umbrella of the Argentine branch of the International Life Sciences Institute (ILSI Argentina) to discuss if the gained scientific knowledge, cumulative experimental evidence, and experience would make advisable a timely review of the RA methodology. Development of a simplified science-based, harmonized RA platform was the main purpose of this exercise, which had the relevant antecedent of a recommendation by a previous harmonization-addressed workshop (Bartholomaeus et al., 2015), were "The importance of making all possible efforts toward more integrated and harmonized regulatory oversight for GM organisms … was strongly emphasized." This previous workshop also concluded that such harmonization was a "feasible goal." At the time, the Argentina's Competent Authority had already implemented a simplified RA for "identical or essentially similar constructs" (MAGyP, 2013), and analogous approaches were underway in other countries (see Fig.6.4.1, Beker et al., 2016), indicating that other harmonization efforts were taken place linking these efforts with innovative RA approaches.

The focus of the tripartite working group was the development of a science-based assessment approach for transgenic crops in cases when the introduced genetic constructs were identical or analogous to those used in previously evaluated or approved GM crops (Beker et al., 2016). Both environmental and food safety aspects were covered in the approach, as well as to whether the new transformation events were within the same or different species. Focusing on the mode of action of the introduced genes, a "construct similarity" concept was developed: "similarity" is identified when constructs are designed to obtain the same phenotypic characteristic(s) in the recipient organism through the same biological mechanism(s). Environmental and dietary exposure, familiarity with both the crop and the trait, as well as the crop biology, were identified as key data required for a construct-based RA process. A case-by-case component will still consider different situations that might trigger different data requirements. Accordingly, a similarity claim would have to be substantiated with the appropriate data, as depicted in Fig. 6.4.1.

A set of guiding questions were developed covering the eligibility for the simplified approach based on the construct identity or similarity, familiarity with the crop and environment combination, and for the trait in this or other species, exposure

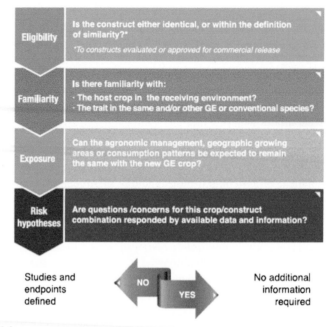

FIGURE 6.4.1

Risk assessment (RA) approach for identical or similar constructs. Affirmative answers to all questions indicate that a simplified risk assessment (SRA) is justified and no additional assessment is required. Any negative answers may call for additional RA. All cases will need to provide a full description of the event and a basic set of data. The type and extent of data will be defined on a case-by-case basis.

Source: Beker, P., Boari, P., Burachik, M., Cuadrado, V., Junco, M., Lede, S. et al., 2016. Development of a construct-based risk assessment framework for genetic engineered crops. Transgenic Research 25, 597–607.

details (agronomic practices, cultivation areas, consumption patterns, or intended uses) and the possibility of plausible new risk hypotheses, see Fig. 6.4.1.

Conclusion of this work was a framework for a simplified RA of a given case, that considers the likelihood of unintended effects from the transformation and the familiarity (with both the crop and the trait), against the background of the construct similarity concept, based on functional characteristics. Eligibility criteria for the RA simplified approach, along with the information that would be required to make a science-based decision about the safety of the new case were defined (Beker et al., 2016).

Based on these kinds of initiatives and results, it is reasonable to expect that the development of simplified, science-based, and agreed-upon RA procedures would contribute to regulatory harmonization.

The genetically modified organisms debate

The complexity

The GMO debate stands as a decades-long controversy, with highly polarized public perceptions, permeating inside social contexts and into national and international institutions. How was that the anti-GMO stance captured public opinion to such an extent? How was that a group of dedicated NGOs, opinion leaders (and even scientists), media, and communicators were able to drive so many people into the distrust of scientific facts? Is really science the issue? The introduction and adoption of GMOs in Argentina was not isolated from this debate (still ongoing), which started in the EU and other countries at the time (see, e.g., Ewen and Pusztai, 1999; Kuiper et al., 1999). Therefore, discussion of some of the conflicting arguments are included here as they had impact on the adoption process.

It is difficult to give a full, satisfactory answer to these questions. The opposition to GMO is a complex phenomenon in which science (and its understanding by the public) as well as a set of social, cultural, economic, and even religious values, together with strong symbolic components, operates and interacts (and eventually clash) simultaneously. A great diversity of arguments is raised within a variety of different contexts: human, animal and plant health, agronomic practices, food, environment, risk perception, legal frameworks, retail markets, and international trade. This landscape lends to confusion: arguments in favor tend to be causal relationships in concrete systems in which risk $=$ hazard $\times$ likelihood or exposure. Opponents, instead, will tend to see risks derived from more complex, putative interactions (Gray, 2004), long range, and more systemic. Risk would now depend also on outrage, while likelihood or exposure are no longer considered (Sandman, 2012; see also Smyth and Phillips, 2014, for scientific, socially constructed, modern and political definitions of risk).

The anti-GMO narrative involves, at least, two categories: arguments amenable to concrete, science-related representation (environment, food safety), and those originating on more abstract concepts and rhetoric (emotion, intuition, bias, commonly held beliefs vs. cognitive processing or reasoning), both within a complex sociopolitical and cultural context (National Research Council, NRC, 2015). The first of these categories will be dealt with below (Pseudoscience and false science and how the peer-review system works)). The second will be briefly outlined at the end of this section (Scientific literacy is not enough. Natural science is not the only issue).

Pseudoscience and false science and how the peer-review system works

The first of the above categories illustrates the false roots of the anti-GMO stance when analyzed under the light of scientific evidence. The arguments below were chosen for the relevance they have (or have had) in these discussions. The basic assumption in this section is the so-called "deficit model" (Ahteensuu, 2012; NRC, 2015; Scheufele, 2013), by which increasing public literacy will lead to a scientific evidence-founded, rational conversation. As will be seen later, this assumption has many limitations.

a. Bt corn is harmful to monarch butterfly

In 1999, a group of researchers found that "transgenic pollen harms monarch larvae" (Losey et al., 1999). Their results were based on laboratory assays showing "that larvae of the monarch butterfly, *Danaus plexippus*, reared on milkweed leaves dusted with pollen from *Bt* corn (GM corn expressing a protein produced by *Bacillus thuringiensis, Bt,* toxic to insects*)*, ate less, grew more slowly and suffered higher mortality than larvae reared on leaves dusted with untransformed corn pollen or on leaves without pollen" (Losey et al., 1999).

As this butterfly has a great symbolic, iconic meaning, this paper reached a great deal of public attention (see for example, https://www.usda.gov/media/blog/2015/06/16/conserving-monarch-butterflies-and-their-habitats; Scheufele, 2013).

Soon after (Beringer, 1999; Shelton and Roush, 1999), several flaws were pointed out in the Losey (1999) publication, which is a "scientific correspondence" piece, not a full, regular paper, and refutations appeared. No evidence was found that pollen from events Bt11 and Mon810, two GM *Bt* corn varieties containing the toxin Cry1Ab from *B.thuringiensis*, affected larvae at pollen densities less than 1000 pollen grains/cm2 (Hellmich et al., 2001). This new research concluded that "The laboratory bioassays used in the Losey et al. (1999) studies produce an extreme artificial environment where larvae are given no choice but to feed on milkweed leaves with high densities of pollen". The results of Hellmich et al. (2001) suggest that pollen with Cry1Ab toxin (events Bt11 and Mon810), Cry1F toxin and experimental Cry9C toxin, other insecticidal proteins from *B.thuringiensis*, (corn) hybrids will have no acute effects on monarch butterfly larvae in field settings.

This incident is often described as a model of the role of the media in disseminating high-impact news lacking adequate verification of their validity, and the harm that this may make (McInerney et al., 2004; Scheufele, 2013). It is interesting to note that the finding of (harmful) effects was obtained by setting artificial conditions addressed at showing what the researcher wishes to find, i.e., the so-called "confirmation bias" (Kunda, 1990; NRC, 2015). This is a strategy commonly used in the false science within the GMO debate (see also below). Although stated in a different discipline (medical research), the following characterization applies: "For many areas of investigation at present, what is presented as scientific evidence often is simply *exact and precise measurements of a prevailing bias*" (Ioannidis, 2005).

b. Antibiotic resistance genes inserted in GM plants can be acquired by bacterial pathogens through the "horizontal gene transfer" (HGT) effect

As the transformation process to generate many of the first GM crops used antibiotic resistance genes to aid in the selection of plant cells receiving the DNA insertion, e.g., corn Bt176 contained an ampicillin resistance gene, the possible transfer of these genes, eventually acquired by bacterial pathogens through plant-to-bacteria recombination-driven *horizontal gene transfer* phenomena was considered a risk, because it would led to a reduction of the therapeutic efficacy of the relevant antibiotics or even antibiotic resistance.

A great deal of research work soon found the risk of this "horizontal gene transfer" was negligible (Schlüter et al., 1995). In fact, HGT of recombinant genes from GM plants to bacteria has never been shown under field conditions with GM plants used in agriculture (EFSA, 2015, 2017). Should such transfer occur, it would be several orders of magnitude lower than naturally occurring gene transfer between bacteria. In the environment, HGT is strongly limited by physical and biological barriers inherent in the transfer process itself (EFSA, 2009; Nielsen et al., 2014; Van den Eede et al., 2004).

Plant-to-bacteria gene transfer phenomena have been only observed under highly artificial laboratory conditions by a process called "homology-facilitated illegitimate recombination," aided by previous deliberate introduction in the recipient bacteria of appropriate homologous sequences (i.e., bacterial sequences flanking the target gene to promote recombination). In one case (Cérémonie et al., 2006; Demanèche et al., 2001), the possible DNA transfer was obtained under laboratory conditions imitating *lightning,* intended to mimic a natural situation. Although HGT phenomena have been induced in laboratory microcosms by artifacts such as homology-facilitated illegitimate recombination, they have never been found under natural conditions (Rizzi et al., 2012) and are highly unlikely to occur in the field. However, European Food Safety Authority (EFSA) still require the GM crop DNA to be searched (by bioinformatic analyses) "to identify plant sequences with sufficient identity (with the DNA present in microbial genomes) to promote homologous recombination as means to increase the probability of HGT" (EFSA, 2017). The basis of this search clearly recognizes these recombinant-prone DNA stretches as an essential condition for HGT to occur (EFSA, 2009, EFSA, 2017; see Box 6.4.1, for EFSA overall data requirements and assessment for GMO approval in the EU).

c. Consumption of GMO-derived food will cause allergy

It has been argued that (1) genetic modification may increase the natural allergenicity of food derived from the GM crop and (2) foreign proteins expressed in GM crops will lead to allergic reactions. The answer to these questions rests on the regulatory review that a GM crop needs to comply for commercial approval. This review includes compositional, bioinformatic, and digestibility assessments as explained below.

(1) The first of these assumptions is questionable: endogenous allergen levels show a wide range of variation due to differences in genetic background and environmental effects. Statistical analyses of these differences and comparisons between GM and non-GM varieties show that, for most allergens, the effects of environment far outweigh the differences between varieties brought about by breeding (Panda et al., 2013). Data obtained using profiling techniques (transcriptomics, proteomics, and metabolomics) support the conclusion that genetic modification presents *less risk* of up-regulating endogenous allergens

Box 6.4.1 TYPICAL INFORMATION REQUIREMENTS AND REPORT OF GMO RISK ASSESSMENT

Example of the components of a typical risk assessment of a GMO
(taken from a "Scientific opinion on an application for the placing on the market"
by the European Food Safety Authority)

Source: *EFSA GMO Panel (EFSA Panel on Genetically Modified Organisms), 2017. Scientific opinion on an application by Dow AgroSciences LLC (EFSAGMO-NL-2012-106) for the placing on the market of genetically modified herbicide-tolerant soybean DAS-44406-6 for food and feed uses, import and processing under Regulation (EC) No 1829/2003. EFSA Journal 2017;15(3):4738, 33 pp. doi:10.2903/j.efsa.2017.4738 www.efsa.europa.eu/efsajournalBox*

compared with traditional breeding (Ricroch et al., 2011). Also, assessment of the mechanisms by which transgenesis could increase the levels of endogenous allergens (insertional mutagenesis, interaction with endogenous biochemical pathways, and gene modulation) has concluded that the likelihood of up-regulating an endogenous allergen due to transgenesis is not greater than from traditional breeding (Herman and Ladics, 2011).

Moreover, full compositional data comparison from materials obtained from field experiments in different environment, where GMO-derived materials are compared with similar materials from the non-GM counterpart, demonstrated compositional equivalency unless nonequivalence is the purpose of the modification, e.g., enhanced nutritional properties. Statistical design and data analysis complying with the best state-of-the-art practices have shown no significant differences in the levels of the plant natural, endogenous allergens.

It must be emphasized that compositional equivalence is a fundamental component of human health safety assessment (Kuiper et al., 2001). For more than 20 years, this assessment has shown that *no unintended compositional effects were derived from the genetic modification*. Accordingly, it has been proposed that compositional equivalence studies required for regulatory approval of GM crops may no longer be justified (Herman, 2013).

(2) Food safety assessment of GM crops demands a bioinformatic analysis where the amino acids sequence of the newly expressed protein is compared, taking 35 amino acids stretches along the whole sequence, with the sequences of known allergens: for approval, no similarity must be confirmed. The power of this requirement can be roughly measured from a simple calculation: the search takes a window of 35 contiguous amino acids sliding through the full sequence of the target protein (some 170 different sequences for a 200 amino-acids protein) which is compared with the sequences of known allergens (some 2000), giving 340,000 comparisons for one given protein, or 429 million comparisons for the ca. 1300 proteins in the transgenic crops currently in the market (Dunn et al., 2017). This is a good measure of the negligible opportunity to reach the consumers for an allergen derived from a genetic modification of the crop.

Many allergenic proteins are resistant to gastric digestion. Although not absolutely correlated to allergenicity potential, digestibility by a human-simulated gastric fluid is also a regulatory requirement: rapid degradation is usually found.

The sum of the above safety requirements, compositional equivalence, absence of sequence homologies with known allergens and rapid digestion, together with the absence of conformational homologies with allergens and of glycosylation sites, build up to a "weight-of-evidence" conclusion on the allergenicity of a newly expressed protein. Only when all these safety conditions are met is a GM crop released for cultivation and consumption.

To date, no human or animal model study has demonstrated that a GMO-derived food was more allergenic than its conventional counterpart. No studies were identified that demonstrated that consumption of a GM food was associated with an increased prevalence of clinical allergy (defined as typical signs or symptoms of IgE-mediated reactivity in human or animal models), compared with its conventional counterpart (Dunn et al., 2017)

d. Long-term effects I (the role of risk assessment)

Long-term effects, derived from consumption of GMO-derived food/feed or infringed to the environment by the release of GMOs, are frequently raised as sources of harm. The answer to this question resides in the central methodology for the approval process of a GMO: the RA. RA is the careful, comprehensive examination of information we have available today as peer-reviewed-quality experimental evidence addressed at identify and characterize potential sources of future harm. It is a scientific activity (the *assessment*), which starts with a risk hypothesis with the identification of the hazard, the *problem formulation* step (Wolt et al., 2010) and develops a conceptual model for a causal relationship (the *harm prediction pathway*) linking: (a) the likelihood and exposure to harm, with (b) critical parameters of the system which are amenable to measurement (the *assessment variables*). Examples would be "effects on nontarget organisms" in an environment or the potential of allergenicity in a food. Further measurement of the critical parameters, i.e., end-point values associated to protection goals (directly or through surrogate variables, the *experimental* phase) will allow to predict the probability and exposure to the future, potential source of harm. With this information, we should reach a level of knowledge (the *regulatory* phase) enough to take an appropriate course of action, i.e., to grant or deny the release/consumption of the GMO, consistent with established criteria of protection goals and values demanded by the statutory level of precaution (the *decision* phase). This RA methodology applies to both, food/feed and the environment and compares the GMO with the nonmodified counterpart, with which we are familiar as having a known long record of safety. A good example of the kind of information, which is processed for taking decision of granting approval for release a GMO into the market, is shown in Box 6.4.1.

Long-term effects are then considered in the comparative approach embodied in the RA: a favorable report will assure that no significant differences exist, with exception of the new introduced trait(s). When no equivalence is sought, as the case of nutritional modifications, all other features must be verified as equivalent to the no-GMO comparator. A good indication of the irrelevant nature of the "long-term effects" argument could be found in the record of GMO approvals in the EU, where the RA done by the EFSA includes approval of a "postmarket monitoring" proposal requested to the applicant. In the period 2004−17, from 26 approval decisions, in 21 cases such monitoring (supposedly to detect putative "long-term effects") was considered "not necessary." Of the other five cases, three were to GMO with modification in their nutritional characteristics, where the recommendation was to follow consumption patterns (not a safety issue) and on the remaining two cases, EFSA were not in position to give opinion because of lack of data. However, in all 26 cases, the overall RA by EFSA did not find reasons of concern and approval was granted.

Long-term effects II (biodiversity)

Biodiversity damage was one of the most effective arguments intended to support the "long-term effects" issue in the GMO debate. This argument has successfully reached international "recognition" and permeated into a complex body of (supposedly) protective regulations: the Cartagena Protocol (CP) on Biosafety to the Convention on Biological Diversity (SCBD, 2000). The Protocol was intended to provide "an adequate level of protection in the field of the safe transfer, handling and use of living modified organisms resulting from modern biotechnology that may have adverse effects on the conservation and sustainable use of biological diversity, taking also into account risks to human health, and specifically focusing on transboundary movements" (SCBD, 2000). The CP is the first environmental international law to address possible problems with GMOs and has greatly contributed to support an anti-GMO stand, as reflected from the choice of the precautionary criterion (see Box 6.4.2). Notably, the Protocol opens the way for nonscientific issues: "Public Awareness and Participation (Article 23)" and "Socio-Economic Considerations (Article 26)," thereby greatly contributing to the weight of social components (see Scientific literacy is not enough. Natural science is not the only issue, below) of the anti-GMO stand. In fact, this support is notably reinforced by the emotional rhetoric prevailing in the text: when referring to GMOs, the CP never uses the expression "genetically modified organisms," but "living modified organisms" (53 times in the English text), where "living" clearly has emotional appeal.

Box 6.4.2 THE CARTAGENA PROTOCOL ROLE IN THE GMO DEBATE

Although the risk assessment of GMOs has proved to be an efficient methodology to provide "long-term" food and environmental safety, the GMO debate has evolved also on which should be the underlying "precautionary" criterion. Two alternatives may be considered:

- The *Agreement on Sanitary and Phytosanitary measures* (SPS): Establishes that any claim of potential harm should be based on scientific evidence; additional information that may be needed and not available for an appropriate decision should be defined and sought. Because of its relevance for undisrupted trade, the SPS agreement is one of the pillars of the WTO rules.
- The Cartagena Protocol, reaffirms the precautionary approach contained in Principle 15 of the Rio Declaration: "lack of full scientific certainty shall not be used as a reason for postponing cost-effective measures to prevent environmental degradation" (UNEP, 1992).

Clearly, the precautionary criterion adopted by the CP (to date having 196 Nations as Parties, with 168 Signatures, https://www.cbd.int/information/parties.shtml) opens the way to nonscientific arguments, which will be strongly reflected in the GMO debate.

Scientific literacy is not enough. Natural science is not the only issue

Despite the benefits to millions of farmers, especially in developing countries, by improving agronomic practices such as herbicide tolerance, insect resistance, lesser use of toxic chemicals and to consumers by enhancing nutritional value and food/feed safety, increasing public scientific literacy (the assumption of the so called "deficit model"), by which "Knowledge Deficits Are Responsible for a Lack of Public Support of Science" (NRC, 2015; Scheufele, 2013) has shown not to drive the overall public attitude toward a rational conversation. Societal debate has moved to other fields, like social sciences, cultural values, and political arenas, complex areas usually little familiar to scientists.

How scientists are (or should be) performing in the GMO debate has been extensively studied within the framework of diverse social disciplines (Blancke et al., 2015, Clancy and Clancy, 2015; Kuntz, 2015, 2018; NRC, 2015; Valentinov et al., 2018, to name a few).

Contributions to this multifaceted issue take views from a diverse array of disciplines and approaches: perceived risks, benefits, and "naturalness" value (Bearth and Siegrist, 2016; Bonny, 2003; Lucht, 2015; Siegrist, 2008); value differences in the definition of risk (Smyth and Phillips, 2014); postmodernist philosophy critique of science (Kuntz, 2018); effects of news media sources ("information equity," Priest, 1995; also McInnerney et al., 2004; Scheufele, 2013); communication failures (Scheufele, 2013; Scholderer and Frewer, 2003); emotional effects (fear, beliefs, experiences, intuition, romantic views of agriculture Blancke et al., 2015, 2017; Hansen et al., 2003; Heilscher, 2016; Laros and Steenkamp, 2004; Marris, 2001); "motivated reasoning" and "confirmation bias" (Kunda, 1990; NRC, 2015), conditioned perceptions episodes of tragedies and damages caused by other factor wrongly related to GMO, Knox, 2000; Kuntz, 2014, 2018; Marris 2001; marketing, the remarkable ability of messages exerting a powerful influence over people and their behavior (e.g., Frankenfood, Hellsten, 2003; powerful visual rhetoric, Clancy and Clancy, 2016); NGOs advocacy (able to shape and manipulate public attitudes and sentiments, EGP, 2005, Valentinov et al., 2018); cultural (Finucane and Holup, 2005; NRC, 2015), social and political contexts (Devos et al., 2008; Pielke, 2007a,b; Sarewitz, 2015; Trewavas and Leaver, 2001); the growing business of non-GMO food (e.g., U\$S 89.7 billion organic food market in 2016, Goodwin et al, 2016, Willer and Lernoud, 2018; Bonny, 2014), and even the business of GMO-free certification (1,58 billion U\$S in 2017, Market and Market, 2018).

What emerges from this rich corpus of knowledge is that to make science and rational thinking to enter and prevail in the transgenics debate seems to be a very complex challenge, and that increasing science literacy, although needed, is not enough (Hansen et al., 2003). Further discussion involving this relevant aspect of the GMO debate is beyond the scope of the present work.

Lessons learned

On regulations

Analysis of the Argentina case has shown the pivotal role of a science-based regulatory framework for GM crops in the inception and development of agricultural biotechnology. Adoption of GM crops allowed to rapidly expand the available breeding tools to achieve beneficial traits, including some with complex genomic basis which resulted in increasing the efficiency of agricultural production.

Central in decision-making process were the risk assessment methodologies, i.e., risk hypotheses formulations based on plausible pathways presumed to result in harm, followed by rational or experimental measurement of the critical variables for their verification. While providing an adequate level of precaution, science-based regulations prepare the road to synchronic approvals between countries. The Argentina case also shows the consequences of changing this scenario: when nonscientific considerations enter in regulations, approval decisions tend to depart from predicted courses between countries, which in turn would have adverse local and trade consequences.

Consequently, science-based regulations are a key step toward harmonization, by avoiding not scientific issues to enter in decision-making processes. Harmonization not only optimizes the use of available professional and material resources but also promotes undisrupted trade avoiding barriers that can damage national economies.

On the genetically modified organism debate

Opposition to GMO resorts to a great deal of false (misleading) statements encompassing a wide array of fields. A diverse set of notorious arguments (often reinforced by clever marketing strategies) are presented as purported scientific evidence which are in fact rooted on biased and/or flawed research.

Confronted with this scenario, scientists are driven to respond with scientific, peer-reviewed arguments addressed to debunk the false statements. This is clearly necessary and consistent with one of the noblest roles of scientists in Society (quote: "One of the most noble tasks of scientists is to make out of facts public opinion." Hannah Arendt, cited in Ammann, 2004). Despite the great efforts put in this exercise, the truth hardly prevails. The assumption behind this kind of conversation, the "deficit model" (i.e., increased public understanding would lead to a rational conversation), does not seem to fit the purpose.

There is a complex underlying background: myths, public perception conditioned by emotional effects, like inner fears, beliefs, and prejudices, are subtly shaping the cognitive process into demonizing GMOs. Outrageous press releases presenting supposed "scientific" results and an efficient, pervasive written and visual rhetoric by some NGOs, all build the context for a market-quality discourse framed to shape public opinion in opposing to GMOs.

A comprehensive, inclusive, and holistic conversation including not only technical issues but also considering people's social and cultural values would be needed to shed light in this debate and fully ripe the benefits of GM technology.

References

Ahteensuu, M., 2012. Assumptions of the deficit model type of thinking: ignorance, attitudes, and science communication in the debate on genetic engineering in agriculture. Journal of Agricultural and Environmental Ethics 25, 295–313.

Ammann, K., 2004. The role of science in the application of the precautionary approach. In: Fischer, R., Schillberg, S. (Eds.), Molecular Farming, Plant-Made Pharmaceuticals and Technical Proteins, vol. 1, pp. 291–302.

Bartholomaeus, A., Batista, J.C., Burachik, M., Parrott, W., 2015. Recommendations from the workshop on comparative approaches to safety assessment of GM plant materials: a road toward harmonized criteria? GM Crops and Food 6, 69–79.

Bearth, A., Siegrist, M., 2016. Are risk or benefit perceptions more important for public acceptance of innovative food technologies: a meta-analysis. Trends in Food Science and Technology 49, 14–23.

Beker, P., Boari, P., Burachik, M., Cuadrado, V., Junco, M., Lede, S., et al., 2016. Development of a construct-based risk assessment framework for genetic engineered crops. Transgenic Research 25, 597–607.

Beringer, J.E., 1999. Cautionary tale on safety of GM crops. Nature 399 (6735), 405.

Blancke, S., Van Breusegem, F., De Jaeger, G., Braeckman, J., Van Montagu, M., 2015. Fatal attraction: the intuitive appeal of GMO opposition. Trends in Plant Science 20 (7), 414–418.

Blancke, S., Grunewald, W., De Jaeger, G., 2017. De-problematizing 'GMOs': suggestions for communicating about genetic engineering. Trends in Biotechnology 35 (3), 185–186.

Bohannon, J., 2002. Zambia rejects GM corn on scientists' advice. News of the week. Food Aid Science 298 (5596), 1153–1154.

Bonny, S., 2003. Why are most Europeans opposed to GMOs? Factors explaining rejection in France and Europe. Electronic Journal of Biotechnology 6 (1). Issue of April 15, 2003.

Bonny, S., 2014. Taking stock of the genetically modified seed sector worldwide: market, stakeholders, and prices. Food Security 4 (6), 525–540.

Burachik, M., 2012. Regulation of GM crops in Argentina. GM Crops and Food: Biotechnology in Agriculture and the Food Chain 3 (1), 48–51.

Burachik, M., 2013. The trade dispute about genetically engineered products: Argentina against the European communities. AgBioforum 16 (2), 170–176.

Cérémonie, H., Buret, F., Simonet, P., Vogel, T.M., 2006. Natural electrotransformation of lightning-competent *Pseudomonas* sp. strain N3 in artificial soil microcosms. Applied and Environmental Microbiology 72 (4), 2385–2389.

Chan, R.L., 2009. Plant transcription factors as biotechnological tools. Phyton 78, 5–10.

Chan, R.L., 2014. Plant science with relevance to biotechnology. Journal of Biotechnology 174, iv. https://doi.org/10.1016/S0168-1656(14)00098-4.

Clancy, K.A., Clancy, B., 2016. Growing monstrous organisms: the construction of anti-GMO visual rhetoric through digital media. Critical Studies in Media Communication 33 (3), 279–292.

Demanèche, S., Bertolla, F., Buret, F., Nalin, R., Sailland, A., Auriol, P., Vogel, T.M., Simonet, P., 2001. Laboratory-scale evidence for lightning-mediated gene transfer in soil. Applied and Environmental Microbiology 67 (8), 3440–3444.

Devos, Y., Maeseele, P., Reheul, D., Van Speybroeck, L., De Waele, D., 2008. Ethics in the societal debate on genetically modified organisms: a (Re)quest for sense and sensibility. Journal of Agricultural and Environmental Ethics 21 (1), 29−61.

Dunn, S.E., Vicini, J.L., Glenn, K.C., Fleischer, D.M., Greenhawt, M.J., 2017. The allergenicity of genetically modified foods from genetically engineered crops. A narrative and systematic review. Annals of Allergy, Asthma, and Immunology 119, 214−222.

EC, 1996. Commission Decision (96/281/EC) of 3 April 1996 concerning the placing on the market of genetically modified soya beans (*Glycine max* L.) with increased tolerance to the herbicide glyphosate, pursuant to Council Directive 90/220/EEC. Official Journal of the European Communities − Legislation 10−11. https://eur-lex.europa.eu/legal-content/EN/TXT/?uri=CELEX%3A31996D0281.

EFSA, 2009. Consolidated presentation of the joint scientific opinion of the GMO and BIO-HAZ panels on the "use of antibiotic resistance genes as marker genes in genetically modified plants" and the scientific opinion of the GMO panel on "consequences of the opinion on the use of antibiotic resistance genes as marker genes in genetically modified plants on previous EFSA assessments of individual GM plants". EFSA Journal 7 (6). https://doi.org/10.2903/j.efsa.2009.1108, 1108, 107 pp.

EFSA, 2015. Explanatory note on DNA sequence similarity searches in the context of the assessment of horizontal gene transfer from plants to microorganisms. European Food Safety Authority. EFSA supporting publication 2015:EN-916. 10 pp.

EFSA, Gennaro, A., Gomes, A., Herman, L., Nogue, F., Papadopoulou, N., Tebbe, C., 2017. Technical report on the explanatory note on DNA sequence similarity searches in the context of the assessment of horizontal gene transfer from plants to microorganisms. European Food Safety Authority. https://doi.org/10.2903/sp.efsa.2017.EN-1273. EFSA supporting publication 2017:EN-1273. 11 pp.

EGP, 2005. Adopted Resolution on GMO. European Green Party/EFGP. 3rd Council Meeting. Kyiv, pp. 21−23. https://europeangreens.eu/content/gmo.

European Parliament and Council, 1997. Regulation (EC) No 258/97 on novel food directive. Official Journal of the European Union L043, 1−6.

European Parliament and Council, 2003a. Regulation (EC) No 1829/2003 on genetically modified food and feed. Official Journal of the European Union L268, 1−23.

European Parliament and Council, 2003b. Regulation (EC) No 1830/2003 on traceability and labelling of genetically modified organisms and the traceability of food and feed products produced from genetically modified organisms and amending Directive 2001/18. Official Journal of the European Union L268, 24−28.

Ewen, S.W., Pusztai, A., 1999. Effect of diets containing genetically modified potatoes expressing *Galanthus nivalis* lectin on rat small intestine. The Lancet Research Letter 354 (9187), 1353−1354.

Finucane, M.L., Holup, J.L., 2005. Psychosocial and cultural factors affecting the perceived risk of genetically modified food: an overview of the literature. Social Science and Medicine 60 (7), 1603−1612.

Goodwin, B.K., Marra, M.C., Piggott, N.E., 2016. The cost of a GMO-free market basket of food in the United States. AgBioforum 19 (1), 25−33. http://www.agbioforum.org.

Gray, A., 2004. Ecology and government policies: the GM crop debate. British Ecological Society (BES) lecture. Journal of Applied Ecology 41, 1−10.

Hansen, J., Holm, L., Frewer, L., Robinson, P., Sandøe, P., 2003. Beyond the knowledge deficit: recent research into lay and expert attitudes to food risks. Appetite 41 (2), 111−121.

Hellmich, R.L., Siegfried, B.D., Sears, M.K., Stanley-Horn, D.E., Daniels, M.J., et al., 2001. Monarch larvae sensitivity to *Bacillus thuringiensis* purified proteins and pollen. Proceedings of the National Academy of Sciences of the United States of America 98 (21), 11925–11930.

Hellsten, L., 2003. Focus on metaphors: the case of "frankenfood" on the web. Journal of Computer-Mediated Communication 8 (4), 1. JCMC841. https://doi.org/10.1111/j.1083-6101.2003.tb00218.x.

Herman, R.A., 2013. Unintended compositional changes in genetically modified (GM) crops: 20 Years of research. Journal of Agricultural and Food Chemistry 61, 11695–11701.

Herman, R.A., Ladics, G.S., 2011. Endogenous allergen upregulation: transgenic vs. traditionally bred crops. Food and Chemical Toxicology 49, 2667–2669.

Hielscher, S., Pies, I., Valentinov, V., Chatalova, L., 2016. Rationalizing the GMO Debate: The Ordonomic Approach to Addressing Agricultural Myths. Int. J. Environ. Res. Public Health 13, 476. https://doi.org/10.3390/ijerph13050476.

Holt, T.A., Phillips, J., 1988. Bovine spongiform encephalopathy. British Medical Journal 296, 1581–1582.

Ioannidis, J.P.S., 2005. Why most published research findings are false. PLoS Medicine 2 (8), e124. https://doi.org/10.1371/journal.pmed.0020124.

ISAAA, 2017. Global Status of Commercialized Biotech/GM Crops in 2017: Biotech Crop Adoption Surges as Economic Benefits Accumulate in 22 Years. ISAAA Brief No. 53. ISAAA, Ithaca, NY.

Knox, B., 2000. Consumer perception and understanding of risk from food. British Medical Bulletin 56 (1), 97–109.

Kuiper, H.A., Noteborn, H.P.J.M., Peijnenburg, A.A.C.M., 1999. Adequacy of methods for testing the safety of genetically modified foods. The Lancet 354, 1315–1316.

Kuiper, H.A., Kleter, G.A., Noteborn, H.P.J.M., Kok, E.J., 2001. Assessment of the food safety issues related to genetically modified foods. The Plant Journal 27, 503–528.

Kunda, Z., 1990. The case for motivated reasoning. Psychological Bulletin 108 (3), 480–498.

Kuntz, M., 2014. The GMO case in France: politics, lawlessness and postmodernism. GM Crops and Food 5 (3), 163–169.

Kuntz, M., 2015. Is it possible to overcome the GMO controversy? Some elements for a philosophical perspective. In: Ricroch, A., Chopra, S., Fleischer, S.J. (Eds.), Plant Biotechnology: Experience and Future Prospects, pp. 107–111 (Chapter 9).

Kuntz, M., 2018. Science and postmodernism: from right-thinking to soft-despotism. Trends in Biotechnology 35 (4), 283–285. https://doi.org/10.1016/j.tibtech.2017.02.006. Epub 2017 Feb 28.

Laros, F.J.M., Steenkamp, J.-B.E.M., 2004. Importance of fear in the case of genetically modified food. Psychology and Marketing 21 (11) (Special Issue: Fear Appeals in Social Marketing Campaigns).

Losey, J.E., Rayor, L.S., Carter, M.E., 1999. Transgenic pollen harms monarch larvae. Nature (Scientific Correspondence) 399, 214.

Lucht,, J.M, 2015. Public Acceptance of Plant Biotechnology and GM Crops. Viruses 7, 4254–4281. https://doi.org/10.3390/v7082819.

MAGyP, 2013. Ministerio de Agricultura, Ganadería y Pesca. Resolución N° 318/2013. servicios.infoleg.gob.ar/infolegInternet/anexos/215000-219999/218394/norma.htm.

MAGyP, 2015. Ministerio de Agricultura, Ganadería y Pesca. Resolución 397/2015. Secretaría de Agricultura, Ganadería y Pesca. Buenos Aires, 01/10/2015.

MAGyP, 2017. Ministerio de Agricultura, Ganadería y Pesca. RESOL-2017-103-APN-SECAV#MA. Secretaría de Agricultura, Ganadería y Pesca. Buenos Aires, 07/12/2017.

Market and Market, 2018. Report FB 4219: GMO Testing Market by Trait (Stacked, Herbicide Tolerance, Insect Resistance), Technology (Polymerase Chain Reaction, Immunoassay), Crop Tested, Processed Food Tested, and Region — Global Forecast to 2022. https://www.marketsandmarkets.com/Market-Reports/genetically-modified-food-safety-testing-market-101319111.html.

McInerney, C., Bird, N., Nucci, M., 2004. The flow of scientific knowledge from lab to the lay public. The case of genetically modified food. Science Communication 26 (1), 44—74.

Marris, C., 2001. Public views on GMOs: deconstructing the myths. Stakeholders in the GMO debate often describe public opinion as irrational. But do they really understand the public? EMBO Reports 2 (7), 545—548.

Minagri, 2017. Ministerio de Agroindustria. Secretaria de Mercados Agroindustriales, Subsecretaría de Mercados Agropecuarios, pp. 51—55. Unregistered Notification dated 30/06/2017, fs.

Minagri, 2018. Ministerio de Agroindustria. RESOL-2018-33-APN-SAYBI#MA, Buenos Aires, 07/06/2018.

MPYT, 2018. Ministerio de Producción y Trabajo. Secretaría de Alimentos y Bioeconomía. Resolución 15/2018. RESOL-2018-15-APN-SAYBI#MPYT, RESOL-2017-103-APN-SECAV#MA. Buenos Aires, 12/10/2018.

Mwale, P.N., 2006. Societal deliberation on genetically modified maize in southern Africa: the debateness and publicness of the Zambian national consultation on genetically modified maize food aid in 2002. Public Understanding of Science 15, 89—102.

Mwale, P.N., 2011. The media and genetically modified organisms (GMOs): 'Talking past each other' in science debate in public: the case of Zambia. Journal of Media and Communication Studies 3 (11), 302—314.

NRC, 2015. Public Engagement on Genetically Modified Organisms: When Science and Citizens Connect: Workshop Summary. How People Think (About Genetically Modified Organisms) Roundtable on Public Interfaces of the Life Sciences; Board on Life Sciences; Division on Earth and Life Studies; Board on Science Education; Division of Behavioral and Social Sciences and Education. National Research Council. National Academies Press (US), Washington (DC). https://www.ncbi.nlm.nih.gov/books/NBK305772/.

Nielsen,, K.M, Bøhn,, T, Townsend,, J.P, 2014. Detecting rare gene transfer events in bacterial populations. Frontiers in Microbiology 4 (415).

Panda, R., Ariyarathna, H., Amnuaycheewa, P., Tetteh, A., Pramod, S.N., Taylor, S.L., Ballmer-Weber, B.K., Goodman, R.E., 2013. Challenges in testing genetically modified crops for potential increases in endogenous allergen expression for safety. Allergy 68, 142—151.

Pielke Jr., R., 2007a. When scientists politicize science. In: The Honest Broker: Making Sense of Science in Policy and Politics. Cambridge University Press, Cambridge, pp. 116—134. https://doi.org/10.1017/CBO9780511818110.008.

Pielke Jr., R., 2007b. Making sense of science in policy and politics. In: The Honest Broker: Making Sense of Science in Policy and Politics. Cambridge University Press, Cambridge, pp. 135—152. https://doi.org/10.1017/CBO9780511818110.009.

Priest, S.H., 1995. Information equity, public understanding of science, and the biotechnology debate. Journal of Communication 45 (1), 39—54.

Ricroch, A.E., Berge, J.B., Kuntz, M., 2011. Evaluation of genetically engineered crops. Plant Physiology 155, 1752—1761.

Rizzi, A., Raddadi, N., Sorlini, C., Nordgrd, L., Nielsen, K.M., Daffonchio, D., 2012. The stability and degradation of dietary DNA in the gastrointestinal tract of mammals:

implications for horizontal gene transfer and the biosafety of GMOs. Critical Reviews in Food Science and Nutrition 52 (2), 142−161. https://doi.org/10.1080/10408398.2010.499480.

SAGPyA, 1997. Argentina Secretariat of Agriculture, Livestock, Fisheries, and Food. Resolution N° 289/1997. Buenos Aires, Argentina.

Sandman, P.M., 2012. Responding to Community Outrage: Strategies for Effective Risk Communication. First published in 1993 by the American Industrial Hygiene Association. Copyright transferred to the author. In: Sandman, P.M. (Ed.). ISBN 0-932627-51-X © 2012.

Sarewitz, D., 2015. Science can't solve it (Comment). Nature 522, 414-414.

SCBD, 2000. Cartagena Protocol on Biosafety to the Convention on Biological Diversity. Secretariat of the Convention on Biological Diversity. Montreal, Canada.

Scheufele, D.A., 2013. Communicating science in social settings. Proceedings of the National Academy of Sciences of the United States of America 110 (Suppl. 3), 14040−14047.

Schlüter, K., Fütterer, J., Potrykus, I., 1995. 'Horizontal' gene transfer from a transgenic potato line to a bacterial pathogen (*Erwinia chrysanthemi*) occurs − if at all − at an extremely low frequency. BioTechnologia 13, 1094−1098.

Scholderer, J., Frewer, L.J., 2003. The biotechnology communication paradox: experimental evidence and the need for a new strategy. Journal of Consumer Policy 26, 125−157.

SENASA, 2015. Servicio Nacional de Sanidad y Calidad Agroalimentaria. Dirección de Calidad Agroalimentaria. Coordinación de Biotecnología y Productos Industrializados. Documento De Decisión. Evaluación de la aptitud alimentaria del evento de soja IND-410-5 (OECD: IND-41Ø-5). 07/10/2015.

SENASA, 2016. Servicio Nacional de Sanidad y Calidad Agroalimentaria. Dirección de Calidad Agroalimentaria. Coordinación de Biotecnología y Productos Industrializados. Documento De Decisión. CTAUGMO, 17/03/2016.

Shelton, A.M., Roush, R.T., 1999. False reports and the ears of men. Nature Biotechnology 17, 832. http://biotech.nature.com.

Siegrist, M., 2008. Factors influencing public acceptance of innovative food technologies and products. Trends in Food Science and Technology 19 (11), 603−660.

Smyth, S.J., 2017. Genetically modified crops, regulatory delays, and international trade. Food and Energy Security 6 (2), 78−86.

Smyth, S.J., Phillips, P.W.B., 2014. Risk, regulation and biotechnology: the case of GM crops. GM Crops and Food 5 (3), 170−177. https://doi.org/10.4161/21645698.2014.945880.

Trewavas, A.J., Leaver, C.J., 2001. Is opposition to GM crops science or Politics? An investigation into the arguments that GM crops pose a particular threat to the environment. EMBO Reports 2 (6), 455−459.

Trigo, E., Cap, E., Malach, V., Villarreal, F., 2009. Innovating in the pampas: zero-tillage soybean cultivation in Argentina. In: Spielman, D.J., Pandya-Lorch, Rajul (Eds.), Millions Fed: Proven Successes in Agricultural Development. International Food Policy Research Institute (IFPRI), Washington, D.C, pp. 59−64. Chatepr 8. http://ebrary.ifpri.org/cdm/ref/collection/p15738coll2/id/130818.

UNEP (United Nations Environment Programme), 1992. Rio Declaration on Environment and Development. The United Nations Conferece on Environment and Development, Rio de Janeiro, Brazil. https://www.jus.uio.no/lm/environmental.development.rio.declaration.1992/portrait.a4.pdf.

van den Eede, G., Aarts, H., Buhk, H.-J., Corthier, G., Flint, H.J.., Hammes, W., Jacobsen, B., Midtvedt, T., van der Vossen, J., von Wright, A., Wackernagel, W., Wilcks, A., 2004. The relevance of gene transfer to the safety of food and feed derived from genetically modified (GM) plants. Food and Chem.Toxicol 42, 1127−1156.

Valentinov, V., Hielscher, S., Everding, S., Pies, I., 2018. The anti-GMO advocacy: an institutionalist and systems-theoretic assessment. Kybernetes. https://doi.org/10.1108/.K-01-2018-0016.

Willer, H., Lernoud, J., 2018. The World of Organic Agriculture. Statistics and Emerging Trends 2018. Research Institute of Organic Agriculture FIBL − IFOAM Organics International. https://www.organic-world.net/yearbook/yearbook-2018.html.

Wolt, J.D., Keese, P., Raybould, A., Fitzpatrick, J.W., Burachik, M., Gray, A., et al., 2010. Problem formulation in the environmental risk assessment for genetically modified plants. Transgenic Research 19, 425−436.

Controversial issues: Brazil case studies

6.5

Andre Nepomuceno Dusi, PhD, Virology [1],
Deise Maria Fontana Capalbo, Bs, MSc, PhD, Food Engineering [2],
Josias Correa de Faria, PhD, Plant Pathology [3]

[1]*Ministry of Agriculture, Livestock and Food Supply, Esplanada dos Ministérios, Brasília, DF, Brazil;* [2]*Embrapa Environment, Jaguariúna, SP, Brazil;* [3]*Embrapa Rice and Beans, Santo Antonio de Goiás, GO, Brazil*

Introduction

Not many years ago, there had been an extensive attempt worldwide to meet a range of economic, environmental, and social challenges of the 21st century. Technological solutions to such problems played a key role in these prognostics. Narratives conflating "knowledge-based" actions, technological advance with societal progress prospered (Delvenne and Hendrickx, 2013). In this respect, the issue "biotechnology" and its enlarged international regime of intellectual property rights surfaced, carrying with it topics related to food safety, healthcare, and environmental aspects.

Exploring some facts and perceptions of these topics related to the safety of genetically modified (GM) organisms (usually named as GMOs) is one objective of this chapter. It requires looking both at regulatory scenarios, the role of private and public research sectors, and a wide range of challenges such as building broad societal support to avoid undervalue of these components. To avoid narrow perspectives, the controversy in this scenario of uncertainties had to be addressed.

Current developments indicate that Brazil is the second player in the global production of GM crops (ISAAA, 2016). This is why the other main objective of this chapter is to focus on one GM staple food crop, developed by a public corporation, which passed the challenge of facing the pertinent regulatory system to obtain an approval for commercial release. Some aspects of its own controversy are also presented.

Anatomy of the controversy

Genetic modification of crops provides a methodology for the agricultural improvement needed to deliver global food security (EASAC, 2013); it is not the only one and it depends on integration with good husbandry practices, nevertheless there is scientific consensus that GM technology is efficient and sustainable (CIB-Agroconsult, 2018; Delaney et al., 2018; Pellegrino et al., 2018; Society of Toxicology, 2017)

Focusing on recent releases in Brazil, this chapter shows how specific legitimizing rhetoric downplays technical uncertainties while emphasizing the societal benefits and national prestige of adopting this innovative technology (Delvenne and Hendrickx, 2013).

Development of Brazilian legislation and the controversy

In Brazil, GMOs are regulated by Biosafety Law (No.11.105/2005)[a]. This Law put an end to the dispute surrounding GMOs in the country, caused by a conflict between the previous Biosafety Law (No. 8974/1995) and the Environmental Law. Surprisingly, the major questioning was not the safety of the event but which instance had the competence to authorize the commercial release. As a result of this controversy, from 1995 to 2004, only three GMOs were approved in Brazil (an herbicide-tolerant soybean and two vaccines). The passing of the new Law granted the National Technical Biosafety Committee (CTNBio) the legitimacy it needed to perform technical analysis and make available innovations that have benefited Brazilian agriculture, healthcare, energy, and several other sectors. Therefore, in the next decade, from 2005 to 2014, 62 GMOs were approved, regarding 38 plants, 18 vaccines, 5 microorganisms, and 1 insect.

The described picture reflects the politicization of the developing process of such technology in the country. It was characterized by an extreme social aversion to risk translated to social demands for public policies to reduce risks. Thus, the regulation of the GM technologies in Brazil reflects the huge weight that social perception of risks had on its establishment.

Another side effect of this politicization was the loss of the opportunity to develop a broad environmental impact study of the first cropping of Roundup Ready soy (RR-soy) in the country: RR-soy was smuggled and grown much before it was definitively authorized in 2005 when several thousands of hectares were already being grown. During this politicized debate, some risk control policies were adopted without any evidence that the alleged risks in fact existed (Arantes et al., 2011). The details of the conflict will not be discussed in this chapter.

During the last two decades, CTNBio could develop, modernize, and propose the best possible scientific criteria to perform its duties. The accumulated learning in 20 years (including the first GM bean and GM mosquito of the world) coupled with the capacity build from the exchange with mature international biosafety legislations, led to an even more efficient process. From 2015 on, with the approvals of new regulations, the rhythm of analysis increased preserving a rigorous scientific

---

[a] details at http://ctnbio.mcti.gov.br/inicio.

approach. Between 2015 and 2018, that is only 4 years, 82 GMOs were approved by the Committee (more than 40 plants, 18 vaccines, 17 microorganisms, and 1 medicine). Among these, it is worth mentioning the first GM eucalyptus (2015) and the first GM sugarcane (2017) of the world. An updated list of commercial GM plants can be obtained at http://ctnbio.mcti.gov.br/inicio.

Additionally, in 2018, CTNBio approved a new normative regarding gene editing: biosafety system deals with evolving concepts and technologies and CTNBio have been working on the adjustment of its procedures and requirements to remain functional.

Until 2018,[b] 79 GM plant cultivars were authorized to be grown in Brazil, mainly commodities as maize (44), cotton (16), and soy (16). Beans (1), eucalyptus (1), and sugarcane (1) recently joined the restricted group of GM species with authorization to be grown in the country. The main characteristics are herbicide tolerance and insect resistance, single or stacked genes. There is only one virus-resistant event (bean) and one wood volumetric increase event (eucalyptus).

Research impact on GM development in Brazil: private and public contributions

GM plants are mainly developed by the private sector in Brazil: they were responsible for 77 GM-approved plant events until 2018, while public sector has one (bean) or shares the property with a private company (e.g., Embrapa—Brazilian Agriculture Research Cooperation—and BASF for the soybean "Cultivance"). On the other side, public institutions play a key role in the biosafety risk assessment process due to its importance on the development of food and environmental biosafety protocols and capacitation of personal to act in this area, besides the influence on public perception that will be discussed later in this chapter.

Embrapa, a public company, has played a major role in the development of GM plants process. In 2002, Embrapa organized the "Biosafety Network: GMO—BioSeg" to produce food, feed, and environmental risk analysis protocols, as well as to produce lacking scientific information necessary for the deregulation of Embrapa's GM plants under development at that time. The network gathered professionals and students from Embrapa, Universities, and other institutes.

The five species developed or studied at Embrapa (used as models) were RR-soy, Bt cotton, *Papaya ringspot virus* (PRSV)-resistant papaya, *Potato virus Y* (PVY)-resistant potato, and *Bean golden mosaic virus* (BGMV)-resistant bean. All were chosen mainly due to the lack of scientific information (at the time) and the need to have evaluation protocols scientifically designed to offer for decision-making and to present to the public trustable study standards as they were developed by a respected public institution (Arantes et al., 2011).

---

[b] www.ctnbio.gov.br acessed on January 2019.

Embrapa Biosafety Network: GMO—BioSeg developed the necessary studies to meet the regulatory requests of CTNBio (food, feed, and environmental safety requests), as well as it identified the needs of capacity building of the network members and other sectors. In this context, between 2003 and 2008, three 40 h courses were held for a total of 80 researchers. Also, 25 officials of the Ministry of Agriculture, Livestock and Food Supply were trained to best perform the auditing and inspection processes under their responsibility. At last, a 40 h discipline for MSc and PhD students of Federal University of Viçosa was held.

The BioSeg project ended in 2008, but several of its members and trainees continue working in the area and some also collaborated with CTNBio.

Public perception

GM organisms (crops, insects, microorganism) have been extremely contentious in scientific, public, or policy realms. While this is a global phenomenon (Delvenne and Hendrickx, 2013), there have been significant regional differences or different framings and controversy across Latin America.

Some attitudinal surveys have been conducted across Europe between 1990 and 2010 (Mallison et al., 2018) with varied focused topics like personal acceptance, benefit and risk, knowledge of GM Science, general attitude to science, and trust governance.

In Brazil, public opinion on GMOs was surveyed in several studies as reviewed by Arantes et al. (2011). Furnival and Pinheiro (2008) showed in a work with focus groups that, with rare exceptions, people are not aware of what GMOs are, but they have shown distrust of the "second intentions" in the "defense" of the GMO—the public understands that where there is smoke (controversy) there is fire (bad intentions). There were also experiences of dissemination and scientific communication in the area of genetics, such as Labjor (at University of Campinas) projects[c] and the "Museu da vida" (Museum of Life, in English)[d] developed by Fiocruz[e] a foundation under the Brazilian Ministry of Health.

More recently, Arantes et al. (2011) and Capalbo et al. (2015), using two different approaches on the same raw data, set up the view of Brazilian stakeholders on GMOs and the implications of these views on communication strategies for agricultural biotechnology in Brazil. In Capalbo et al. (2015), they highlighted how information sources, trust in institutions, and socioeconomic characteristics (such as age and occupational qualifications) play important roles in defining patterns of attitudes toward GMOs. In Arantes et al. (2011), they pointed out that respondents hear about GMOs and biosafety through the media (TV, radio, magazines, etc.), although they rely less on these means. Information is considered more reliable

---

[c] http://www.labjor.unicamp.br/?status_projeto=projetos-concluidos.
[d] http://www.museudavida.fiocruz.br/.
[e] https://portal.fiocruz.br/en.

when supplied by scientists and experts. This attitude could be explained by the process of people's knowledge acquisition: it depends on trust and confidence they have in the source of information (Costa-Font et al., 2008). The results obtained are also in agreement with data from other studies, such as Vogt and Polino (2003) where they found elevated levels of confidence in Brazilian science and scientists. Another more recent study developed through online survey,[f] conducted in 18 countries, including Brazil, also indicated that the credibility of science and scientists tends to be high.

A very broad study developed for the Brazilian scenario and attitudes in 2018 (CIB/Agroconsult), available in Portuguese, shows social and economic benefits, environmental, and food safety of the approved products.

As indicated by Capalbo et al. (2015), GMOs for food production are in the spotlight, meaning that it is the main source of disagreement among respondents, as opposed to biotechnology in general. The groups with positive attitudes toward biotechnology, primarily that of transgenic crops, are predominantly composed of males, senior citizens, and individuals who trust in experts as sources of information, even regarding biosafety. By contrast, the groups of respondents with negative attitudes toward GM crops tend to be young people who are under the age of 25, particularly students. These groups primarily consist of individuals who rely on nongovernmental organizations (NGOs) as an information source about GMOs and biotechnology. Since many of the members of these latter groups are unfamiliar with the use of GMOs, communication on the subject is targeted at these members to improve the level of knowledge on GMOs in Brazil.

Public perception and the GM bean case study

Brazil is one of the largest growers and consumers of common beans (*Phaseolus vulgaris*) with a total yield of 2.6 million metric tons on 1.7 million hectares in 2017 (Conab, 2019). Common beans are a well-known source of protein, carbohydrates, and micronutrients for millions of people, considering Brazil and other tropical areas worldwide.[g] The simple way of preparation and excellent nutritional qualities associated to social aspects make common bean an important diet component, especially for those families dependent on agriculture for their living, such as in Africa and in Latin America countries (Broughton et al., 2003).

The Brazilian per capita consumption is around 17 kg/year. From 1985 until 2017, there was a reduction in growing area of common bean, with an increase in total yield due to strong research programs. On the other hand, since the 1970s, the incidence of BGMV has probably been the most devastating viral disease of common beans, especially in the second growing season, defined at Faria et al.

---

[f] Available at http://www.revistapesquisa.fapesp.br/index.php?art=6744&bd=2 &pg=1&lg.

[g] http://www.cgiar.org/our-strategy/crop-factsheets/beans/.

(2016). The effect of this disease, alone, may account for the importation needs of the country.

Breeding for disease resistance using traditional techniques is difficult. Also, chemical control of the vector, the whitefly *Bemisia tabaci* is inefficient, due to the whitefly's transmission ability. Considering this, a GM bean program for resistance to BGMV began in early 1990 after the molecular characterization of the virus (Gilbertson et al., 1993; Faria and Maxwell, 1999) and the development of a genetic transformation system of *Phaseolus vulgaris* (a recalcitrant species to manipulate via genetic engineering) (Aragão et al., 1996).

Due to public opposition to transgenic technology in that period, it was realized that, to be successful, a GMO bean needed to be completely absent of disease symptoms. So, in 2004, the concept of RNA interference (RNAi) to silence the *rep* viral gene was explored (Bonfim et al., 2007). Homozygous plants generated and tested showed 100% immunity under field conditions, while nontransgenic plants showed severe symptoms characteristic of golden mosaic disease (Aragão and Faria, 2009).

In March 2008, an unprecedented experiment took place under the coordination of a group of scientists from University of Santa Catarina and Embrapa. The study aimed at detecting the stakeholders' feelings regarding the eminence of a deregulation of a GM staple food. The consultation model was formatted as a 2-day workshop, in a neutral environment (unrelated to technology), coordinated by a professional mediator, with the presence of stakeholders: small, medium, and large bean producers; consumers (households organization); the sectors of the food industry, including the processing and marketing areas; the business sector in biotechnology, including the product and seed development industries; environmental nongovernmental organizations (NGOs), consumer advocacy; and the promotion of biotechnology.

The stakeholders selected were not spokespersons for social organizations or government sectors. The results, presented in Guivant et al. (2009a,b), showed, among other points, that:

- From the consumer perspective, concerns were identified about the supply, price, and appearance of the product. Environmental concerns were only mentioned by one critical representative to transgenics. More weight was given to price in decision scale.
- It was practically consensus that any health or environmental risk is greater in regard to the application of agrochemicals than to the transgenic use.
- Also a consensus pointed significant advantages in favor to the GM bean, at least in the short term, in reducing the use of pesticides, protecting the health of rural producers and reducing the cost of production.
- There is credibility and trust in the scientific criteria that underlie the Biosafety Law and CTNBio's actions.
- Embrapa has a positive image as a public institution, free from bias in the results of its research.

The field and laboratory studies continued to be developed. The transgenic line Embrapa 5.1 biosafety analysis was carried out by the Biosafety Network of Embrapa. All risk assessment data demonstrated no differences between transgenic lines and parental plants. Line Embrapa 5.1 was considered safe for the environment and human consumption (Aragão and Faria, 2010; Aragão et al., 2013; Carvalho et al., 2015; Faria et al., 2014), and in 2011, CTNBio approved this line for cultivation and human consumption in Brazil[h].

Results from 31 locations (from West-Central Brazil to the South) after 2012 confirmed that no grain yield or commercial grain quality penalties have been observed when the transgenic lines were compared with their respective recurrent parents, and the lines maintained their resistance to BGMV across all tested field conditions and years. The transgenic common bean line, with superior agronomic performance in the field trials, was selected and registered as cultivar BRS FC401 RMD, becoming the first transgenic common bean cultivar in the world (Souza et al., 2018).

Controversy on commercialization of GM bean

The controversy of commercializing a transgenic common bean, harboring an important trait, seems like an insurmountable problem so far. The GM line registered and protected by the Brazilian Ministry of Agriculture, Livestock and Food Supply,[i] although ready for commercialization, is not in the market because Embrapa's directive board was considering the best timing for its release.

In one of the Embrapa's directive board meeting in March of 2019, it was decided to start the process of producing seeds for commercialization to the growers interested. This means that in 2020 the bean cultivar named BRS FC401 RMD will be in the market for consumers.

Final remarks

GM technologies for the control of viruses in common beans in Brazil is an example of a public research GM plant developed that succeed in gathering its commercial release approval in the country. Although immunity to BGMV has been demonstrated in GM bean, other whitefly-transmitted viruses must be addressed. So, GM technology proved to be a good option, but it should be used in a context of good pest control practices directed by the principles of Integrated Pest Management (IPM), which must take into consideration the integration of all available pest control methods that are socially and economically acceptable. Consequently, the

---

[h] http://ctnbio.mcti.gov.br/liberacao-comercial#/liberacao-comercial/consultar-processo.
[i] under the name BRS FC401 RMD, number 34432, on Sept. 14, 2015, and placed under protection on Jan. 15, 2016 under the number 20160006.

management of whiteflies continues to be extremely important, even if its population is below the economically damaging levels of insect damage (Anderson et al., 2019).

We tried to present in this chapter the various aspects that made the scenario of controversies about GMOs in Brazil and focused on the descriptions of the most important aspects during the development of a staple food—the bean—by a public institution—Embrapa. Certainly other points could be reported, but we are sure that the panel presented demonstrates how much still needs to be internalized in teaching and research institutions so that new products (not just GMOs) can quickly reach the market with safety assurance.

If confidence is an indicator of social health, whether trust should be preserved by the institutions, and if the public points to the scientist is the greatest depository of his trust about biosafety of the transgenic plants (as they did in Brazilian studies indicated in this chapter), then the researchers of public institutions should take on such responsibility to dialog on the subject. Moreover, the importance that people place on scientists suggests that there is a need for a sound strategy of communication that combines media resources with scientifically qualified and accessible knowledge to ensure trust and confidence. This highlights the responsibility of representatives of public institutions involved in GMOs research in Brazil that are numerous and important; they have the obligation to be part of the process and bear responsibility for the confidence of the population in their institutions, supporting research, and innovation effectively.

These institutions also have an important function as source of scientific information, and policy makers should ensure the dissemination of this knowledge and to frame it within their regulations.

The most appropriate communication strategy should be developed based on the public's perception and its needs.

References

Arantes, O.M.N., Silveira, J. M. F. J. da, Borges, I.C., Capalbo, D.M.F., Schneider, D.R.S., Gattaz, N.C., Lima, E. de S., 2011. Desenvolvimento de comunicação estratégica sobre biossegurança de plantas geneticamente modificadas — o caso do projeto LAC Biosafety no Brasil. Jaguariúna: Embrapa Meio Ambiente, 33 pp. (Embrapa Meio Ambiente. Documentos, 85), See http://www.cnpma.embrapa.br/download/documentos_85.pdf.

Anderson, J.A., Ellsworth, P.C., Faria, J.C., Head, G.P., Owen, M.D.K., Pilcher, C.D., Shelton, A.M., Michael Meissle, M., 2019. Genetically engineered crops: importance of diversified integrated pest management for agricultural sustainability. Frontiers in Bioengineering and Biotechnology. https://doi.org/10.3389/fbioe.2019.00024.

Aragão, F.J.L., Barros, L.M.G., Brasileiro, A.C.M., Ribeiro, S.G., Smith, F.D., Sanford, J.C., Faria, J.C., Rech, E.L., 1996. Inheritance of foreign genes in transgenic bean (*Phaseolus vulgaris*) co-transformed via particle bombardment. Theoretical and Applied Genetics 93, 142—150.

Aragão, F.J.L., Faria, J.C., 2009. First transgenic geminivirus-resistant plant in the field. Nature Biotechnology 27, 1086—1088.

Aragão, F.J.L., Nogueira, E.O.P.E.L., Tinoco, M.L.P., Faria, J.C., 2013. Molecular characterization of the first commercial transgenic common bean immune to the Bean golden mosaic virus. Journal of Biotechnology 166, 42−50.

Aragão, F.J.L., Faria, J.C., 2010. Proposta de liberação comercial de feijoeiro geneticamente modificado resistente ao mosaico dourado − Evento Embrapa 5.1 (EMB-PV051-1), CTNBio. http://ctnbio.mcti.gov.br/liberacao-comercial#/liberacao-comercial/consultar-processo.

Bonfim, K., Faria, J.C., Nogueira, E.O.P.L., Mendes, E.A., Aragão, F.J.L., 2007. RNAi-mediated resistance to bean golden mosaic virus in genetically engineered common bean (*Phaseolus vulgaris*). Molecular Plant-Microbe Interactions.

Broughton, W.J., Hernández, G., Blair, M., Beeb, S., Gepts, P., Vanderleyden, J., 2003. Beans (*Phaseolus* spp.) − model food legumes. Plant and Soil 252, 55−128.

Capalbo, D.M.F., Arantes, O.M.N., Maia, A.G., Borges, I.C., Silveira, J. M. F. J. da, 2015. A study of stakeholder views to shape a communication strategy for GMO in Brazil. Frontiers in Bioengineering and Biotechnology 3. Article 179. 10 pp.

Carvalho, J.L.V., Santos, J.O., Conte, C., Pacheco, S., Nogueira, E.O.P.E.L., Souza, T.L.P.O., Faria, J.C., Aragão, F.J.L., 2015. Comparative analysis of nutritional compositions of transgenic RNAi-mediated virus-resistant bean (event EMB-PV051-1) with its nontransgenic counterpart. Transgenic Research 24, 813−819.

CIB − Agroconsult, 2018. 20 anos de transgênicos: benefícios ambientais, econômicos e sociais. Available at: https://cib.org.br/20-anos-de-transgenicos/.

Conab, 2019. Acompanhamento da safra brasileira: grãos, pp. 1−127. Available at: http://www.conab.gov.br/conteudos.php?a=1253&t=2.

Costa-Font, M., Gil, J.M., Traill, W.B., 2008. Consumer acceptance, valuation of and attitudes towards genetically modified food: review and implications for food policy. Food Policy 33 (2), 99−111.

Delaney, B., Goodman, R.E., Ladics, G.S., 2018. Food and feed safety of genetically engineered food crops. Toxicological Sciences 162 (2), 361−371. https://doi.org/10.1093/toxsci/kfx249.

Delvenne, P., Hendrickx, K., 2013. The multifaceted struggle for power in the bioeconomy: introduction to the special issue. Technology in Society 35 (2), 75−78.

EASAC − European Academies Science Advisory Council, 2013. Planting the Future: Opportunities and Challenges for Using Crop Genetic Improvement Techonologies for Sustainable Agriculture. EASAC Policy report 21.

Faria, J.C., Maxwell, D.P., 1999. Variability in geminivirus isolates associated with *Phaseolus* spp. in Brazil. Phytopathology 89, 262−268.

Faria, J.C., Valdisser, P.A.M.R., Nogueira, E.O.P.L., Aragão, F.J.L., 2014. RNAi-based Bean golden mosaic virus-resistant common bean (Embrapa 5.1) shows simple inheritance for both transgene and disease resistance. Plant Breeding 133, 649−653.

Faria, J.C., Aragão, F.J.L., Souza, T.L.P.O., Quintela, E.D., Kitajima, E.W., Ribeiro, S.G., 2016. Golden mosaic of common beans in Brazil: management with a transgenic approach. APS Features. https://doi.org/10.1094/APSFeature-2016-10.

Furnival, A., Pinheiro, S., 2008. A percepção publica da informação sobre os potenciais riscos dos transgênicos na cadeia alimentar. História, Ciências, Saúde-Manguinhos 15, 277−291.

Gilbertson, R.L., Faria, J.C., Ahlquist, P., Maxwell, D.P., 1993. Genetic diversity in geminiviruses causing bean golden mosaic disease: the nucleotide-sequence of the infectious cloned DNA components of a Brazilian isolate of bean golden mosaic geminivirus. Phytopathology 83, 709—715.

Guivant, J., Capalbo, D.M.F., Dusi, A.N., Fontes, E., Pires, C.S.S., 2009a. Acima dos confrontos sobre os transgênicos: uma experiência piloto de consulta pública. Cadernos de Ciência and Tecnologia 26 (1/3), 11—37.

Guivant, J., Capalbo, D.M.F., Dusi, A.N., Fontes, E., Pires, C.S.S., Wander, A.E., 2009b. Uma experiência de consulta a setores de interesse no caso do feijão transgênico. In: Biossegurança de OGM: uma visão integrada, Organizers: Marco Antonio F. da Costa, Maria de Fátima Barrozo da Costa, vol. I. Publit, Rio de Janeiro, pp. 158—189. ISBN: 978-85-7773-187-9.

ISAAA, 2016. Global Status of Commercialized Biotech/GM Crops: 2016. ISAAA Brief No. 52. ISAAA, Ithaca, NY.

Mallison, L., Russell, J., Cameron, D.D., Ton, J., Horton, P., Barker, M.E., 2018. Why rational arguments fails the genetic modification (GM) debate. Food Security 10, 1145—1161. https://doi.org/10.1007/s12571-018-0832-1.

Pellegrino, E., Bedini, S., Nuti, M., Ercoli, L., 2018. Impact of genetically engineered maize on agronomic, environmental and toxicological traits: a meta-analysis of 21 years of field data. Scientific Reports 8, 3113. https://doi.org/10.1038/s41598-018-21284-2 12.

Society of Toxicology, Issue Statement, 2017. Food and Feed Safety of Genetically Engineered Food Crops, Approved by SOT Council. Available at: https://www.toxicology.org/pubs/statements/SOT_Safety_of_GE_Food_Crops_Issue_Statement_FINAL.pdf.

Souza, T.L.P.O., Faria, J.C., Aragão, F.J.L., Del Peloso, M.J., Faria, L.C., Wendland, A., Aguiar, M.S., Quintela, E.D., Melo, C.L.P., Hungria, M., Vianello, R.P., Pereira, H.S., melo, L.C., 2018. Agronomic performance and yield stability of the RNA interference-based *Bean golden mosaic virus*-resistant common bean. Crop Science 58, 1—13. https://doi.org/10.2135/cropsci2017.06.0355.

Vogt, C., Polino, C., 2003. Percepção pública da ciência. Editora Unicamp, Campinas.

GM crops and conventional or organic agriculture coexistence in EU regulation

Luc Bodiguel

Director of Research, National Center of Scientific Research (CNRS), UMR 6297 "Droit et Changement Social" (Law and Social Change) Associated Professor, Faculty of Law of Nantes and IHEDREA (Paris), France

From coexistence to GM definition

Coexisting means living together, one with or next to the other. It is directly related to freedom. Freedom to live differently, to make a different choice, as, for example, to cultivate organic, conventional, or genetically modified (GM) crops. That is exactly what the European Commission said in the "2003 Recommendation on guidelines for the development of national strategies and best practices to ensure the co-existence of genetically modified crops with conventional and organic farming" (Commission Recommendation, 2003) (1) No form of agriculture, be it conventional, organic, or agriculture using genetically modified organisms (GMOs), should be excluded in the European Union. (2) The ability to maintain different agricultural production systems is a prerequisite for providing a high degree of consumer choice. (3) Co-existence refers to the ability of farmers to make a practical choice between conventional, organic, and GM-crop production, in compliance with the legal obligations for labeling and/or purity standards. "Even if this recommendation is now removed, it is still the spirit of the European Union (EU) Legislator as said by Recommendation 2010: "(3) It may be necessary for Member States' public authorities to define, in the areas where GMOs are cultivated, appropriate measures to allow consumers and producers a choice between conventional, organic and GM production (hereinafter referred to as 'co-existence measures')".

But freedom is a difficult fellow because it supposes that you have to respect the freedom of the others with whom you have to coexist, a fact that people often find difficult to accept. For crops, it is the same. As written, "'Coexistence' implies two or more things existing in the same place at the same time; and in an ideal world, coexistence should be regarded as essentially 'passive.' It is difficult to argue that this can be achieved when one thing prejudices the viability of another; and inevitably the question arises whether the simultaneous growing of genetically modified

Genetically Modified and Irradiated Food. https://doi.org/10.1016/B978-0-12-817240-7.00011-5

(GM), conventional, and organic crops can satisfy such a definition" (Bodiguel et al., 2010). In other words, crop freedom is just a principle, a legal fiction, "in the sense that it supposedly offers farmers an unfettered choice on the form of agriculture that they wish to adopt, free from interference from other forms of agriculture" (Bodiguel et al., 2010). Numerous scientific reports and policy documents have already shown that the simultaneous growing of genetically modified (GM), conventional, and organic crops can stay together in the same place at the same time with no negative interactions between them, particularly cross-contamination and subsequent standardization of seeds and plants (INRA, 2006; GM Science Review Panel, 2003; Assemblée Nationale Française, 2005; Messean, 2006).

This principle has to be relativized considering EU Law. Firstly because the legal definition of Organic Agriculture is clearly incompatible with GM: "Organic production is a sustainable management system that [required] (…) an appropriate design and management of biological processes, based on ecological systems and using natural resources that are internal to the management system, using methods that (…) exclude the use of GMOs, products produced from GMOs, and products produced by GMOs, other than veterinary medicinal products" (Regulation, 2018/848). Secondly, conventional agriculture is also indirectly incompatible with GM crops because of EU GM labeling rules. If there are traces of authorized GMOs in proportions higher than 0.9% (or even lower national thresholds), even if these traces are adventitious or technically unavoidable, you have no more conventional product but a GM product and you have to sell it in accordance with the GM Regulation (Directive, 2001/18/EC). Thus, in other words, the EU GM crops Regulation is based on the fact that neutral coexistence is impossible.

That is why most of the seed industry tries to escape from the GM definition.

A GMO is defined by EU Directive 2011/18/EC as "an organism, with the exception of human beings, in which the genetic material has been altered in a way that does not occur naturally by mating and/or natural recombination" (art. 2.2). The fact that transgenesis cannot be born from a natural process is the fundamental criterion. The definition is completed by a list of techniques that result (or not) in genetic modification (art. 2-2a and 2b.) and by a list of methods and techniques that are excluded from the application of Directive 2001/18/EC such as mutagenesis (art 3 and annex I B).

That is the point that has been discussed lately, with emergence and multiplication of new plant breeding techniques (NPBTs) that according to the seed industry belongs to mutagenesis. The seed industry has developed various new techniques targeted at changes in the genome or exploiting the epigenetic mechanisms and certain specific processes related to the use of genetic modification techniques. These techniques make it possible to extinguish genes, activate them, mutate them, and replicate them, thus offering new modalities of genome modification. As underlined by French experts from the High Council of Biotechnology (HCB) in 2017, "Molecular targeting of genetic modifications in the genome (…), traits likely to be finally obtained being of comparable nature" (HCB, Scientific Committee Advise, 2017a), but techniques and organisms obtained by mutagenesis are very diverse, "Some of them can be traced and identified, sometimes as GMOs, others—perhaps the majority—remaining unrecognizable" (HCB, Economic, Ethic and Social Committee Recommendation, 2017b).

Considering that some of the most recently developed techniques present risks for health and the environment, several French organizations (Confédération paysanne, Réseau Semences Paysannes …) asked the French Prime Minister and Agricultural Ministry to "revoke the national legislation according to which organisms obtained by mutagenesis are not, in principle, considered to result in genetic modification, and the refusal to ban the cultivation and marketing of herbicide-tolerant rape varieties obtained by mutagenesis." As the Government refused, they went on trial until the high administrative court of the State Council (Conseil d'Etat) that decided to request to the European Court of Justice (ECJ) for a preliminary ruling (interpretation and validity of Articles 2 and 3 of; and the Annexes I A and I B to, Directive, 2001/18/EC, as well as the interpretation of Article 4 of Council Directive, 2002/53/EC of 13 June 2002 on the common catalog of varieties of agricultural plant species). The European Court delivered its judgment on 25 July 2018 (ECJ, 25 July 2018, Case C-528/16, Confédération Paysanne).

After the decision, a press release of the ECJ was titled: "Organisms obtained by mutagenesis are GMOs and are in principle subject to the obligations laid down by the GMO Directive" (ECJ Press Release No 111/18, Luxembourg, 25 July 2018). In Law, however, the solution is neither so simple nor so radical, as some commentators (Brosset and Hermon 2018) had already anticipated when the Advocate General's Opinion was published (ECJ, Opinion of Advocate General Bobek, 18 January 2018). Three alternatives were on the judges' table. The first defended the idea that all mutagenized organisms have to be authorized in respect to Directive 2001/18/EC. The second considered that organisms resulting from mutagenesis techniques born before this Directive should be exempted from authorization and that only the new processes have to be submitted to it; finally, the third solution, promoted by the Advocate General, was based on the sole criterion of the techniques employed (exemption only if the mutagenesis techniques do not involve the use of recombinant nucleic acid or GMOs other than those resulting from mutagenesis).

The ECJ opted for the second approach, with an analysis a contrario of recital 17 of the directive: as "This Directive should not apply to organisms obtained through certain techniques of genetic modification which have conventionally been used in a number of applications and have a long safety record," all the organisms obtained through certain techniques of genetic modification, in particular those "obtained by means of techniques/methods of mutagenesis," which have not conventionally been used in a number of applications and have not a long safety record, have to be considered as GMOs because they meet the definition of GMOs within the meaning of Article 2(2) of Directive 2001/18/EC (Judgment, §30).

This solution has the merit of taking into consideration the evolution of scientific knowledge and techniques. However, it remains a source of uncertainty. On one hand, it is simple only in appearance because the term "mutagenesis" brings together very disparate techniques and the solution offered by the EU judges opens the door to a case-by-case analysis. On the other hand, the distinctions between new and old techniques may hold surprises, as we have already seen with the Novel Food Regulation. It should also be noted that the Court has not really decided the question of what is or is not a "technique/method that modifies the genetic material of an organism in a way that does not occur naturally" Finally, the "old mutagenesis" organisms could be the subject of special legal regimes, different in different EU countries, since the ECJ has confirmed their competence subject to respect of EU law.

More specifically, this solution impact directly our topic because even crops from mutagenesis will have to respect authorization, control, and obviously coexistence rules according to Directive 2001/18.

From GM crops regulation to coexistence measures

Discussion about genetically modified (GM) crops and conventional agriculture coexistence requires understanding of the legal structure of European Union (EU) Regulation in this matter. Directive 2001/18/EC is the main legal pillar.

Based on a precautionary and science-based approach (Bodiguel and Di Lauro, 2016), it distinguishes two different but related uses of GMOs: deliberate release (cultivation for the main) and placing on the market (products circulation for trade). Our theme has only concerns about deliberate release because it focusses on crops as vegetal products used for agriculture and not on trade or on food or feed. That is why there will be no development on labeling of products, that guarantee that GM crops can be sold without causing confusion in the mind of professionals or consumers (art. 21 Labeling; art. 22 Free circulation), or on specific aspect of GM food or feed (Regulation (EC), 1829/2003 and Regulation (EC), 1830/2003).

Directive 2001/18/EC provides for each use three types of rules: at first, rules on the authorization procedure; then rules on coexistence; and finally rules on traceability, alert, and control after deliberate release of GMOs (Bodiguel and Cardwell, 2010). During the authorization phase, EU institutions have to assess if new GM crops do not have any effects on human health and the environment (Directive, 2001/18/EC, art. 6 and 17). It is important to underline that the assessment corresponds to a "cumulative long-term effects analysis, thatrefers to the accumulated effects of consents on human health and the environment, including inter alia flora and fauna, soil fertility, soil degradation of organic material, the feed/food chain, biological diversity, animal health and resistance problems in relation to antibiotics" (Directive, 2001/18/EC, annex II). After authorization, a mandatory monitoring process is set. The key of this process is to allow State members and EU institutions to react in case of new information that calls into question about the scientific basis of the authorization: experts speak about emergency procedure or safeguard clause (Directive, 2001/18/EC, Part B, art. 8 on "Handling of modifications and new information"; also, part C, art. 20 on "Monitoring and handling of new information" and art 23 on "Safeguard clause"). Reports from notifiers and from institutions are also required in order to ensure maximum transparency (Directive, 2001/18/EC, Part B, art 10 on "Reporting by notifiers on releases"; art. 11 on "Exchange of information between competent authorities and the Commission"; annex VI on "Guidelines for the assessment reports" and annex VII on "Monitoring plan").

That is to say that GM and non-GM crops coexistence issue is neither about to know how new GM organisms (GMOs) may be authorized or how they can be renewed, nor to analyze control dimension. EU approach of coexistence measure is narrow: the "question of coexistence is confined by the Community legislature to matters of potential economic loss, on the basis that matters of environmental protection and human health have already been addressed at the authorization stage. (…) As a consequence, it could be argued that all that remains for any coexistence regime is the reduction (rather than total prevention) of cross-contamination" (Bodiguel et al., 2010; Lee, 2008a,b). It is exactly what was said by Commission in Recital 5 of 2003 Recommendation and what repeated by Recommendation 2010: "(4) The objective of co-existence measures in areas where GMOs are cultivated is to avoid unintended presence of GMOs in other products, preventing the potential economic loss and impact of the admixture of GM and non-GM crops (including organic crops)." In other words, coexistence phase might be understood as a period during which an authorized GM vegetal is cultivated at the same time and next to another type of crops. Its "scope extends from agricultural crop production on the farm up to the first point of sale, i.e., from the seed to the silo" (Commission Recommendation, 2003, Recital 6 and point 1.5). In term of Law, this EU conception of coexistence limits the discussion to only one dimension: rules to ensure that GM crops do not affect other crops.

According to Article (26a1) of Directive 2001/18/EC, "Member States may take appropriate measures to avoid the unintended presence of GMOs in other products." This provision gives to Member States the responsibility of coexistence measure, according to EU subsidiarity principle. This choice is officially justified because "Farm structures and farming systems, and the economic and natural conditions under which farmers in the European Union operate, are extremely diverse [and because the] diversity of farming systems and natural and economic conditions in the EU needs to be taken into consideration when designing measures to avoid the unintended presence of GM crops in other crops" (Commission Recommendation, 2010 Recital 2 as in Recommendation, 2013 Recital 6 and point 1.4). No EU binding measure is provided and there is no sanction in case of inaction of a member. Moreover, the inexistence of local coexistence measure cannot justify a Member State who refused the cultivation of authorized GMO crops as said by ECJ in "Pioneer Hi Bred Italia Srl affair" (ECJ, 2013).

Maybe to compensate this fragility, Directive 2001/18/EC provided that "The Commission shall gather and coordinate information based on studies at Community and national level, observe the developments regarding coexistence in the Member States and, on the basis of the information and observations, develop guidelines on the coexistence of genetically modified, conventional and organic crops" (Art. 26a2). In accordance with that, the Commission state the already mentioned 2003 Recommendation. It provided "a list of general principles and factors that Member

States are advised to take into account in developing national strategies and best practices for coexistence" (Recital 6. and point 2). It "did not insist on any particular form of policy instrument for coexistence, but instead welcomed voluntary agreements, legislation, soft law, or a combination of these instruments, as long as they would achieve effective implementation, monitoring, evaluation, and control" (Rosso Grossman, 2010). However, it gave an "open-ended catalog of farm management" (Recital 6 and point 3) in which it was about isolation distances between GM and non-GM fields; buffer zones; pollen traps or barriers; suitable crop rotation systems; planning the crop production cycle; cleaning of seed drills before and after use; sharing seed drills only with farmers using the same production type; preventing seed spillage when traveling to and from the field and on field boundaries; cleaning of harvesting machinery before and after use; sharing harvest machinery only with farmers using the same production type; during transport and storage, ensuring the physical segregation of GM and non-GM crops after the harvest up to the first point of sale and using adequate seed storage arrangements and practices … Recommendation 2010 (Recital 7) made no substantial change on the typology of coexistence measures but gave more space to Member States as an application of subsidiarity principle (as we will see in part 4). State members implemented the coexistence measure in very different ways (Bodiguel et al., 2010, 163−197). In April 2009, only 15 had adopted specific legislation on coexistence (COM, 2006, 2009). The impact of 2013 Commission Recommendation was not very significant and positive. The subsidiarity approach was unsuitable for local pressures, usually leading to minimal measures or to coexistence measures dictated by seed industry or big crops producers. In conclusion, all the indicators of feasibility were flashing red!

Anyway, in 2009, debate was not any more to know what could be coexistence measures but to give to State members the possibility to escape from GM crops, what lead to abandon of the 2013 Recommendation (see below part 4). However, another conception of coexistence could have been developed.

Another conception for crops coexistence: local governance

Instead of thinking to establish a GM and non-GM coexistence everywhere or to ban GM crops in most of the EU states, it would have been opportune to think about the possibility of GM zones: a true paradigm shift from diffused coexistence to concentrated coexistence as announced by the research program CoExtra (2009).

We have already tried to explain what we called our "hope for local governance" (Bodiguel, 2016). The year 2010 would have been the time of a reform encouraging a politically based approach in which the legitimacy of the decision depends more on the democratic process, eventually participative, than on its scientific basis.

Thus, the idea was to overtake this old and sterile debate to provide the opportunity of a reform to invent, experiment, and instigate local governance in the domain of GM crop cultivation (Fig. 7.2). Concretely, it would have been a deal with a new decision-making procedure, which would give more room for authorities

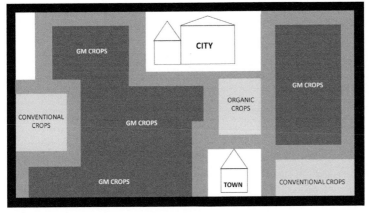

FIGURE 7.1

Schematic Map of genetically modified (GM) Zones and their Environment.

(local authorities), or local actors (individuals, associations, businesses). For example, in an area where crops used already a big part of the space and were the main economic activity, it would have been easy to delimitate a zone for GMOs. Inside, accordingly to a multigovernance approach, different stakeholders would have discussed and established by private and public contracts or convention, the condition for the development of this type of crops (Lee, 2010).

As reveals by Fig. 7.1, stakeholders would have to discuss particularly about buffer zones:

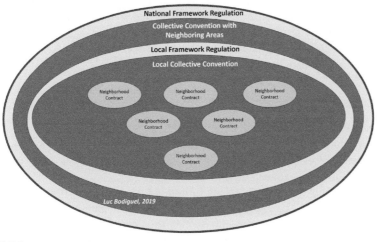

FIGURE 7.2

Overview of multiscale governance of genetically modified (GM) zones.

between GM crops and non-GM crops;

between GM crops and city or town; and

between GM zone and non-GM zone.

They should especially focus on phytosanitary issues, water use, ways of transportation of agricultural products and on agricultural machinery, storage seeds, and agricultural product areas.

Based on a National Regulation, all the stakeholders inside the zone and at the frontier of the zone have to sign a collective convention in which everyone is engaged to respect the National Framework and standards they decide to follow.

Then inside the GM zone, a local Regulation might be provided and a collective convention signed by private and public actors.

At intralevel, each GM farmer has to sign a contract with his non-GM neighbors in which local modalities of protection are planned and specified.

In view of the resistance to GM crops, this type of organization provides an opportunity to avoid centralizing decisions and to develop a decentralized and participative approach based on clear rules of territorial governance. This process would improve social adhesion and acceptability.

Developing this type of strategy could also be beneficial to Member States that are in position to give to local authorities the responsibility of a GM debate. In other words, to find a way out of the issue of GMOs, the States could have unloaded the problem onto the shoulders of local authorities and let a real process of local governance slowly emerge, relative to land use, environmental impact, and sanitary considerations in accordance with different agronomic processes.

Our hopes were quickly dashed in 2010. Member States, those that have strongly resisted GMOs, those that have tried to find an exit by invoking safety clauses or the provisions of the Treaty, did not want to see discussions start again. They quite simply pushed for a general prohibition on growing these crops in their national territory. It was the easiest way, at least politically, but it was a pity for innovation, not only genetic and agronomic (that still have to be proved), but also legal, political, and social; maybe also a pity for the proponents of "GMO free" who, although they were heard, are perhaps not always understood.

The end of the debate on coexistence?

Rebellion against GM crops was powerful and efficient because it concerned not only marginal actors but also numerous people representing various groups of society and institutions (Bodiguel, 2016).

Territorial rebellion was, above all, an individual and local activity, since they were excluded from GMO governance. Indeed, as we have already written, in techno food Regulation and in more particularly GM Regulation, the public and local authorities could only submit the decisions to authorize the cultivation of GM crops: even if there is information likely to invoke the principle of precaution and lead to a safety clause or emergency measure, only States and scientists could take action, the public having only the right to be informed (Bodiguel, 2016-2). This point was source of frustration and action. In France for example, these movements, which were popularized following the destruction of a Mc Donald's outlet, have gradually spread to the point where they influence public authorities, from towns to governments and the European Union. This reaction by the "man in the street" and through action, which was promulgated in France by "voluntary reapers" (crop destruction campaigners, Charte des faucheurs volontaires (2013), was discussed and backed up by claims, which sometimes lead to being classified as civil disobedience (Bodiguel, 2010).

Local authorities quickly followed the movement. Some had been in favor since the outset. This was the case in the Gers department in France and the Land Oberösterreich in Austria. In France, communities (Communal Councils) also reacted by applying orders to prohibit the cultivation of GMO crops on their land; more than 2000 communities were involved. However, the movement affects a large part of the EU, such as the "GMO-free" regions Charter signed in Florence on 4 February 2005, a text which is less operational but has had significant effect (Carta delle Regioni e delle autorità locali d'Europa sulla coesistenza tra colture, transgeniche e convenzionali, 2005).

Placed under pressure by the public and local authorities, Member States also escaped these legal limits on the grounds of various processes, ready to come under fire from the Court of Justice. Hungary included its refusal of GMO crops in its constitution (art. XX from Fundamental Law, 25 April 2011); Poland has promulgated a law prohibiting GMOs (EJC, 18 July 2013, Case C-313/11), Italy tried to ovoid GM crops invoking the lack of local decision on coexistence (EJC, 6 September 2013, Case C-36/11). As for France, after wandering about for a long time among the edicts prohibiting the cultivation of MON 810 maize, generally rejected by the Court (Conseil d'État, ord., 28 mars 2014, n° 376,808 s, Assoc. générale des producteurs de maïs et al.) (Billet, 2014), it passed a law with a single article: the "cultivation of GM varieties of maize is prohibited" (Loi n° 2014-567, 2 June 2014, relative à l'interdiction de la mise en culture des variétés de maïs GM, *JORF* n° 0127 3 June 2014 p. 9208).

All these attempts of resistance came up against European and national jurisdictions and failed (Bodiguel and Cardwell, 2011). Similarly, declarations of local independence (GMO-free zone) have been reduced to nothing (Portugal: Commission Decision of 3 November 2009 relating to the draft Regional Legislative Decree declaring the Autonomous Region of Madeira to be an Area Free of Genetically Modified Organisms. Austria: ECJ, 13 September 2007, case C-439/05 P and 0454/05 *Land Oberösterreich.* France: EJC, 8 September 2011, cases C-58/10 à C-68/10 *Monsanto SAS*) (Bodiguel, 2009). This systematically disapproved resistance led to a real political crisis, involving the paralysis of European documents to the point where the European legislature was not attempting to resolve the situation.

Face to generalized frustrations and disillusions, the European Parliament and Council modified directive 2001/18 by Directive 2015/412 and the 2003 Recommendation was canceled. It did not call the general system of authorization into question, it did not organize a new governance with participative approach, but it just modulated its geographical scope (Directive (EU) 2015/412).

From then, "During the authorisation procedure of a given GMO or during the renewal of consent/authorisation, a Member State may demand that the geographical scope of the written consent or authorisation be adjusted to the effect that all or part of the territory of that Member State is to be excluded from cultivation" (ordinary procedure: Directive, 2001/18, article 26b1 on "Cultivation".) This faculty of "opt out" of the GM Regulation implies the notifier who "Within 30 days from the presentation by the Commission of that demand, (…) may adjust or confirm the geographical scope of its initial notification/application" (Directive, 2001/18, article 26b2). If he doesn't maintain the initial geographical scope, its adjustment will be implemented by Commission. But, if he "confirmed the geographical scope of its initial notification/application," or if the authorization/renewal procedure is completed, "a Member State may adopt measures restricting or prohibiting the cultivation in all or part of its territory of a [authorised] GMO" only if he provides "that such measures are in conformity with Union law, reasoned, proportional and nondiscriminatory and, in addition, are based on compelling grounds such as those related to: (a) environmental policy objectives; (b) town and country planning; (c) land use; (d) socioeconomic impacts; (e) avoidance of GMO presence in other products without prejudice to Article 26a; (f) agricultural policy objectives; (g) public policy" (special procedure: Directive, 2001/18,/EC article 26b3 and procedure 26b4). Underline that a Member State can ask to reintegrate all or part of its territory into the geographical scope of the initial consent/authorization (Directive, 2001/18/EC, article 26b5).

The spirit of the reform is clear: avoid any debate on GMOs and put an end to public, local, and national authorities' rebellion. Thus now, each Member State who does not want to have GM crops on its territory is able to ask and to have it. There is no experimentation of the special procedure, but the subjectivity of criteria leads to a global acceptation of the demand. Consequently, the question of coexistence remains only for those who decide to keep GMOs, like Spain, where the debate on GMOs is less strong and hard.

References

Assemblée Nationale Française, 2005. Rapport sur les Enjeux des Essais et de l'Utilisation des OGM: No 2254, vol. 1, p. 57. http://www.assemblee-nationale.fr/12/pdf/rap-info/i2254-t2.pdf.

Billet, P., 2014. L'interdiction de la mise en culture du maïs GM. Environnement, 2014-12, comm. 78.

Bodiguel, L., Di Lauro, A., 2016. Food safety policy in a time of technofoods: risk, governance and legal issues of nanofoods. In: Mcmahon, J., Cardwell, M. (Eds.), Research Handbook on EU Agriculture Law. Edward Elgar Pub, p. 375, 31 January 2016.

Bodiguel, L., 2009. La coesistenza delle colture: lo Stato ai comandi. Rivista di Diritto Alimentare 5, 2009-4.

Bodiguel, L., 2010. Conclusion (on GMO and civil disobedience). In: Bodiguel, L., Cardwell, M. (Eds.), The Regulation of Genetically Modified Organisms: Comparative Approaches. Oxford University Press, p. 375.

Bodiguel, L., 2016. Local governance of GMOs: from hope to pragmatism. In: Ragionieri, M.P. (Ed.), GMO's in the EU law, Wolters Kluwer Italia (WKI), Collana di Diritto agrario e dell'ambiente, p. 265.

Bodiguel, L., Cardwell, M. (Eds.), 2010. The Regulation of Genetically Modified Organisms: Comparative Approaches. Oxford University Press, p. 410.

Bodiguel, L., Cardwell, M., 2011. Les juridictions pénales britanniques et françaises face aux Anti- OGM: au-delà des différences, une communauté d'esprit. Revue Juridique de l'Environnement 267–279, 2011/2.

Bodiguel, L., Cardwell, M., Carretero, G.A., Viti, D., 2010. Coexistence of genetically modified and non-genetically modified crops: national implementation in Europe. In: Bodiguel, L., Cardwell, M. (Eds.), The Regulation of Genetically Modified Organisms: Comparative Approaches. Oxford University Press, pp. 163–197.

Brosset, E., Hermon, C., 2018. Les nouvelles techniques de sélection des plantes:les perspectives ouvertes par le renvoi du Conseil d'État à la Cour de justice de l'Union Européenne. Droit de l'Environnement, p. 219.

Carta, 2005. delle Regioni e delle autorità locali d'Europa sulla coesistenza tra colture, transgenichee convenzionali. https://www.agri.marche.it.

Charte, 2013. des faucheurs volontaires d'OGM. https://www.combat-monsanto.org.pdf.

CoExtra, 2009. Growing Number of Genetically Modified Crops Worldwide Could Disrupt International Trade (07/09/2009. http://www.coextra.eu/news/news1435.html.

COM, 2006. Report on the Implementation of National Measures on the Coexistence of Genetically Modified Crops with Conventional and Organic Farming, vol. 104.

COM, 2009. Report from the Commission to the Council and the European Parliament on t he Coexistence of Genetically Modified Crops with Conventional and Organic Farming, vol. 153.

Directive, 17 April 2001. 2001/18/EC of the European Parliament and of the Council on the deliberate release into the environment of genetically modified organisms and repealing Council Directive 90/220/EEC,12. Official Journal. L106.

Directive, 13 March 2015. (EU) 2015/412 amending Directive 2001/18/EC as regards the possibility for the Member States to restrict or prohibit the cultivation of GMOs in their territory. Official Journal 1–8. L68.

ECJ, 2013. Pioneer Hi Bred Italia Srl Affair. 6 September 2013. Case C-36/11.

GM Science Review Panel, 2003. GM Science Review: First Report – an Open Review of the Science Relevant to GM Crops and Food Based on Interests and Concerns of the Public, London,, p. 18.

HCB Economic, Ethic and Social Committee Recommendation, 2017b. Recommandation sur les nouvelles techniques d'obtention de plantes (New Plant Breeding Techniques NPBT), Paris, 2 Nov, 2017, p. 6. http://www.hautconseildesbiotechnologies.fr/www.hautconseildesbiotechnologies.fr.

HCB Scientific Committee Advice, 2017a. Avis sur les nouvelles techniques d'obtention de plantes (New Plant Breeding Techniques- NPBT), Paris, 2 Nov. 2017, p. 17. http://www.hautconseildesbiotechnologies.fr/www.hautconseildesbiotechnologies.fr.

INRA (Institut National de la Recherche Agronomique), 2006. Coexistence: entre cultures OGM et non OGM en Europe. Paris. http://www.inra.fr/en/Scientists-Students/Agricultural-systems/All-the-news/Coexistence-GM-and-non-GM.

Lee, M., 2008a. EU Regulation of GMOs: Law and Decision Making for a New Technology. Edward Elgar, Cheltenham, pp. 105–127, 2008.

Lee, M., 2008b. The governance of coexistence between GMOs and other forms of agriculture: a purely economic issue? Journal of Environmental Law 2008–20, 193.

Lee, M., April 2010. Multi-level governance of Gmos in the European Union: ambiguity and hierarchy. In: Bodiguel, L., Cardwell, M. (Eds.), The Regulation of Genetically Modified Organisms: Comparative Approaches. Oxford University Press, p. 101.

Messean, A., Angevin, F., Gomez- Barbero, M., Menrad, K., Rodriguez- Cerezo, E., January, 2006. New case studies on the coexistence of GM and non-GM crops in: European agriculture. Tech. Rep. EUR 22012 (European Commission Joint Research Centre. EUR22102EN), 116 p. https://scholarworks.iupui.edu/handle/1805/775.

Commission Recommendation, July 23, 2003. Guidelines for the development of national strategies and best practices to ensure the co-existence of genetically modified crops with conventional and organic farming, Brussels. Official Journal L189/36.

Regulation (EC) 1829/2003, 22/09/2003. Regulation (EC) 1829/2003 Of the Parliament and of the Council on genetically modified food and feed. Official Journal L268/1.

Regulation (EC) 1830/2003, 22/09/2003. Regulation (EC) 1830/2003 of the Parliament and of the Council concerning the traceability and labelling of genetically modified organisms and the traceability of food and feed products produced from genetically modified organisms. Official Journal L268/24.

Regulation, 14/06/2018, 2018/848 of the European Parliament and of the council on organic production and labelling of organic products and repealing council regulation (EC) No 834/2007. Official Journal L150/1.

Rosso Grossman, M., April 2010. Coexistence of conventional and organic cropsin the European Union. In: Bodiguel, L., Cardwell, M. (Eds.), The Regulation of Genetically Modified Organisms: Comparative Approaches. Oxford University Press.

The impact of GM crops on agriculture

Alan H. Schulman[1,2]

*Professor, Production Research, Natural Resources Institute (Luke), Helsinki, Finland[1]; Institute of
Biotechnology and Viikki Plant Science Centre, University of Helsinki, Helsinki, Finland[2]*

Introduction

Genetically modified (GM) crops, meaning those containing transgenes or which are
regulated as such, arrived into commercial use at the turn of the 1990s and became
widespread by the middle of that decade. While field tests of engineered tobacco
began in 1986 in France and the United States, a virus-resistant GM tobacco was
commercialized in China in 1992 (Huang et al., 2002). The Flavr Savr tomato
was approved in 1994 (Kramer and Redenbaugh, 1994) in the United States and
herbicide-resistant tobacco in the European Union also in 1994 (Saeglitz and
Bartsch, 2003). In the 25 years since then, GM crops have been sown and harvested
more and more extensively throughout the world. The 1.7 M ha of GM crops in 1996
expanded to about 190 million hectares by 2017 (ISAAA, 2017), comprising about
13.5% (FAOStat) of global arable land (Fig. 8.1). More than 18 million farmers, 90%
of whom on subsistence or small farms, have grown GM crops; 19 of the 24 countries that grew GMs in 2017 were classified as developing (ISAAA, 2017). Penetration has been particularly great in the United States, where 40% of the cropland
produces GM crops; 96% of the cotton, 94% of the soybean, and 93% of the maize
area are covered by GM varieties (ISAAA, 2017). The greatest proportion of GM
crops consists of soybean, maize, cotton, and oilseed rape (canola), with herbicide
and disease resistance being the most common traits conferred by the transgenes.

Within the context of area planted, GM crops have made great inroads into conventional agriculture in the sense of replacing the cultivation of non-GM varieties, in
regions where field release and marketing of GM varieties have been generally
permitted. Given that the farmer's field is poised between the seed industry and a
very long value chain extending both directly and indirectly (via domestic livestock)
to the dinner plate, the true impact of GM crops on conventional agriculture is much
greater than the area under cultivation. One needs to consider as well: the economic
impact along the value chain; the impact on farming practice; the impact on crop
genetic diversity and on the biodiversity of noncrop species; impact on soil; the
impact on food production, marketing, and distribution; the impact on the secondary
stakeholders, the consumers.

Genetically Modified and Irradiated Food. https://doi.org/10.1016/B978-0-12-817240-7.00012-7

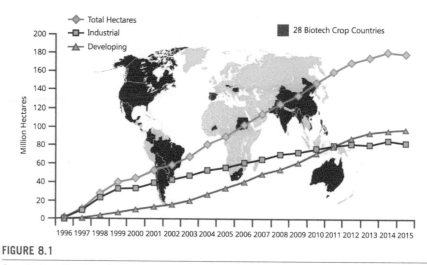

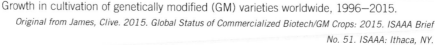

FIGURE 8.1

Growth in cultivation of genetically modified (GM) varieties worldwide, 1996–2015.

Original from James, Clive. 2015. Global Status of Commercialized Biotech/GM Crops: 2015. ISAAA Brief

No. 51. ISAAA: Ithaca, NY.

The economic impact of GM crops and their traits for farmers and consumers

GM approaches have been used for crop plants in the main to achieve pest resistance, particularly to viruses, insects, and fungi, as well as herbicide and antibiotic tolerance (Kamthan et al., 2016). However, the list of traits conferred by GM events is long and growing (ISAAA, 2019). Beyond the ones just mentioned, others include improved stress tolerance, such as to drought; altered plant development such as reduced lignin production, higher yield, higher biomass, delayed fruit ripening; improved quality, such as reduced allergenicity, nonbrowning tubers, more healthful fatty acids, and longer shelf life. All of these traits either improve the yield of the crop or its value, adding value along the production chain from the farmer to the consumer. As a share of the total area under the crops for which GM varieties are most commonly available (Fig. 8.2A), GM soy and cotton may have reached near market saturation in countries where they are grown, even for maize despite the lower GM adoption rate globally. For example GM cotton, maize, and soy cover, respectively, 96%, 93.4%, and 94% of the areas planted for these crops (ISAAA, 2017). Globally, the overwhelming majority of GM crops confer either herbicide tolerance, insect resistance, or both stacked in combination (Fig. 8.2B).

Without doubt, GM crops would not have become so prevalent if not for some benefit to the farmer. Given that farming is ultimately a livelihood and a business and farmers in essence place bets on what crop and variety to grow against future sales revenues over the cost of their inputs (their break-even), it makes sense to analyze the impact of GM crops in economic terms. In a meta-analysis of earlier

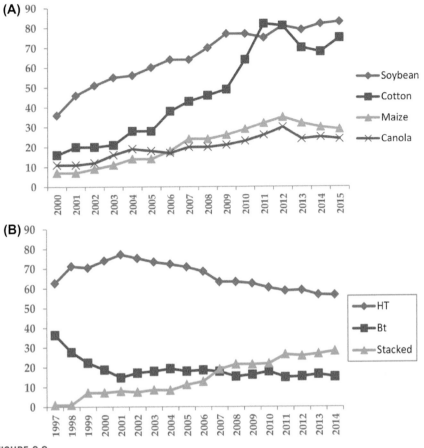

FIGURE 8.2

Global adoption of genetically modified (GM) crops and traits. (A) Adoption rate of GM varieties as a percent of total hectares planted. (B) Share of most abundant GM traits as percent total GM area. HT, herbicide tolerance; Bt, insect-resistant Bt-producing crops; Stacked, both HT and Bt traits present in the variety.

Source: Brankov, T., et al., 2016. Gene Revolution in Agriculture: 20 Years of Controversy. Genetic Engineering — An Insight into the Strategies and Applications. Jamal, F. IntechOpen Limited, London, UK, figures provided under Creative Commons License (https://creativecommons.org/licenses/by/4.0/).

studies focused on cultivation of GM varieties of maize and cotton conferring insect-resistance, as well as on herbicide-tolerant GM soybean, maize, and cotton, Klumper and Qaim (Klumper and Qaim, 2014) found striking benefits for farmers, whose profits increased overall by 68% through GM cultivation. For example, based on 36 primary datasets, the authors found that insect-resistant crops increased profit margins by 68.8% with 99% statistical confidence.

Although GM cultivation is often associated in the public mind with agribusiness and corporate farms, strikingly, the positive impact of GMs on farmer's profits has been much greater in developing countries than in developed ones, primarily due to yield differential and high pesticide costs in the developing world (Klumper and Qaim, 2014). In the most recent effort to aggregate and quantify the impact of GM crops on farm impact and production, Brookes and Barfoot (2018) found that these crops conferred a benefit of 186.1 billion USD over the period 1996–2016, with the benefit in 2016 alone being 18.2 billion USD. While the impact varied widely between crops and regions, overall 48% of the gains went to farmers in developed countries and 52% to those in developing countries, an impact seen by others as well (Finger et al., 2011). Field trials by Oxfam at various locations in India demonstrated that use of cotton-producing *Bacillus thuringiensis* insecticidal proteins (Bt cotton) conferred yield gains of 80%−87%, while reducing insecticide use by 70% (Qaim and Zilberman, 2003); these results for India have been confirmed and extended to elsewhere in the developing world more recently (Smyth et al., 2015).

Perhaps the most striking example of the social and economic impact of GM varieties on conventional farming and agriculture is that of the papaya and the development of GM varieties resistant to papaya ringspot virus (PRSV). PRSV spreads rapidly through Hawaii's papaya plantations in the early 1990s, devastating the industry (Fuchs and Gonsalves, 2007). The adoption by Hawaiian papaya farmers of the GM Rainbow papaya, resistant to PRSV by virtue of its carrying the PRSV coat protein gene, saved the industry on the islands (Fuchs and Gonsalves, 2007). In practice, GM papayas offered farmers a sustainable solution for providing locally produced food that is also available for export. More generally, engineering virus resistance has been one of the biggest success stories for GM, even if currently the majority of the hectares in GM crops are represented by insect-resistant and herbicide-tolerant varieties. The idea and implementation of viral resistance, particularly for coat-protein-mediated resistance, was already well developed by 1990 (Beachy et al., 1990). In addition, several other strategies have been effective, involving incorporation of resistance (R) genes, constructs to mediate posttranscriptional gene silencing, and antiviral antibodies, among others (Kamthan et al., 2016). Given the promise and success of engineered virus resistance and the multiple threats to the staple crops of low-income subsistence farmers, efforts are underway to deliver virus-resistant GMs aimed particularly at banana, cassava, maize, rice, and yams (Kreuze and Valkonen, 2017).

A side-effect of the advent of GM foodstuffs moving through the supply chain, combined with the effect on consumer preferences of anti-GM campaigns, has been the demands for labeling of GM-derived products. Labeling has economic impact. While the costs of the labels per se are negligible, the costs of certifying the ingredients' non-GM status and of tracking the ingredients through to the final product increase the food prices (Winfree and McCluskey, 2017). Mandatory labeling in the state of California was estimated at 400 USD per household in 2012 and was one important factor in defeat of the labeling referendum (Zilberman, 2012). Hence, mandatory labeling, which could be triggered by public response to the advent of

GM foods in the marketplace, would pass on increased costs on to all consumers. Consistent with this observation, the per-capita GDP of the 63 countries that require labeling of GM foods is 28,914 USD, compared with 19,077 USD for those that do not (McCluskey et al., 2018). If the added costs of tracking and labeling for export to developed countries were to decrease the cultivation of GM crops in poorer countries that supply the market, those poorer countries would suffer from the loss of the 22% higher yields conferred by the most commonly cultivated GM crops (Klumper and Qaim, 2014), as well as the decreased profitability of conventional crops cited above. The trends regarding economic impact of GM crops on conventional agriculture would be all the greater from a yield perspective when considering organic cultivation, which has been shown to give 13%—34% lower yields than do conventional crops (Seufert et al., 2012).

Impact of GM crops on farming practice

The impact of GM crops on conventional farming has brought a variety of changes to farm practice, as well as benefits to farmers, both in developed and developing countries. Two major changes have been the expansion of no-tillage methods and reductions in pesticide use, as consequences respectively of efficient weed killing through glyphosate-tolerant GM varieties and insect resistance from Bt-producing varieties. These are discussed in more depth below. One overlooked consequence of the drop in insecticide use is the health benefit for farmers in developing countries, due to the drop in the skin and respiratory exposure from unprotected use of toxic pesticides (Smyth et al., 2015). In India alone, several million annual cases of acute pesticide poisoning have been thereby avoided, realizing a savings to the health authorities of 14—51 M USD (Kouser and Qaim, 2011).

Contrary to the simplistic view that biological pest control and GM cultivation are opposing approaches, they may well complement each other if intelligently managed (Lundgren et al., 2009). Integrated pest management is not in conflict with GMs, because the careful tracking of pest populations, interventions scaled to potential losses, and a diverse suite of tools for response, which are typical of integrated approaches, can include GMs as part of the package. Biological control agents may increase the durability of GM pest resistance both by delaying emergence of the resistance and by suppressing pests to which the GM crops are not resistant. Likewise, herbicide tolerance can simplify the task of using biological control agents against some of the target species.

Low-tillage agriculture, or conservation tillage, another outcome of the use of herbicide-tolerant GM crops, aside from benefits to soil structure, offers enormous savings in labor, particularly in underdeveloped economies where weeding is done by hand. In North America, between 1999 and 2015, use of conservation tillage as the oilseed rape producers' favored method increased from 11% to 64%, in parallel with the transition from 30% (1996) to 63% (2015) among the soybean producers (Smyth et al., 2015). In Africa, labor-intensive hand weeding, generally the work of women, is the main factor limiting farm size (Kent et al., 2001). Field studies found that herbicide-resistant GM maize freed up 10–12 days of labor per season (Smyth et al., 2015). Detailed analyses indicate that the benefit for Africa would be very great for smallholders if GM bananas that were resistant to *Xanthomonas* wilt disease were available. In the Great Lakes Region of Africa (Burundi, the Democratic Republic of the Congo, Kenya, Malawi, Rwanda, Tanzania, and Uganda), GM bananas could save 51%–83% of the harvest from being lost, given initial adoption rates between 21% and 70% (Ainembabazi et al., 2015).

A key question regarding the impact of GM crops on conventional agriculture is the possibility for coexistence, meaning the presence, side-by-side or nearby, of fields with GM and conventional varieties. Traits such as self-fertilization, low-outcrossing rates, poor pollen mobility, lack of cross-fertile crop species, annual growth habit, poor overwintering of seed, and low seed shattering rates all increase the likelihood of successful coexistence. Oilseed rape is notoriously difficult in this regard, due to its high pollen mobility, cross-fertility with other *Brassica spp.*, and seed shattering. Efforts to model these processes and the growth patterns of oilseed rape indicate that gene flow from GM to non-GM fields is virtually inevitable (Colbach, 2009) and that sampling strategies for GM detection possibly problematic (Begg et al., 2008). Nevertheless, field trials in the United Kingdom indicated that with moderate separation distances and buffer crops, bulked samples would remain below declarable levels (0.9%) despite gene flow (Weekes et al., 2005). Azadi and coauthors examined coexistence specifically in developing countries and concluded that it is not easy but also not impossible (Azadi et al., 2018).

A striking, positive example of coexistence is that of GM and conventional papaya varieties in Hawaii described above (Fuchs and Gonsalves, 2007). The supplanting of non-GM papaya, which was susceptible to the PRSV virus, by the resistant GM Rainbow variety greatly reduced the viral load in the growing areas. This, in turn, has made it possible to cultivate non-GM papayas for the market in Japan, which will not import the GM variety, albeit at some risk of crop loss due to the PRSV. There is still risk of loss due to viral infection of the non-GM papayas, but it is considerably less due to the presence of the GM varieties.

A major consideration in the implementation of coexistence concerns the legislative framework. Strict minimum distance rules and difficulties in marketing agricultural products that are legally GM (i.e., above 0.9% detectability of a transgenic event) would tend to drive GM cultivation down, through a "domino effect," to a low level (Demont et al., 2008). On the other hand, the increased yield and profitability of GM cultivation, combined with geneflow into conventional crops that may change the legal status of the conventional crops to GM even if their yield remains at conventional (lower) levels, would lead to the dominos falling in the other direction, i.e., driving most farmers to adopt GM varieties.

Impact of GM varieties on crop genetic diversity

The introduction of GM crops has raised concerns that crop genetic diversity might decrease as breeding programs narrowed around expensively produced and priced cultivars with high genetic gain and high market value. Studies on this issue show quite variable results depending on the crop, ranging from 28% reduction of diversity in cotton varieties in the United States, but only a small effect in India (Carpenter, 2011). In conventional agriculture as well, single elite varieties may come to dominate nationally and regionally if they offer winning traits to the farmer, processor, or consumer. As GM cultivation has both spread and matured over the last couple of decades, however, many GM varieties carrying the same trait and transgene, but in different genetic backgrounds, have been introduced into each agricultural region (Qaim, 2009).

Case studies for soybean and cotton show that GM-based herbicide tolerance has, if anything, increased genetic diversity among the cultivars in use, because it enabled various lines with local adaptations to carry as well the herbicide tolerance (Ammann, 2005). In another analysis of GM cotton (Krishna et al., 2016), the authors found that to the extent that a GM variety reduces production risk, it also reduces demand for varietal diversity as an alternative strategy to reducing risk. However, as more GM varieties become available, on-farm diversity again rises. Currently, GM technology has been adopted by over 90% of the cotton growers in India. However, varietal diversity is the same as it was before GM technology came onto the scene in that country.

GM approaches are, in essence, ways to increase genetic diversity where conventional sexual crossing cannot introduce the traits needed, because they are lacking in compatible germplasm. Returning to the case of GM papaya discussed earlier, it is also relevant to the question of the impact of a GM variety on cultivar diversity. Back in 1998, indeed 95% of the papaya area was covered by a single variety, Kapoho, which was the favored nontransgenic variety, and less than 5% comprised Sunrise and Kamiya (Fuchs and Gonsalves, 2007). As the PRSV crisis intensified, first the PRSV-resistant GM variety SunUp was introduced. This was followed by Rainbow (which had the preferred standard flesh color of Kapoho) and then Laie Gold. Hence, the ability to move the PRSV resistance into other varieties by crossing in fact increased varietal diversity because the essential trait was not tied to a complex set of minor genes.

In summary, GM varieties do not, in and of themselves, lead to lower crop genetic diversity. The integrated transgenes are but one of the approximately 30,000 genes in a crop plant, which together determine the genetic diversity of the plant; the transgene can be moved between varieties of diverse genetic backgrounds by conventional crosses. Rather, the diversity question is a more general, applying as well to conventional varieties, and is based on intellectual property right (IPR) regulatory structures, the economics of the breeding and seed industries, various national policies on distribution of improved seed, and also cultural practices surrounding use of the crop.

Impact on biodiversity of noncrop species

Since the advent of GM crops, various academic researchers and advocacy groups have been interested in the risk and impact of these crops' cultivation on wild plants bordering cultivated areas, for example through gene transfer into the gene pool of wild relatives or through seed dispersal or spillage on the local biome. However, the past 20 years of extensive cultivation has, if anything, indicated a generally positive effect from GM cultivation. First, adoption of GM technology has reduced chemical pesticide use by 37% overall (Klumper and Qaim, 2014), corresponding to more than 618 million kg of chemicals (Brookes and Barfoot, 2017). This reduction has thereby decreased the corresponding pollution and risk to nontarget insects, some of which are also pollinators, in surrounding areas. Using the Environmental Impact Quotient (EIQ) (Gallivan et al., 2001) indicator, this suggests a reduced hazard of 18.6% (Brookes and Barfoot, 2017) as a result of GM technologies.

A field study was carried out directly assessing the impact of GM-based resistance to the potato late blight organism, *Phytophthora infestans* (Lazebnik et al., 2017). Cultivation site, year, potato genotype, and fungicide management regimes were analyzed regarding their impact on the arthropod community. Because the study included two varieties that differed only by the presence of the transgene, it was able to establish that the impact on community structure was due to cultivar differences rather than to the GM event (A15-31) itself. Likewise, extensive studies and risk analyses on the impact of GM varieties producing Bt insecticidal proteins on nontarget species overwhelmingly indicate that there is none and that Bt crops can be an effective component of integrated pest management as described above (Carzoli et al., 2018; Romeis et al., 2019).

Reduced weed production and associated farming intensification, an impact of glyphosate-tolerant GM crops, could be viewed as a risk for birds and wildlife that depend, directly or indirectly, on those weeds for food. However, an analysis in the United Kingdom indicated that leaving margins of at most 2% of the field area that are left unsprayed is sufficient to mitigate loss of weed seed production (e.g., for birds). Margins of 4% are enough to mitigate weed biomass production (supporting insects that birds feed on), equivalent to a 1 meter increase in field margins (Pidgeon et al., 2007).

Use of the herbicide glyphosate has increased in general, both due to its effectiveness and to the availability of glyphosate-tolerant GM crops. A widely recognized consequence is the advent of glyphosate resistance (Brookes and Barfoot, 2017); www.weedscience.org (accessed 26 September, 2019). So far, glyphosate resistance has been reported in 44 weed species across 37 countries (Heap and Duke, 2018). The problem has been caused not by the transgene or the GM plant per se, but rather by the pest management strategy, whereby use of glyphosate as the sole agent of weed control led to strong selective pressure for resistance. In parallel, resistance to the herbicide atrazine, which is not present in GM crops, has been reported so far in 239 weed species (www.weedscience.org, 2019). Rather than treating glyphosate as the magic bullet to eradicate weeds, an integrated approach using several herbicides in combination with crop rotation, buffer strips, and other altered cultivation practices provides a sustainable solution not only for GM but also for conventional agriculture (Green et al., 2008; Dewar, 2009). A drop has been seen in the proportion of glyphosate in the herbicide mix used on herbicide-tolerant GM crops from 82% in 1998 to 67% in 2015 (Brookes and Barfoot, 2017). Specific design criteria for stacks of multiple resistance genes in GM crops have been elaborated, which could also help delay the advent of glyphosate resistance (Gressel et al., 2017), as indeed gene stacking does for fungal resistance genes in conventional varieties.

Besides glyphosate resistance being driven by selection for mutations, the trait has also spread via pollen flow from GM crops, particularly in *Brassica spp.* In a case study in Argentina, the transgene has been shown to persist at least 4 years in nature (Pandolfo et al., 2018). Nevertheless, in the absence of selection, natural mutational rates will eventually lead to inactivation of resistance genes, whether the resistance is of transgenic or mutational origin. Moreover, for the resistant allele or transgene to be maintained, the selective pressure for the trait it confers must be greater than the fitness cost of the trait or gene.

The potential fitness cost of glyphosate resistance has been demonstrated in a greenhouse experiment with the dicot *Bassia scoparia* (Martin et al., 2017) and of sulfonylurea (acetolactate synthase [ALS]) herbicides in the monocot *Alopecurus myosuroides*, a common weed among cereals (Comont et al., 2019). Beyond pesticide tolerance, physiological traits such as drought tolerance might be selectively advantageous. An early example is Monsanto's DroughtGard maize hybrids (event MON 87460) (Castiglioni et al., 2008). The potential environmental risks associated with its cultivation were assessed, regarding increased weediness inside or outside agricultural areas, impact on nontarget organisms, and risks to the rhizosphere, but none was found (Sammons et al., 2014). Generalizing, the risk of the spread and persistence of transgenes or weediness, either into conventional cultivation or bordering natural areas, as an impact of GM crops must be viewed against the trade-offs associated with the specific traits conferred by the transgenes outside the GM agronomic system.

Given that field crops are for the most part grown in monocultures and not in complex mixtures of species, cultivated fields will generally have a lower biodiversity than surrounding natural areas, except perhaps for irrigated fields in deserts. Hence, the fewer the hectares under cultivation, the greater the overall biodiversity. This being the case, perhaps the largest positive impact conferred by GM crops on the biodiversity of noncrop species has been through the number of hectares their use has kept out of cultivation while still delivering the same yield. Overall, GM technology has contributed a gain in yield of 22% to the most commonly cultivated crops (Klumper and Qaim, 2014). Between 1996 and 2016, the use of GM technology for soybean and maize alone is estimated to have delivered a total yield gain, respectively, of 213 million tons and 405 million tons (Brookes and Barfoot, 2018). For soybean, maize, cotton, and oilseed rape together, maintaining production at 2016 levels without the yield gain conferred by the GM transgenes would have required an additional 22.4 million hectares (Brookes and Barfoot, 2018). For comparison, this is greater than the total 21.5 M ha of arable land in France. In the case of papaya cultivation in Hawaii, before the advent of GM-based virus resistance, growers were clearing forests, where the virus had not yet taken hold, to make new fields (Fuchs and Gonsalves, 2007). The PRSV-resistant GM varieties enabled the farms to grow papaya on existing land where the virus had become endemic, thereby preserving the surrounding forests.

Impact of GMs on food production, marketing, and distribution of agricultural products

Particularly in the large single market of the EU, uncertainty from consumers largely generated by media campaigns of various nongovernmental organizations (NGOs), together with the stiff resistance of the NGOs themselves to GMs, has fragmented the marketing of agricultural products into GM and non-GM streams, complicating the lives of producers and leading to a de facto ban on GM food products (Doh and Guay, 2006; Paarlberg, 2014). The distrust of GM food products shows little signs of abating, although 20 years of study have failed to find unintended compositional changes between GM and conventional foodstuffs, which are a consequence of the GM technology per se (Herman and Price, 2013). In the United States, too, GM food products have led to calls for mandatory labeling. The first unconditional mandatory labeling law went into effect in Vermont, USA, in 2014. Modeling of the impact of labeling indicates that producers of non-GM foodstuffs benefit weakly from voluntary labeling but more strongly when it is mandatory, if consumers see non-GM as a positive quality (McCluskey and Winfree, 2017). This is especially the case both because consumers tend to see GM labeling as a warning and because the costs of labeling are borne by the producers.

A recent study, one of the few empirical studies on the added cost to consumers of *non*-GM foods, found that US consumers, during 2009–16, paid a premium of 9.8% −61.8% for non-GM food products (Kalaitzandonakes et al., 2018). For organic foods, this premium jumped to between 13.8% and 91%. The price premium is derived from multiple sources. Reformulation to avoid GM ingredients can be expensive, and non-GM, especially organic, ingredients themselves are generally more costly than GM due to lower yields (Seufert et al., 2012). Moreover, the segregation costs of certified non-GM harvests also leads to higher prices for them (Varacca and Soregaroli, 2016). This may well explain why European consumers look the other way when the question is GM-based feed for livestock rather than labeled foods themselves.

Impact of GMs in Europe, a special case

The impact of GM crops in Europe has been brought about by their general absence from cultivation, rather than by their widespread adoption. The various food scandals in recent decades, such as bovine spongiform encephalopathy (BSE) and foot-and-mouth disease, combined with effective lobbying by NGOs and the freighting of breeding technologies with opposition to large corporations engaged in agribusiness, led to the growth in suspicions of food production in general and of anti-GM sentiments among the general public (Varzakas et al., 2007). These in turn resulted in a host of EU regulations, including Directive 2001/18 on deliberate release of GMOs, as well as Regulations 1829/2003 on GM food and feed, 1830/2003 on traceability and labeling, and 1946/2003 on transboundary movement of GMOs. Altogether, as they were transposed into the national laws of EU member states, these decisions were implemented as a very tight regime of restrictions on the release within the EU of GM varieties, as well as on commerce of GM-derived food and feed.

Currently only a single GM event, Bt maize MON810, is authorized for cultivation in Europe, with only Spain growing it in significant quantities. More than 30% of the Spanish maize crop carries this transgene (Gomez-Barbero et al., 2008). In 2017, a total of 124,000 ha of GM maize were grown in Spain, supplemented by 7000 ha in Portugal, comprising all GM crops that were grown that year in Europe (ISAAA, 2017). Earlier, small quantities had been grown in Czech Republic, Germany, Poland, Romania, and Slovakia, altogether peaking at 144,000 ha in 2013, but by 2017, Spain and Portugal remained the only countries growing a GM crop (ISAAA, 2017). Nevertheless, even under the current regulations, since 1998, as more than 100 GM crop events have been approved for import as food or feed into the EU. What is striking given this number, and tantamount to an NGO-led boycott of GM products at the retail level, is that virtually no GM-labeled foods can be found on European grocery shelves. While GM crops have largely so far failed to penetrate into agriculture in the European Union (EU), that is not true for the markets for agricultural products. In contrast to the limited amount of GM maize cultivated in Europe, the EU imported over 62 million metric tons of maize in 2017, of which over 20%, or about 12.5 million metric tons, was GM (ISAAA, 2017). Europe also imports over 30 million tons of soy for feed supplements yearly (ISAAA, 2017), but only 15% is certified as GM-free (Lucht, 2015). Given that more than 90% of soybeans traded globally are from GM varieties, Europe is bringing in massive amounts of what it will not allow or encourage its own farmers to cultivate (Van Eenennaam and Young, 2014).

A good example of what GM varieties could mean for Europe can be found in the case of Romania (Lucht, 2015). Herbicide-tolerant GM soybeans came under cultivation in Romania starting in 1999, which gave farmers new weed control options, increased average yields by over 30%, and made this crop the most profitable arable crop grown in that country. In 2006, the GM soy varieties were grown on 137,000 ha in Romania and had reached an adoption rate of 68% compared with the total soy production area. Because of increased yields and plantings, Romania's soy production soared and surplus soybeans could be exported to other European countries while soybean meal imports decreased substantially. When Romania joined the European Union in 2007, where GM soybeans do not have a cultivation authorization, farmers were forced to return to conventional varieties. Because of strongly reduced profitability, the area planted with soybeans shrank by 70% within just 2 years, and Romania became a net importer of soy.

Similar to their fellow farmers in Romania, surveys indicate that at least a third of Spanish, French, and Hungarian farmers would grow GM crops if they could, as well as half the farmers in the United Kingdom (Areal et al., 2011). Recently, stakeholders in the EU were surveyed concerning the prospective impact of GM crops in Europe, were they to become available by 2025 (Jones et al., 2017). The study focused on crops providing traits that were both suited to cultivation conditions in the EU, would provide benefits to both farmers and consumers, and were already either available or would soon be. For farmers, herbicide-tolerant and insect-resistant maize, soy, and sugar beet was most desired and most likely to be adopted. Whereas oilseed rape with improved fatty acid composition would offer benefits to consumers, it was expected to be at most a niche product. The stakeholders were generally pessimistic that the current restrictive EU policies would change in the foreseeable future, so the benefits of GM crops for farmers and consumers the world over would largely be foregone in Europe. Because European consumers have no chance to become familiar with GM foodstuffs through consumption, it is likely that their general squeamishness toward them will continue.

Aside from the negative impact the lack of GM varieties have had on agriculture, the lack of easy commercialization paths have had a chilling effect on transgene research in Europe, which was a pioneer in the subject. Field trials have been curtailed, abetted by attacks on them by vandals (Nausch et al., 2015). Efforts in Europe were abandoned to register a GM potato variety that carried genes from wild potatoes than conferred effective resistance to *Phytophthora*-induced late blight, which would replace the use of fungicides (Dixelius et al., 2012). In 2012, BASF, one of the largest European biotechnology companies, abandoned development of GM varieties for Europe, shut down its corresponding facilities, and shifted its focus to America and Asia (Lucht, 2015). Although the overall framework is not promising, there are distinct differences between individual European countries and regions in the potential willingness of their farmers and public to grow and to eat GM foods (Dunwell, 2014). Aside from the countries currently already growing GM maize, mentioned above, Denmark, Estonia, Finland, the region of Flanders, the Netherlands, Sweden, and the United Kingdom are most positive to GM technologies, whereas Austria, Croatia, Cyprus, Greece, Hungary, Italy, Malta, and Slovenia are the most negative. While these differences may not affect the impact of GM crops inside Europe, they may become important for GE-derived foodstuffs, as described below.

Concluding comments

Over the last 30 or so years, where farmers have been free to choose whether to grow GM or conventional varieties, they have overwhelmingly chosen GM. Whether we consider maize, cotton, and soybean in the United States, or soybean in Argentina and Brazil, or cotton in India, or oilseed rape in Canada, the answer is the same:

over 90% adoption (ISAAA, 2017). The reasons for the nearly universal use of GM varieties where they are available are similar in both developed and developing countries: they permit farmers to grow more food with fewer inputs and less labor, primarily by controlling pests and weeds better than conventional varieties and approaches, thereby increasing farmers' income. The widespread adoption of GM crops has had a range of positive environmental effects as well. These range from reduced agricultural impact on biodiversity via conservation tillage, lower insecticide use, more environmentally friendly herbicides, and less pressure to expand agricultural areas (Carpenter, 2011). Replacement of older insecticides with Bt-carrying varieties has reduced human pesticide poisoning, particularly in the developing world.

The advent and adoption of GM crops have not only increased the profits and yields of those farmers who took GM varieties into use but also changed their agronomic practices, for example by expanding no-tillage cultivation. Depending on the local regulatory framework, GM crops have complicated for farmers their postharvest treatment of fields and harvests, due to coexistence and traceability requirements. Part of the overall impact of GMs may be attributable to leveraging, whereby the early-adopting farmers may have been more effective in any case in achieving higher yields and profits than their neighbors. This, combined in certain crops such as oilseed rape with a domino effect, may drive conversion of most farms to GM varieties. The widespread benefit of GM varieties for farmers is perceived even among European farmers, despite their not being able to cultivate GMs in most places and despite the widespread negative perception of foods derived from GM crops among the general public in Europe. Perhaps no technology has been more thoroughly investigated regarding impact than the use of transgenes in agriculture. The literature, which is extensive (Dale et al., 2002; Gianessi et al., 2002; Sanvido et al., 2007; National Research Council, 2010), generally concludes that GM crops have had little or no negative impact on the environment and moreover, that any adverse effects have been smaller and fewer than those of conventional varieties.

Nevertheless, public perception of GM crops continues to be, at least in Europe, quite negative. Overall, among the public, the risks, if any, of GM crops are vastly overrated, while the benefits are drastically underrated. The global contributions currently being made by GM crops to food security and farm sustainability seem to be ignored entirely in public discourse. The one group of consumers in Europe that has overwhelmingly taken to eating GM crops is the livestock. Globally, 70% −90% of GM crops are used to produce feed (Lucht, 2015). This GM feed is sustaining no fewer than 100 billion animals or 13 times the human population on the planet. No evidence has emerged of detrimental effects linked to the GM feed.

Prospects: the impact of gene editing

A major difference between agriculturalists and hunter-gatherers is that the former group are generally growing and consuming plants that have been somehow GM, in the scientific rather than legal sense of the words (without the "G" and "M"), through their own actions (Doebley et al., 2006). Among the earliest examples of genetic modifications being fixed into agricultural species by humans was the loss of seed shattering in cereals (Lin et al., 2012). Over the last 10,000 or 15,000 years, farmers have propagated plants with desired traits, i.e., selected and fixed genes and alleles, modifying the genetic structure of the species. Over the last 100 years, breeders have employed sexual crosses to introduce and combine these.

Almost 80 years ago, Stadler described the use of X-rays to mutagenize and introduce new variation from which selections could be made for desired traits (Stadler, 1930). In this chapter, the focus here has been on the impact of new variation produced by *Agrobacterium*-mediated introduction of genes or forms thereof not found in the host plant, as a way of creating specific novel traits. The basic methodology, involving the use of T-DNA from the Ti-plasmid, was described already 35 years ago (Joos et al., 1983). However, the real revolution of today concerns "gene editing" (GE), which is a form of mutagenesis that directs changes to specific genes already in the host (Hilscher et al., 2017). The revolution got well underway about 7 years ago, with publication of the CRISPR-*Cas9* system (Jinek et al., 2012; Cong et al., 2013), which is simpler to set up than the earlier site-directed mutagenesis methods. While chemical and radiation mutagenesis might generate 100,000 more or less random changes in the genome (Hussain et al., 2018), GE generates one or very few at specific, targeted sites (Feng et al., 2018; Lee et al., 2019).

GE will have, if anything, a greater impact on agriculture than GM has had. This is because GE methods offer a reliable way to alter crop traits associated with any of the genes in a plant genome. The first implementation of CRISPR-*Cas9* created deletions that knocked out gene activity. More recently, a variation of GE, base editing, allows individual nucleotides to be changed for subtle alterations in gene function, creating finely targeted allelic variation (Kim, 2018). In essence, any of the 30,000 or so genes found in a monoploid plant genome could be edited, either alone or in combination with, in essence, any number of others. The greater the number of genomes sequenced, the greater the knowledge of the relationship between gene structure and function and between genes and traits, the more useful the technique will be. The ratchet of growth in scientific knowledge will make GE an increasingly subtle and powerful tool.

Plant biologists and breeders in both the public and private sectors are extremely excited about GE, because of the range of traits that will become accessible to improvement. These range from sustainability traits such as disease resistance and drought tolerance to increase in yield to removal of allergens and improvement of nutritional qualities (Kumlehn et al., 2018). Many products are already undergoing commercialization, particularly in the United States, including high-oleic-acid soy oil, high-fiber wheat, cold-storable potatoes, reduced-browning potatoes, celiac-friendly wheat, and maize with waxy starch (Schulman et al., 2019). It is widely understood that crop wild relatives hold the key to sustainability traits due to their high genetic diversity, much of which has been lost through domestication, as well as due to their survival without the inputs and interventions of agriculture (Mascher et al.,

2019). It has now been shown that GE offers the potential to redomesticate the wild relatives, without the difficult and lengthy process of backcrossing the exotic germplasm (assuming genetic compatibility) to an elite domesticated cultivar (Zsögön et al., 2018).

In light of its potential, GE methods are currently in use by researchers worldwide. However, the impact of GE on agriculture will be strongly affected by the regulatory framework around its use, as has that of GM. Currently, most of the American countries either does not regulate GE as if they were GMs or use product-based, rather than process-based, approaches on a case-by-case basis (Smyth, 2017; Schulman et al., 2019). Russia, China, Japan, and New Zealand appear to be heading as well toward a regulatory regime considerably more liberal than for GMs.

Nevertheless, the European Court of Justice (ECJ) confirmed in 2018, in their ruling (Case C-528/16; http://curia.europa.eu/juris/documents.jsf?num=c-528/162018), that all methods of mutagenesis create genetically modified organisms; "conventional" mutagenesis, meaning the inaccurate chemical and radiation methods of Stadler's time, is however exempted from regulation. Nevertheless, the plant lines created by the accurate, targeted GE methods nonetheless have to be regulated as GMs in Europe, even those that carry only deletions or single-nucleotide changes. The ruling, which flies in the face of both logic and scientific knowledge, has generated an enormous backlash among European scientists, not only at an individual level, but also at an institutional level, with more than 400 institutions having come forward in protest and demanding a remedy in the year following the ruling (Schulman et al., 2019). The ruling will generate enormous problems for national authorities in the EU regulating import and movement of GE food, feed, and plants because of the lack of traceability where the method is unregulated and due to the lack of detection methods that can distinguish foodstuffs from GEs without insertions from those derived from plants carrying other forms of genetic variation. While the final status of GEs in Europe remains contested, it is safe to say that worldwide the method will likely have enormous impact on agriculture and foodstuffs, limited only by what is possible in plants biochemically, physiologically, and developmentally.

References

Ainembabazi, J.H., et al., 2015. Ex-ante economic impact assessment of genetically modified banana resistant to xanthomonas wilt in the great Lakes region of Africa. PLoS One 10 (9).

Ammann, K., 2005. Effects of biotechnology on biodiversity: herbicide-tolerant and insect-resistant GM crops. Trends in Biotechnology 23 (8), 388−394.

Areal, F.J., Riesgo, L., Rodriguez-Cerezo, E., 2011. Attitudes of European farmers towards GM crop adoption. Plant Biotechnology Journal 9 (9), 945−957.

Azadi, H., Taube, F., Taheri, F., 2018. Co-existence of GM, conventional and organic crops in developing countries: main debates and concerns. Critical Reviews in Food Science and Nutrition 58 (16), 2677−2688.

Beachy, R.N., Loesch-Fries, S., Tumer, N.E., 1990. Coat protein-mediated resistance against virus infection. Annual Review of Phytopathology 28, 451–474.

Begg, G.S., et al., 2008. Heterogeneity in the distribution of genetically modified and conventional oilseed rape within fields and seed lots. Transgenic Research 17 (5), 805–816.

Brankov, T., et al., 2016. Gene revolution in agriculture: 20 years of controversy. In: Jamal, F. (Ed.), Genetic Engineering – an Insight into the Strategies and Applications. IntechOpen Limited, London, UK.

Brookes, G., Barfoot, P., 2017. Environmental impacts of genetically modified (GM) crop use 1996–2015: impacts on pesticide use and carbon emissions. GM Crops and Food 8 (2), 117–147.

Brookes, G., Barfoot, P., 2018. Farm income and production impacts of using GM crop technology 1996–2016. GM Crops and Food 9 (2), 59–89.

Carpenter, J.E., 2011. Impact of GM crops on biodiversity. GM Crops 2 (1), 7–23.

Carzoli, A.K., et al., 2018. Risks and opportunities of GM crops: Bt maize example. Global Food Security 19, 84–91.

Castiglioni, P., et al., 2008. Bacterial RNA chaperones confer abiotic stress tolerance in plants and improved grain yield in maize under water-limited conditions. Plant Physiology 147 (2), 446–455.

Colbach, N., 2009. How to model and simulate the effects of cropping systems on population dynamics and gene flow at the landscape level: example of oilseed rape volunteers and their role for co-existence of GM and non-GM crops. Environmental Science and Pollution Research International 16 (3), 348–360.

Comont, D., et al., 2019. Alterations in life-history associated with non-target-site herbicide resistance in Alopecurus myosuroides. Frontiers of Plant Science 10, 837.

Cong, L., et al., 2013. Multiplex genome engineering using CRISPR/Cas systems. Science 339 (6121), 819–823.

Dale, P.J., Clarke, B., Fontes, E.M., 2002. Potential for the environmental impact of transgenic crops. Nature Biotechnology 20 (6), 567–574.

Demont, M., et al., 2008. Regulating coexistence in europe: beware of the domino-effect! Ecological Genomics 64, 683–689.

Dewar, A.M., 2009. Weed control in glyphosate-tolerant maize in Europe. Pest Management Science 65 (10), 1047–1058.

Dixelius, C., Fagerstrom, T., Sundstrom, J.F., 2012. European agricultural policy goes down the tubers. Nature Biotechnology 30 (6), 492–493.

Doebley, J.F., Gaut, B.S., Smith, B.D., 2006. The molecular genetics of crop domestication. Cell 127 (7), 1309–1321.

Doh, J.P., Guay, T.R., 2006. Corporate social responsibility, public policy, and NGO activism in europe and the United States: an institutional-stakeholder perspective. Journal of Management Studies 43 (1), 47–73.

Dunwell, J.M., 2014. Genetically modified (GM) crops: European and transatlantic divisions. Molecular Plant Pathology 15 (2), 119–121.

Feng, C., et al., 2018. High-efficiency genome editing using a dmc1 promoter-controlled CRISPR/Cas9 system in maize. Plant Biotechnology Journal 16 (11), 1848–1857.

Finger, R., et al., 2011. Meta analysis on farm-level costs and benefits of GM crops. Sustainability 3, 743–762.

Fuchs, M., Gonsalves, D., 2007. Safety of virus-resistant transgenic plants two decades after their introduction: lessons from realistic field risk assessment studies. Annual Review of Phytopathology 45, 173–202.

Gallivan, G.J., Surgeoner, G.A., Kovach, J., 2001. Pesticide risk reduction on crops in the Province of Ontario. Journal of Environmental Quality 30 (3), 798–813.

Gianessi, L.P., et al., 2002. Plant Biotechnology: Current and Potential Impact for Improving Pest Management in US Agriculture: An Analysis of 40 Case Studies, vol. 75. National Center for Food and Agricultural Policy, Washington, DC.

Gomez-Barbero, M., Berbel, J., Rodriguez-Cerezo, E., 2008. Bt corn in Spain—the performance of the EU's first GM crop. Nature Biotechnology 26 (4), 384–386.

Green, J.M., et al., 2008. New multiple-herbicide crop resistance and formulation technology to augment the utility of glyphosate. Pest Management Science 64 (4), 332–339.

Gressel, J., Gassmann, A.J., Owen, M.D., 2017. How well will stacked transgenic pest/herbicide resistances delay pests from evolving resistance? Pest Management Science 73 (1), 22–34.

Heap, I., Duke, S.O., 2018. Overview of glyphosate-resistant weeds worldwide. Pest Management Science 74 (5), 1040–1049.

Herman, R.A., Price, W.D., 2013. Unintended compositional changes in genetically modified (GM) crops: 20 years of research. Journal of Agricultural and Food Chemistry 61 (48), 11695–11701.

Hilscher, J., Burstmayr, H., Stoger, E., 2017. Targeted modification of plant genomes for precision crop breeding. Biotechnology Journal 12 (1).

Huang, J., et al., 2002. Plant biotechnology in China. Science 295 (5555), 674–676.

Hussain, M., et al., 2018. Identification of induced mutations in hexaploid wheat genome using exome capture assay. PLoS One 13 (8), e0201918.

ISAAA, 2017. Global status of commercialized biotech/GM crops. In: 2017: Biotech Crop Adoption Surges as Economic Benefits Accumulate in 22 Years. ISAAA Brief No. 53. ISAAA. ISAAA, Ithaca, NY.

ISAAA, 2019. GM Traits List. Retrieved 26.09.2019, 2019, from. https://www.isaaa.org/gmapprovaldatabase/gmtraitslist/default.asp.

Jinek, M., et al., 2012. A programmable dual-RNA-guided DNA endonuclease in adaptive bacterial immunity. Science 337 (6096), 816–821.

Jones, P.J., et al., 2017. Assessing the potential economic benefits to farmers from various GM crops becoming available in the European Union by 2025: results from an expert survey. Agricultural Systems 155, 158–167.

Joos, H., et al., 1983. Genetic analysis of transfer and stabilization of agrobacterium DNA in plant cells. The EMBO Journal 2 (12), 2151–2160.

Kalaitzandonakes, N., Lusk, J., Magnier, A., 2018. The price of non-genetically modified (non-GM) food. Food Policy 78, 38–50.

Kamthan, A., et al., 2016. Genetically modified (GM) crops: milestones and new advances in crop improvement. Theoretical and Applied Genetics 129 (9), 1639–1655.

Kent, R.J., Johnson, D.E., Becker, M., 2001. The influences of cropping system on weed communities of rice in Côte d'Ivoire, West Africa. Agriculture, Ecosystems and Environment 87, 299–307.

Kim, J.S., 2018. Precision genome engineering through adenine and cytosine base editing. Native Plants 4 (3), 148–151.

Klumper, W., Qaim, M., 2014. A meta-analysis of the impacts of genetically modified crops. PLoS One 9 (11).

Kouser, S., Qaim, M., 2011. Impact of Bt cotton on pesticide poisoning in smallholder agriculture: a panel data analysis. Ecological Economics 70, 2105–2113.

Kramer, M.G., Redenbaugh, K., 1994. Commercialization of a tomato with an antisense poly-galacturonase gene - the flavr savr(Tm) tomato story. Euphytica 79 (3), 293–297.

Kreuze, J.F., Valkonen, J.P., 2017. Utilization of engineered resistance to viruses in crops of the developing world, with emphasis on sub-Saharan Africa. Current Opinion in Virology 26, 90–97.

Krishna, V., Qaim, M., Zilberman, D., 2016. Transgenic crops, production risk and agrobiodiversity. European Review of Agricultural Economics 43 (1), 137–164.

Kumlehn, J., et al., 2018. The CRISPR/Cas revolution continues: from efficient gene editing for crop breeding to plant synthetic biology. Journal of Integrative Plant Biology 60 (12), 1127–1153.

Lazebnik, J., et al., 2017. Biodiversity analyses for risk assessment of genetically modified potato. Agriculture, Ecosystems and Environment 249, 196–205.

Lee, K., et al., 2019. Activities and specificities of CRISPR/Cas9 and Cas12a nucleases for targeted mutagenesis in maize. Plant Biotechnology Journal 17 (2), 362–372.

Lin, Z., et al., 2012. Parallel domestication of the Shattering1 genes in cereals. Nature Genetics 44 (6), 720–724.

Lucht, J.M., 2015. Public acceptance of plant biotechnology and GM crops. Viruses 7 (8), 4254–4281.

Lundgren, J.G., et al., 2009. Ecological compatibility of GM crops and biological control. Crop Protection 28, 1017–1030.

Martin, S.L., et al., 2017. Glyphosate resistance reduces kochia fitness: comparison of segregating resistant and susceptible F2 populations. Plant Science 261, 69–79.

Mascher, M., et al., 2019. Genebank genomics bridges the gap between the conservation of crop diversity and plant breeding. Nature Genetics 51 (7), 1076–1081.

McCluskey, J.J., Wesseler, J., Winfree, J.A., 2018. The economics and politics GM food labeling: an introduction to the special issue. Food Policy 78, 1–5.

McCluskey, J.J., Winfree, J., 2017. The economics of GM labeling and implications for trade. Journal of Agricultural and Food Industrial Organization 15, 20160017.

National Research Council, 2010. The Impact of Genetically Engineered Crops on Farm Sustainability in the United States. The National Academies Press, Washington, DC.

Nausch, H., et al., 2015. Public funded field trials with transgenic plants in Europe: a comparison between Germany and Switzerland. Current Opinion in Biotechnology 32, 171–178.

Paarlberg, R., 2014. A dubious success: the NGO campaign against GMOs. GM Crops and Food 5 (3), 223–228.

Pandolfo, C.E., et al., 2018. Transgene escape and persistence in an agroecosystem: the case of glyphosate-resistant Brassica rapa L. in central Argentina. Environmental Science and Pollution Research International 25 (7), 6251–6264.

Pidgeon, J.D., et al., 2007. Mitigation of indirect environmental effects of GM crops. Proceedings, Biological Sciences 274 (1617), 1475–1479.

Qaim, M., 2009. The economics of genetically modified crops. Annual Review of Resource Economics 1, 6665–6693.

Qaim, M., Zilberman, D., 2003. Yield effects of genetically modified crops in developing countries. Science 299 (5608), 900–902.

Romeis, J., et al., 2019. Genetically engineered crops help support conservation biological control. Biological Control 130, 136–154.

Saeglitz, C., Bartsch, D., 2003. Regulatory and associated political issues with respect to Bt transgenic maize in the European Union. Journal of Invertebrate Pathology 83 (2), 107–109.

Sammons, B., et al., 2014. Characterization of drought-tolerant maize Mon 87460 for use in environmental risk assessment. Crop Science 54, 719–729.

Sanvido, O., Romeis, J., Bigler, F., 2007. Ecological impacts of genetically modified crops: ten years of field research and commercial cultivation. Advances in Biochemical Engineering 107, 235–278.

Schulman, A.H., Oksman-Caldentey, K.M., Teeri, T.H., July 2019. European court of justice delivers no justice to Europe on genome-edited crops. Plant Biotechnology Journal pp. 1–3. https://doi.org/10.1111/pbi.13200.

Seufert, V., Ramankutty, N., Foley, J.A., 2012. Comparing the yields of organic and conventional agriculture. Nature 485 (7397), 229–232.

Smyth, S.J., 2017. Canadian regulatory perspectives on genome engineered crops. GM Crops and Food 8 (1), 35–43.

Smyth, S.J., Kerr, W.A., Phillips, P.W.B., 2015. Global economic, environmental and health benefits from GM crop adoption. Global Food Security 7, 24–29.

Stadler, L.J., 1930. Some genetic effects of X-rays in plants. Journal of Heredity 21, 3–19.

Taheri, F., Azadi, H., D'Haese, M., 2017. A world without hunger: organic or GM crops? Sustainability 9 (4).

Van Eenennaam, A.L., Young, A.E., 2014. Prevalence and impacts of genetically engineered feedstuffs on livestock populations. Journal of Animal Science 92 (10), 4255–4278.

Varacca, A., Soregaroli, C., 2016. Identity preservation in international feed supply chains. EuroChoices 15 (1), 38–43.

Varzakas, T.H., Arvanitoyannis, I.S., Baltas, H., 2007. The politics and science behind GMO acceptance. Critical Reviews in Food Science and Nutrition 47 (4), 335–361.

Weekes, R., et al., 2005. Crop-to-crop gene flow using farm scale sites of oilseed rape (Brassica napus) in the UK. Transgenic Research 14 (5), 749–759.

Winfree, J.A., McCluskey, J.J., 2017. The economics of GM labeling and implications for trade. Journal of Agricultural and Food Industrial Organization 15 (1). https://doi.org/10.1515/jafio-2016-0017.

Zilberman, D., 2012. Lessons from Prop 37 and the Future of Genetic Engineering in Agriculture. The Berkeley Blog, Energy and Environment 2012. Retrieved 28.08, 2019, from. https://blogs.berkeley.edu/2012/12/20/lessons-from-prop-37-and-the-future-of-genetic-engineering-in-agriculture/.

Zsögön, A., et al., 2018. De novo domestication of wild tomato using genome editing. Nature Biotechnology 36, 1211–1216.

Irradiated food

What is the benefit of irradiation compared to other methods of food preservation?

Anuradha Prakash, PhD

Food Science Program, Schmid College of Science and Technology, Chapman University, One University Drive, Orange, CA, United States

Introduction

Commercially available food products are processed using a range of technologies ranging from as minimal as cleaning and peeling to extensive processing involving multiple treatments to meet consumer preferences in terms of sensory attributes, price, or lifestyle needs and to extend shelf-life and/or assure safety. Conventional methods include thermal processing, dehydration, refrigeration and freezing, and extrusion. Consumers are increasingly interested in products that are minimally processed and formulated without chemical preservatives, and the food industry has responded by developing nonthermal technologies such as high-pressure processing (HPP), pulsed electric field (PEF), and thermal technologies such as ohmic heating, which maximize retention of quality and nutrition while achieving pasteurization goals. In fact, processors have available an arsenal of food processing technologies that singly or in combination can be used to preserve food products. Many products are preserved using a hurdle approach, where several sublethal treatments, such as mild heat, refrigeration, pH control, water activity, and redox potential, used in combination, can effectively suppress microbial growth.

Irradiation processing of food cannot be classified as conventional nor can it be considered novel. It has been used for various food ingredients and products since the 1950s, yet its use has not been widespread enough to be considered conventional. In large part, irradiation processing has been stymied by its categorization as a food additive requiring that irradiated foods be labeled as such and thus contributing to consumer wariness about this technology (Koutchma et al., 2018). So while irradiation of certain ingredients, spices, and dehydrated seasonings in particular, which as minor ingredients in foods are not required to be labeled, has been common, irradiation of finished products has not achieved commercial success, except in China where irradiated snacks are commonly found in the marketplace. Nevertheless, keeping in mind that consumers are increasingly educated and interested in nonchemical forms of food preservation, we should consider the particular benefits

Genetically Modified and Irradiated Food. https://doi.org/10.1016/B978-0-12-817240-7.00013-9

that irradiation offers related to its mode of action on microorganisms, parasites, and insect pests that spoil our food and cause disease. Current commercial uses of food irradiation include pasteurization and sterilization, insect disinfestation and sprout inhibition. Table 9.1 shows the technologies currently used for these applications and the sections below discuss the benefits and limitations of these technologies and the specific advantages that irradiation offers.

Pasteurization and sterilization
Thermal

Heat processing is probably the most commonly used technology to achieve microbial reduction and enzyme inactivation in foods (Floros et al., 2010). Thermal pasteurization and sterilization equipment is widely available and the process is economical. In-container or canned food sterilization has a long history of use dating back to the early 1800s (Ramaswamy and Marcotte, 2005), and recent advances in retorts and packaging have maintained interest in the technology. Aseptic processing allows for quicker heating and cooling of the product prior to packaging in sterile containers and confers better quality and nutrient retention than conventionally canned products. Consumer emphasis on minimal processing products has encouraged development of newer thermal processes such as microwaves and radiofrequency technology, which utilize dielectric heating to raise the temperature of products rapidly and volumetrically. Ohmic heating, which relies on the heat generated by resistance of the food to the flow of electricity, is currently used in the processing or pasteurization/sterilization of various food products such as sliced and whole fruit in syrup, soup, panko bread, surimi products, tofu, and meat (Sastry, personal communication).

Regardless of the thermal process used, the basis of microbial destruction is the same. Heating affects the bonds necessary for stable protein structures. At temperatures specific to each protein, enzymes and membrane proteins start to unfold (denature), affecting vital functions and ultimately leading to cell death. Adequate microbial destruction is dependent upon process temperature and time. Achieving process temperature can be challenging in solid foods where heat is transferred by conduction, and there can be a large temperature gradient between the surface and center of the food. In the time required for the center of the product to reach processing temperature, the surface of the food can be overly heated, resulting in degradation of quality. For products that can flow, heat transfer occurs via convection and process temperatures can be achieved more uniformly, helping preserve quality. These products can be heated to high temperature for short times (HTST) or ultrahigh temperature (UHT), which also contributes to better retention of quality factors. For spices, nuts, and other granular food materials, steam sterilization may be used. While steam at 100°C will destroy most vegetative pathogens, inactivation of spores requires saturated steam at temperatures closer to 118–120°C and

Table 9.1 Commercial food technologies currently used to achieve pasteurization, sterilization, insect disinfestation, and sprouting.

Technology	Products
I. Pasteurization and sterilization	
a. Thermal	
i. Canning	Fruit and vegetables, beans, fish and seafood, meat, milk and cream, soups, broths, condiments, pet food
ii. Aseptic	Fruit and vegetable purees, juice, milk, cream, creamers, soups, broths, pet food
iii. Microwave/ radiofrequency/ohmic	Prepared meals
b. Nonthermal	
i. High-Pressure Processing	Juices, salad dressings, fruit and vegetable pastes, purees, preserves, deli meat, prepared meals, salads
ii. Pulsed electric field	Juice
iii. Irradiation	Spices, seasonings, dehydrated vegetables, refrigerated and frozen ground beef and poultry, fermented chicken feet and wings, snack foods, NASA meals, oysters, frog legs
c. Chemical	
a. Ethylene oxide and propylene oxide	Spices, seeds, nuts, dehydrated vegetables
II. Insect disinfestation	
a. Thermal	
i. Hot water immersion	Mangoes, papayas, lime
ii. Vapor heat	Bell pepper, aubergine, papaya, pineapple, squash, tomato, courgette, citrus, lychee, mango, pitaya, rambutan
iii. High-temperature forced air	Citrus, mango, papaya, rambutan
b. Nonthermal	
i. Cold treatment or quick freeze	Citrus, apples, pear, stone fruit, kiwifruit, carambola, loquats, papaya, quince, pomegranate
c. Chemical	
i. Fumigants	
a. Methyl bromide	Quarantine and preshipment treatments of fresh fruits and durables (e.g., grain, flour, nuts, dried fruit)
b. Phosphine	Fresh fruits and durables
c. Sulfuryl fluoride	Durables
d. Ethyl formate	Possibly dried fruit, cereals, tobacco
ii. Insecticidal dips and sprays (Fenthion[a], dimethoate[a], pyrethrins)	Fresh fruit
III. Inhibition of sprouting	
a. Chemical	
i. CIPC (Chlorpropham)	Potatoes, onions, garlic
ii. Maleic hydrazide	Onions, garlic

[a] *Phased out in many countries.*

pressures of 10–15 psi. For spices, seeds, and nuts, vacuum-assisted steam pasteurization or sterilization has become increasingly popular although the high temperatures can cause discoloration and reduction of volatile oil content in some spices (Almela et al., 2002).

Heating causes irreversible changes in food components (Fellows, 2016a). For example, starches hydrate and gelatinize and proteins denature, resulting in changes in viscosity and mouthfeel. Caramelization and Maillard reactions lead to production of flavor and aroma compounds and color changes. In some cases, these changes in product attributes are desirable and make the food edible and palatable; but depending on the extent of processing, undesirable changes may be manifested in the product. Pigments present in cellular matrices change so that color intensity is decreased or color is modified. Lipid and protein oxidation reactions may be accelerated leading to the production of off-flavors and off-odors. Almost always, heat processing changes the characteristics of the product so that the processed product is significantly different from the fresh product. Heating also impacts nutritional value, both positively and negatively. By destroying antinutritive factors, heating increases availability of certain nutrients in various foods including beans, cereal grains, eggs, fish, and soybeans (IFT, 1975). However, heating can reduce nutrient content of foods. Vitamin B1 (thiamin) and vitamin C (ascorbic acid) are particularly heat labile and used as indices of the extent of heat processing. Loss of these vitamins into processing water as would occur during washing, blanching, and cooling for example, further exaggerates the loss (Reddy and Love, 1999). Extensive heat processing can also destroy essential amino acids (IFT, 1975).

Because of these heat-induced changes in product quality, there is great interest in nonthermal technologies that can maintain freshness but deliver the safety and shelf life needed in a product offered for retail sale. Refrigeration and freezing do not destroy microorganisms but the low temperatures reduce microbial growth and increase shelf life. There is renewed interest in this market segment due to the perception that refrigerated food is less processed. Refrigeration is also commonly used as part of a hurdle approach but is not by itself able to deliver the microbial reduction needed for pasteurized foods.

Nonthermal

In the last decade, the use of HPP in the United States and Europe has exploded. HPP involves applications of 400–1000 MPa of pressure applied to food, usually prepackaged, using water as the pressure conveying medium. The increase in pressure within the food is instantaneous and isostatic and destroys microbial cells by disrupting noncovalent bonds which are important to maintain structures of large macromolecules such as enzymes and damage the cell membrane. The transfer of pressure requires a certain amount of moisture, generally considered to be 40%, thus treatment is limited to moist and semimoist foods. At this time, HPP is used for pasteurization purposes for a variety of foods including juices, salad dressings, jams, fruit and vegetables pastes, deli meat, prepared meals, and salads. Inactivation of vegetative cells is achieved at 400–600 MPa, but spore inactivation requires pulsing of pressure or combination with heat (Balasubramaniam and Farkas, 2008).

PEFs, which involve the application of high-intensity electric pulses, 10–80 kV/cm, for a short period of time (1–100 μs), have only recently been commercialized. The mechanisms of inactivation include electroporation of the cell membrane, activity of reactive oxygen species, oxidation and reduction reactions within the cell, and transient temperature increase, which can be up to $\sim 30°C$, depending upon the field strength and frequency and number of pulses (Fellows, 2016b). Pasteurization can be achieved but spores are not inactivated. Continuous pasteurization is limited to liquid foods and particles, if present, need to be small. The liquid should be of relatively low conductivity and able to withstand high electric field and absent of any bubbles.

Chemical

Dry and granular products such as spices, seeds, nuts, and dehydrated vegetables can be sterilized by fumigating with ethylene oxide (EtO) or propylene oxide (PPO) (Atungulu and Pan, 2012). Despite low moisture content, these products tend to be highly contaminated because they are often dried or fermented under the sun in open air and subject to contamination from soil, insects, rodents, birds, and humans (Duncan et al., 2017). *Salmonella* is the major bacterial concern associated with spices, and the vast majority of illnesses are associated with consumption of foods to which spices have been added after the processing (Van Doren et al., 2013). Thus, it is especially critical that decontaminated spices are used on ready-to-eat products not subject to further microbial reducing processes. EtO is not allowed in the EU and in the United States; it is allowed as a reconditioning technology on detained spices or spice blends that do not contain salt (US CFR, 1996). EtO and PPO processing involves a preconditioning step to preheat and humidify the product prior to sterilization following by aeration to accelerate out gassing and eliminate any residual EtO or PPO from the product. The process generally requires a day or more. Some EtO-processed spices exhibit changes in color, flavor, and volatile oils related to the partial vacuum necessary during off gassing (Vajdi and Pereira, 1973).

Irradiation

Irradiation is a nonthermal technology but has vastly greater versatility than the thermal and nonthermal processes described above, in that it can be used on a wide range of products from dry such as spices and seasonings to higher moisture products such as meat and poultry. Because irradiation is a volumetric treatment, the irregular shape of many foods is much less of a problem than with conventional treatments. At present, it is used to extend the shelf life and safety of spices, seasonings, dehydrated vegetables, refrigerated and frozen ground beef and poultry, fermented chicken feet and wings, NASA meals, oysters, and frog legs. The minimal increase in temperature allows irradiation to be used on products at room temperature, as well as refrigerated or frozen without requiring that they be thawed for processing.

Ionizing irradiation uses gamma, e-beams, or X-rays to inactivate microorganisms and insects. The direct impact of photons or electrons and the indirect effects of generated reactive oxygen species and free ions lead to damage to cellular DNA and RNA and cell membranes. Enzyme activity is also affected impacting normal functioning of the cell eventually causing devitalization or death of the organism. The sensitivity to irradiation is expressed as D value which is the dose required for a one log or 90% reduction of microbial cells. D values of bacterial pathogens range from 0.24 kGy for *Escherichia coli* O157:H7 to 0.45 kGy for *Salmonella* spp. to 2–4 kGy for spore-forming bacteria such as *Clostridium botulinum* (Sommers and Fan, 2008). Thus doses of 1–7 kGy are used to provide pasteurization treatment for chicken, beef, and seafood, while higher doses, >10 kGy, are used to sterilize spices, seasonings, pet treats, NASA meals, hospital food, and snack products. Simultaneous reductions of spoilage organisms help to extend shelf-life commensurate with safety.

In addition to bacterial pathogens, parasite control could be a valuable use of irradiation. A 2014 report issued by the Food and Agriculture Organization (FAO/WHO, 2014) ranked the 10 most important parasites worldwide based on multiple criteria (number of global foodborne illnesses, global distribution, morbidity severity, case fatality ratio, likelihood of increased human burden, relevance to international trade, and impact on economically vulnerable commodities). Parasite occurrence in fresh produce is the cause for heightened concern especially since these commodities are often consumed in the raw state and also because of increased global trade in such products. Common sanitation approaches such as chlorination and acidification used to clean fruits and vegetables are ineffective against common parasites. The US Food and Drug Administration allows use of 0.3–1 kGy to control *Trichinella spiralis* in pork. These doses would also be effective to control *Anisakis* spp. in fish, *Toxoplasma gondii* in meat and poultry, and *Cryptosporidium* in fresh fruit and vegetables (Anonymous, 1993).

As a nonthermal treatment, irradiation offers particular benefits for products that may be consumed without further processing such as fresh or minimally processed lettuce and spinach that may be used in salads, oysters that are eaten raw, herbs that are used as garnish, ready-to-eat snacks and treats that are not heated before consumption, meat products that may be consumed "rare" or not cooked sufficiently to inactivate bacterial pathogens, and spices or seasonings which may lose flavor, color, or aroma by heat processing or EtO.

In recent years, there has been a huge demand for ready-to-eat foods that not only meet the criteria for convenience and cost but also satisfy consumer demand for freshness and notion of healthfulness. Ready-to-eat foods include complete single or multicomponent meals, snacks, salads, cereals, nuts, seasonings, fish, shellfish, deli meats, and fruits and vegetables that can be consumed directly without further cooking or other processing. Some ready-to-eat products such as canned foods have been traditionally sterilized and pose low risk of foodborne illness. Similarly, fully cooked snacks with low water activity such as potato chips present low risk of microbial hazards. However, refrigerated foods that are heat processed but not sterilized present a higher risk of foodborne illness. Of particular concern are extended shelf life refrigerated foods, which have received none or some treatment but may contain sufficient numbers of pathogens that can multiply during extended storage. These products include salads, pasta products, seafood, soups, ready-to-heat meals, fruit purees, and juices. These are products whose safety could be significantly enhanced with irradiation.

From a nutritional point of view, proteins are resistant to irradiation, with little effect on digestibility and amino acid composition, thus meat-, poultry- and fish-based foods are good candidates for irradiation. Carbohydrates such as pectins and starches may be hydrolyzed or depolymerized leading to changes in viscosity or firmness in fruits and vegetables limiting the irradiation dose that they can tolerate. Lipids are the most sensitive macromolecule to food irradiation because of irradiation-induced autoxidation or the direct or indirect impact of irradiation on lipid molecules (Molins, 2001). In mixed foods, these effects are limited and similar to the effects of heat processing, but foods that are very high in fat may not be suitable for irradiation.

The extent of vitamin loss is not different from heat processing, but the specific vitamins affected by irradiation are somewhat different from heat-sensitive vitamins. Among the fat-soluble vitamins, vitamin E is sensitive to irradiation followed by vitamin A and carotenoids. However, the major sources of food for these vitamins, milk and dairy products for vitamin A, and oils, nuts, and butter for vitamin E, are unlikely candidates for irradiation. Fruits and vegetables, which are good sources of carotenes and vitamin E, would be treated at doses too low to affect dietary intake. Among the water-soluble vitamins, B1 and C, both highly heat labile, are also the most sensitive to irradiation. The destruction of these vitamins is limited when the food is refrigerated or frozen during irradiation processing. In general, food irradiation is considered unlikely to have an impact on population nutritional adequacy (Woodside, 2015).

Insect disinfestation
Thermal

Fresh foods, particularly fruits and vegetables, grains, nuts, and spices, traded between countries are subject to phytosanitary measures that are designed to inactivate pests that otherwise could harm agriculture or the environment if they were to be established in new areas (Hallman and Blackburn, 2016). The International Plant Protection Convention (IPPC) supports phytosanitary treatments that are effective in killing, inactivating or removing pests, or rendering pests infertile or for devitalization. Treatments should be proven feasible and not cause adverse effects (IPPC, 2016). Conventional thermal treatments include hot water immersion, vapor heat, and forced hot air. Nonthermal treatments used for fresh produce include cold fumigation with methyl bromide or phosphine and irradiation (Tang et al., 2007).

Heat treatments are generally easy to apply and to control, do not leave a chemical residue, and are relatively low cost. Hot water dips require the fruit to be dipped in water and be heated to an internal temperature of >40°C for up to 90 min. Hot water provides uniform heating and simultaneous cleaning of the fruit. The fruit may or may not be cooled following the hot water dip. This treatment is commonly used for mangoes from Mexico, Puerto Rico, Virgin Islands, and the West Indies and requires the mangoes to be heated to 43–46.7°C for 35–90 min in a batch or continuous system (Collin et al., 2007). While hot water treatment offers the advantages of easy installation in packing houses and much lower cost than most other phytosanitary treatments, it can cause significant internal and external damage to the fruit, particularly skin scalding, darkened lenticels, and internal cavities. Fruit maturation is also accelerated, so fruit subjected to hot water dips are usually treated while fairly unripe to provide sufficient shelf life (Tang et al., 2007).

Vapor heat treatment uses saturated steam to increase the temperature of the fruit as the steam condenses on its surface. Heat transfer into the fruit is slower with vapor heat than it is with hot water requiring 6–8 h for the internal temperature of 43–44°C to be achieved which is then maintained for an additional 6–8 h (Tang et al., 2007). In high-temperature forced-air treatments, hot (40–50°C) air is circulated through cases of fruit. The hot air is humidified which helps to reduce dehydration of the fruit surface.

With all heat treatments, the major concern is the effect on fruit quality and while only heat-tolerant fruit are subjected to this treatment, examples of heat-damaged fruit are abundant in the market. Heat treatments are also used for spices, grains, nuts, and dried fruits (Tang et al., 2007).

Nonthermal

Cold treatment is probably among the easiest of treatments; exposure to cold temperatures, 0–3.3°C, for an extended period can achieve satisfactory disinfestation for cold-tolerant fruit such as apples and grapes. The treatment can be applied to fruit following packing and during transit. The disadvantage of this method is the long treatment time necessary and also the treatment does not destroy all pests adequately (Sharp, 1993). Quick freezing may be used for thick-skinned fruit such as durian or coconuts and because of impacts on quality; it is not common and only used for commodities that will be further processed to make puree or juice (USDA-APHIS, 2016).

Chemical

Fumigation utilizes gaseous forms of chemicals that at certain temperature, pressure, and time combinations can satisfactorily eliminate pest risk. While several compounds can achieve pest destruction, the challenges lie with toxicity, chemical instability, and environmental effects (Bond, 1989). The most common fumigant in use today is methyl bromide, a broad-spectrum fumigant. Advantages of methyl bromide include its high penetration rate into the commodity and ability to vaporize readily following treatment. However, methyl bromide releases elemental bromine in the stratosphere, which is highly destructive to the ozone layer. Methyl bromide is a class 1 ozone-depleting substance, and for this reason its use has been increasingly restricted as specified by the Montreal Protocol (UNEP, 2018). While critical use exceptions remain for its use as a quarantine treatment, it is expected to be phased out for postharvest use as soon as viable alternate treatments are identified.

Phosphine or hydrogen phosphide (PH_3), a gas usually produced from aluminum or magnesium phosphide, also has a high penetration depth into tightly packed bulk materials. It is highly toxic to insect pests but requires a long exposure time, several days, for sufficient destruction of insects (Jobling et al., 2002). The effectiveness of phosphine is low at refrigerated temperatures, thus for fruit products that need to be maintained at low temperatures to maintain quality, long exposure times would be needed. Unlike methyl bromide, phosphine is flammable, but like methyl bromide, it is toxic and leaves a residue. Sulfuryl fluoride is another fumigant; however, its use is generally limited to wood pests (USDA-APHIS, 2016).

Irradiation

Irradiation has been used as a phytosanitary treatment for fresh fruit and vegetables continuously since 1996, and since 2000, its global use has increased by $\sim 10\%$ per year due to reduced use of chemical fumigants and its broad efficacy (Hallman and Blackburn, 2016). In contrast to other phytosanitary measures, acute mortality is not the goal, rather it is the prevention of adult emergence. Another point of differentiation is the use of generic doses, a set of specific doses used for groups of quarantine pests and/or commodities rather than specific doses for each insect/commodity pairing. The irradiation doses used for most insect groups are fairly low. For example, a generic dose of 150 Gy is used against Tephritid fruit flies, which is a significant and common regulated pest group, and 400 Gy is used as a generic dose against all insects except pupae and adults of Lepidoptera (moths and butterflies). In New Zealand, 500 Gy is the generic dose for mites other than Tetranychidae (Hallman and Blackburn, 2016). For fruit from certain countries that present a high risk of invasive pests, irradiation is the only accepted phytosanitary treatment. For mangoes from India, as an example, irradiation is the only accepted treatment by the United States and Australia. In contrast to heat, cold, or fumigants which need to diffuse through the tissue by conduction or diffusion, irradiation is a volumetric treatment resulting in target doses being achieved quickly and efficiently eradicating internal and surface pests. In addition to the broad efficacy of irradiation against insect pests, the doses used are tolerated well by many fruits and vegetables with little to no loss of quality. In fact, the tolerance to irradiation is greater than to fumigation or thermal treatments which can cause disorders due to the high temperatures and long times used for the treatments. Irradiation facilities, especially newer ones are refrigerated so there is no break in the cold chain, and the treatment is quick. A truckload of product can generally be treated within a few hours. It is important to note that the treatment is applied to fresh produce that is already packaged in its final, pest-proof container, minimizing the possibility of pest infestation following treatment. This feature is very important to reduce pest risk and has helped develop a robust global trade in irradiated fresh produce.

Commodities that are highly tolerant to the dose distribution achieved in commercial processing include apples, bell peppers, blueberries, dragon fruit, grape, grapefruit, guava, lime, longan, lychee, mango, manzano pepper, papaya, peach, persimmon, plum, pummelo, rambutan, sweet cherries, sweet potato, and tomato (Hallman and Blackburn, 2016). Some fruit such as certain varieties of citrus and avocadoes are less tolerant and develop disorders especially at the higher than target doses that may be experienced in some parts of the pallet or case of fruit. Other fruit can experience loss of firmness at higher doses. Generally, the tolerance to irradiation varies by variety, maturity stage, harvest season, and pre- and postharvest conditions such as water and temperature stresses; thus, growers and shippers must ensure that the specific cultivar/variety is tolerant of the doses under commercial conditions of distribution (Prakash and Foley, 2004). Radiation can be considered to be an abiotic stress, and it can affect physiological processes, especially in climacteric fruit. In mangoes and papayas for example, irradiation treatment can delay ripening, but it does so without affecting final eating quality. For some fruit, the delay in ripening can serve as an advantage in terms of shelf life (Prakash, 2016). Additionally, spoilage by decay organisms might be inhibited albeit to a small extent, but for some fruit, an extension of even a few days can provide an economic benefit (Fan et al., 2008).

Inhibition of sprouting
Chemical

Potatoes: Cold temperature storage (2–4°C) is effective at extending the dormancy period of potatoes, but these potatoes will sprout at once after being brought to warmer temperatures. Cold temperature storage is not used for potatoes destined for consumer consumption or the processing market because cold storage increases the concentration of reducing sugars resulting in increased sweetness and a darker color when processed at high temperatures such as frying. Isopropyl N-(3 chlorophenyl) carbonate (CIPC), also known as chlorpropham, is the most commonly used chemical to inhibit sprouting in potatoes in the world (Paul et al., 2016) and many other countries. It interferes with cell division and long-term sprout inhibition can be achieved with a single application. When CIPC is applied using a process called thermal fogging, CIPC is degraded to form aniline-based derivatives, one of which is 3-chloroaniline (3-CA). This compound is of increasing health concern due to its similarity in structure to 2-CA and 4-CA which are considered carcinogenic to humans (Paul et al., 2016). In addition, other metabolites of CIPC are also considered to be harmful to human and animal health and the environment. Because of the lack of alternative effective sprout suppressants and the long history of use, the potato industry is dependent on the use of CIPC. However, as health concerns related to CIPC become clearer, alternatives to CIPC will be needed.

For garlic and onions, sprouting and rooting are major reasons for postharvest loss during storage. In addition to CIPC, maleic hydrazide, an herbicide and plant growth regulator, is commonly used as a preharvest foliar spray or postharvest bulb treatment to reduce sprouting during dormancy. It effectively stops cell division but does not affect cell expansion. A residue of maleic hydrazide on the bulb is necessary to prevent sprouting. Similar to CIPC, maleic hydrazide is also being evaluated by regulators for its effect on human health (Petropoulos et al., 2016).

Irradiation

Irradiation at very low doses, generally 60−120 Gy, is used commercially on potatoes shortly after harvest while they are in their dormant state (Ogata, 1973). In Japan, potatoes are the only commodity that can be treated with irradiation and have been treated as such since 1973 (Prakash, 2016), although the amounts have been steadily declining. Treating the potatoes as close to harvest helps ensure high efficacy in sprout inhibition as well as minimal increase in reducing sugars. China treats garlic and India treats onions and garlic at 60 Gy (Prakash, 2016). The high quality of the irradiated product, inhibition of sprouting, and increase in shelf life, lack of chemical residues, make this is a valuable technology for extending the shelf life of potatoes, onions, and garlic. However, similar to other food applications of irradiation, the use of this technology remains underutilized.

Conclusion

Compared to established treatments, irradiation offers tremendous benefits in terms of efficacy on microorganisms, parasites, and insects, the lack of quality and nutritional defects, and the versatility of products that can be treated. Particularly for products such as fresh foods, for which no other treatments exist, there is a compelling rationale for using irradiation.

Table 9.2 is an SWOT analysis for food irradiation, which highlights the major advantages of using irradiation. As the weakness section points out, the technology is not suitable for all foods and all applications, but where appropriate, it can play a major role in making our food safer, reducing food waste, and fostering trade. The use of irradiation treatment for food remains hampered mainly due to labeling requirements and policy constraints in terms of regulatory approvals needed and lack of harmonization in irradiation-related regulations between countries. Other barriers, such as lack of facilities and costs, will be addressed by the market as demand for the technology increases. There is a continued need, however, for

Table 9.2 SWOT Analysis of food irradiation.

Strengths

- Efficacy
  - Highly effective against pathogens and pests
  - Volumetric treatment allows penetration through solid food and efficacy on irregular shapes
- Safety
  - No health concerns related to irradiated food
  - Postpackaging treatment reduces chances of postprocessing microbial contamination
  - Established history of safe use
- Nonthermal/nonchemical treatment
  - Can be used on fresh produce, raw meat, poultry, and fish
  - Maintains quality and nutritional value
- Environmentally friendly
  - Does not deplete the ozone layer
  - No chemical residues
- Process control
  - Continuous
  - Dose distribution can be measured
- Facilitates trade
  - Physical alternative to use of chemicals
  - Generic treatments facilitate treatment
  - Only treatment option in some cases (phytosanitary, for example)
  - Best treatment option in many cases

Weaknesses

- Certain irradiation-resistant pathogens and toxins require high doses:
- Clostridium botulinum, viruses such as hepatitis A
- Not configured for use on liquid products
- Certain foods are radiosensitive: high-lipid-containing products, some fruit
- Regulations
  - Considered to be an additive in many countries, requires labeling
  - Each new product requires approval
  - The FDA limit of 1 kGy on fresh produce is difficult to maintain for certain processors
  - Lack of harmonized global standards
- Logistical
  - ost: adequate product volume must be treated in order to maximize the use of the facility and minimize the unit cost of treatment
  - Lack of facilities at locations where irradiation may be used
  - Supply chain logistics—extra transportation, handling
  - Lack of packaging options—regulations only approved for a few basic packaging options
- Consumer acceptance
  - Lack of understanding and the negative connotation of the term "radiation"
  - Distributor and retailer apprehension of consumer acceptance
  - Labeling requirement perceived as a warning rather than simply information

Table 9.2 SWOT Analysis of food irradiation.—*cont'd*

Opportunities

- Equipment: smaller scale or self-shielded in-line units
- Low-energy electron beam for surface treatment
- Multilateral harmonization of standards
- Can be used to comply with the Food Safety Modernization Act as a validated preventive control
- Information literacy:
  - Create education platforms that are easy to access and use
  - Provide guidance to growers, distributors, retailers through application briefs and case studies
  - Develop cost benefit and feasibility evaluations
  - Provide training
- Consumer Education
  - Focus on the product
  - Highlight the benefits
- Identify niche applications—where other technologies are not (or not as) effective, such as for phytosanitary uses, efficacy in reducing parasite load on foods, or in situations where there is a cost or trade benefit.
- Estimate the economic benefits of irradiating food due to reduced foodborne disease outbreaks, increased trade, and associated benefits

Threats

- Negative events
  - Accidents
  - Loss of process control
- Not doing enough
  - Not taking the initiative
  - Losing momentum
- Doing too much
  - Overpromising on safety and quality

information literacy regarding food irradiation. Comprehensive application scenarios should be made available to potential users complete with cost benefit analyses that highlight the benefits of irradiation for their products and feasibility of commercial irradiation processing. To be effective, this information must be easy to locate, access, and apply to solve the challenge on hand. Such an endeavor would require all stakeholders processors, users, educators, and regulators to work together.

References

Almela, L., Nieto-Sandoval, J.M., Fernandez Lopez, J.A., 2002. Microbial inactivation of paprika by a high-temperature short-X time treatment. Influence on color properties. Journal of Agricultural and Food Chemistry 50 (6), 1435—1440.

Anonymous, 1993. Use of irradiation to control infectivity of food-borne parasites. In: Proceedings of a Final Research Co-ordination Meeting. International Atomic Energy Agency, 24–28 June 1991, Mexico City, Mexico. STI/PUB/93 Panel Proceedings Series, Vienna, Austria.

Atungulu, G., Pan, Z., 2012. Microbial decontamination of nuts and spices. Microbial Decontamination in the Food Industry: Novel Methods and Applications 125–162. https://doi.org/10.1533/9780857095756.1.125.

Balasubramaniam, V.M., Farkas, D., 2008. High-pressure food processing. SAGE Journal 14 (5), 413–418. https://doi.org/10.1177/1082013208098812.

Bond, E.J., 1989. Manual of Fumigation for Insect Control. FAO Plant Production and Protection Paper 54, FAO, Rome, Italy. www.fao.org/docrep/X5042E/x5042E00.htm.

Collin, M.N.D., Arnaud, C., Kagy, V., Didier, C., 2007. Fruit flies: disinfestation, techniques used, possible application to mango. Fruit 62 (4), 223–236. https://doi.org/10.1051/fruits:2007018.

Duncan, S.E., Moberg, K., Amin, K.N., Wright, M., Newkirk, J.J., Ponder, M.A., et al., 2017. Processes to preserve spice and herb quality and sensory integrity during pathogen inactivation. Journal of Food Science 82 (5), 1208–1215. https://doi.org/10.1111/1750-3841.13702.

Fan, X., Niemira, B.A., Prakash, A., 2008. Irradiation of fresh fruits and vegetables. Food Technology 3, 37–43.

FAO\WHO [Food and Agriculture Organization of the United Nations/World Health Organization], 2014. Multicriteria-based ranking for risk management of food-borne parasites. Microbiological Risk Assessment Series No 23, 302.

Fellows, P.J., 2016a. Food Processing Technology: Principles and Practice, fourth ed. Elsevier, Cambridge, MA (Chapter 12).

Fellows, P.J., 2016b. Food Processing Technology: Principles and Practice, fourth ed. Elsevier, Cambridge, MA (Chapter 7).

Floros, J.D., Newsome, R., Fisher, W., Barbosa-Canovas, G.V., Chen, H., Dunne, C.P., et al., 2010. Feeding the World Today and Tomorrow: The Importance of Food Science and Technology. Comprehensive Reviews in Food Science and Food Safety, vol. 0. Institute of Food Technologists, pp. 1–28. https://doi.org/10.1111/j.1541-4337.2010.00127.x.

Hallman, G.J., Blackburn, C.M., 2016. Phytosanitary irradiation. Foods 5 (1), 8. https://doi.org/10.3390/foods5010008.

IFT, 1975. The effects of food processing on nutritional values. Nutrition Reviews 33 (4), 123–126. https://doi.org/10.1111/j.1753-4887.1975.tb07435.x.

IPPC, 2016. International Plant Protection Convention, ISPM 28 Phytosanitary Treatments for Regulated Pests. FAO, Rome, Italy. www.ippc.int/en/publications/84488/.

Jobling, J., Morris, S., James, H., 2002. Methyl Bromide Usage and Alternatives for Disinfestation Treatments. Horticultural Australia Ltd, Sydney, Australia. https://ausveg.com.au/app/data/technical-insights/docs/AH01034.pdf.

Koutchma, T., Keener, L., Kotilainen, H., 2018. Discordant International Regulations of Food Irradiation Are a Public Health Impediment and a Barrier to Global Trade. Global Harmonization Initiative 1-18. www.globalharmonization.net/share-sheets-and-consensus-documents.

Molins, R.A., 2001. Food Irradiation: Principles and Application. John Wiley & Sons Inc., Canada (Chapter 2).

Ogata, K., 1973. Improved storage life of fruits and vegetables by ionizing radiation. Japan Agricultural Research Quarterly 7, 55−60. https://www.jircas.go.jp/ja/file/7253/download?token=zJwBSfXK.

Paul, V., Ezekiel, R., Pandey, R., 2016. Sprout suppression on potato: need to look beyond CIPC for more effective and safer alternatives. Journal of Food Science and Technology 52 (1), 1−18. https://doi.org/10.1007/s13197-015-1980-3.

Petropoulos, S.A., Ntatsi, G., Ferreira, I.C.F.R., 2016. Long-term storage of onion and the factors that affect its quality: a critical review. Food Reviews International 33 (1), 62−83. https://doi.org/10.1080/87559129.1137312.

Prakash, A., 2016. Particular applications of food irradiation: fresh produce. Radiation Physics and Chemistry 129, 50−52. https://doi.org/10.1016/j.radphyschem.2016.07.017.

Prakash, A., Foley, D., 2004. Improving safety and shelf-life of fresh-cut fruits and vegetables using irradiation. In: Komolprasert, V., Morehouse, K.M. (Eds.), Irradiation of Food and Packaging: Recent Developments. ACS Symposium Series 875, vol. 875. Oxford University Press, United States, pp. 90−106.

Ramaswamy, H.S., Marcotte, M., 2005. Food Processing: Principles and Applications, first ed. CRC Press, FL (Chapter 3).

Reddy, M.B., Love, M., 1999. The impact of food processing on the nutritional quality of vitamins and minerals. In: Jackson, L.S., Knize, M.G., Morgan, J.N. (Eds.), Impact of Processing on Food Safety. Advances in Experimental Medicine and Biology, vol. 459. Springer, Boston, MA, pp. 96−106.

Sharp, J.L., 1993. Heat and cold treatments for postharvest quarantine disinfestation of fruit flies (Diptera: Tephritidae) and other quarantine pests. Florida Entomologist 76 (2), 212−218. https://doi.org/10.2307/3495716.

Sommers, C.H., Fan, X., 2008. Food Irradiation Research and Technology, second ed. Blackwell Publishing and Institute of Food Technologists Series, Ames, IA (Chapter 10).

Tang, J., Mitcham, E., Wang, S., Lurie, S., 2007. Heat Treatments for Postharvest Pest Control: Theory and Practice. CABI International, Cambridge, MA (Chapter 1).

UNEP, 2018. United Nations Environment Programme. Methyl Bromide. http://web.unep.org/ozonaction/what-we-do/methyl-bromide.

US CFR, 2018. United States Code of Federal Regulations 40CFR Section 185.2850 − Ethylene Oxide. https://www.govinfo.gov/app/collection/cfr/2018/.

USDA-APHIS, 2016. PPQ Treatment Manual. https://www.aphis.usda.gov/aphis/ourfocus/planthealth/import-information/SA_Quarantine_Treatments/CT_Quarantine-treatment.

Vajdi, M., Pereira, R.R., 1973. Comparative effects of ethylene oxide, gamma radiation and microwave treatments on selected spices. Journal of Food Science 38 (5), 893−895. https://doi.org/10.1111/j.1365-2621.1973.tb02102.x.

Van Doren, J.M., Neil, K.P., Parish, M., Gieraltowski, L., Gould, L.H., Gombas, K.L., 2013. Foodborne illness outbreaks from microbial contaminants in spices, 1973−2010. Food Microbiology 36 (2), 456−464. https://doi.org/10.1016/j.fm.2013.04.014.

Woodside, J.V., 2015. Nutritional aspects of irradiated food. Stewart Postharvest Review 2015 3 (2), 1−6. https://doi.org/10.2212/spr.2015.3.2.

Irradiation kills microbes: can it do anything harmful to the food?

10

Franco Pedreschi, PhD[1], María Salomé Mariotti-Celis, PhD[2]

[1]*Departamento de Ingeniería Química y Bioprocesos, Pontificia Universidad Católica de Chile, Santiago, Chile;* [2]*Programa Institucional de Fomento a la Investigación, Desarrollo e Innovación, Universidad Tecnológica Metropolitana, Santiago, Chile*

Introduction

Food irradiation is an efficient technology that can be used to ensure food safety by eliminating insects and pathogens. Food irradiation is a process exposing food to ionizing radiations such as gamma rays emitted from the radioisotopes 60Co and 137Cs or high-energy electrons and X-rays produced by machine sources (Farkas, 2004). This process can be applied to fresh or frozen foods to prolong their shelf life without affecting significantly the nutritional value and sensorial properties of the irradiated products (Maherani et al., 2016).

The potential application of ionizing radiation in food processing is based mainly on the fact that ionizing radiations damage very effectively the DNA so that living cells become inactivated. Therefore microorganisms, insect gametes, and plant meristems are prevented from reproducing, resulting in various preservative effects as a function of the absorbed radiation dose. At the same time, radiation-induced other chemical changes in food are minimal (Thayer, 1990). Radiation can be applied through packaging materials including those that cannot withstand heat (Farkas, 2004; Farkas and Mohacsi-Farkas, 2011).

Differences in food radiation sensitivities among the microorganisms are related to differences in their chemical and physical structure and in their ability to recover from radiation injury (Kilcast, 1995). Besides such inherent abilities, several factors such as composition of the medium, the moisture content, the temperature during irradiation, presence or absence of oxygen, the fresh or frozen state influence radiation resistance, particularly in case of vegetative cells (Farkas, 2004).

Market requirements are driving the need for radiation facility capacities, and dedicated food irradiation facilities may not deliver the return of investment in an acceptable time frame (Mittendorfe, 2016). Wholesomeness and legislation of irradiated food (toxicological safety, nutritional adequacy, and microbiological safety) have been carefully evaluated by an unprecedented width of research and testing over more than 50 years (Diehl, 1995; WHO, 1999). Nowadays, national and international organizations and regulatory agencies have concluded that irradiated food is

Genetically Modified and Irradiated Food. https://doi.org/10.1016/B978-0-12-817240-7.00014-0

safe and wholesome. This approval led to numerous studies on a variety of food irradiation applications (Junqueira - Goncalves et al., 2011). This book chapter describes how the irradiation process is used practically, including the benefits and limitations, especially focused on killing microbes and the chemical consequences over treated foods.

Current status of food irradiation in the world

Food irradiation is a "cold" process for preserving food that has been extensively used for over 50 years (Junqueira -Goncalves et al., 2011). Immediately after the discovery of ionizing radiation, speculations arose to use it not only for therapeutic treatment but also for food preservation. However, at that time, no radiation sources suitable for such applications had been available. With the development of military nuclear technologies, suitable radiation sources became more and more available and food irradiation has become a standard technology worldwide. Main potential applications and general dose requirements of food irradiation are listed in Table 10.1 (Farkas and Mohacsi-Farkas, 2011), where the unit of absorbed radiation doses are given in kilo gray (kGy) unit (1 Gy is equal to 1 J/kg absorbed energy).

Food irradiation is approved for use in over 60 countries for various applications and purposes in a wide variety of foodstuffs, mostly as a postharvest phytosanitary measure (Breidbach and Ulberth, 2016). Activities of food irradiation at commercial scale have increased significantly in these countries during the last few years. Attention is also focused on the phytosanitary treatment of fruits and vegetables. The main advantage of food irradiation is that it can be used to treat packaged foods, which will remain safe and protected from microbial contamination after treatment. Packaging material can either affect the irradiation process by barrier properties or can

Table 10.1 Main potential applications and general dose requirements of food irradiation.

Application	Dose requirement (kGy)
Inhibition of sprouting	0.03—0.12
Insect disinfestation	0.2—0.8
Parasite disinfestation	0.1—3.0
Shelf-life extension ("radurization")	0.5—3.0
Elimination of non—spore-forming pathogenic bacteria ("radicidation")	1.5—7.0
Reduction of microbial population in dry food ingredients	3.0—2.0
Production of meat, poultry, and fishery products shelf-stable at ambient temperature ("radappertization")	25—60

Original from J. Farkas, Food irradiation A. Mozumder, Y. Hatano (Eds.), Charged particle and photon interactions with matter, Marcel Dekker, Inc, New York, Basel (2004), pp. 785-812.

add radiolysis products into the product (Hammad, Abo-elnour, and Salah, 2006). This subject area has been discussed under "high-dose irradiation: Wholesomeness of food irradiated with doses above 10 kGy" (WHO, 1999). US-FDA enforces pre-evaluation and approval of packaging material prior to irradiation.

Radiation of food products and ingredients must be indicated by proper labeling in accordance with the Codex General Standard for the Labeling of Pre-packaged Food (WHO, 1999). The use of the international food irradiation symbol Radura is optional, but when it is used it shall be in close proximity to the name of the food. When an irradiated product is used as an ingredient in another food, this shall be so declared in the list of ingredients. When a single ingredient product is prepared from a raw material which has been irradiated, the label of the product shall contain a statement indicating the treatment.

The current status of activities of food irradiation at commercial scale has increased significantly in the United States of America (USA) and European Union (EU). Attention is also focused on the phytosanitary treatment of fruits and vegetables (Ihsanullah and Azhar, 2017). Food irradiation has the potential to answer global challenges in the way foods are processed and preserved, providing issues related to food safety and shelf life can be overcome effectively. Currently, food irradiation is approved in more than 60 countries, and there has been a notable growth in production and trade of irradiated foods since 2010 (Eustice, 2017).

Regarding research advances, the role, contribution, and impact of irradiation technology to control the presence of fungi and mycotoxins in food and in feed have been deeply evaluated (Calado et al., 2014; Junqueira-Goncalves et al., 2011). The effect of this technology on the viability of mold spores and on preventing the formation of mycotoxins was reviewed, and a critical evaluation of the advantages and disadvantages of irradiation in this context has been presented.

On fresh fruits and vegetables, irradiation at low- and medium-dose levels can effectively reduce microbial counts which can enhance safety, inhibit sprouting to extend shelf life, and eliminate insect pests which can serve to facilitate trade between countries (Farkas and Mohacsi-Farkas, 2011). At the dose levels used for these purposes, the impact on quality is negligible. Despite the fact that regulations in many countries allow the use of irradiation for fresh produce, the technology remains underutilized, even in the light of an increase in produce-related disease outbreaks and the economic benefits of extended shelf life and reduced food waste.

From a nutritional point of view, trace elements and minerals are not affected by irradiation. Macronutrients such as protein, carbohydrates, and fats are not affected significantly by doses up to 10 KGy (Maherani et al., 2016; Pauli and Tarantino, 1995; Woodside, 2015). Different studies on meat irradiation and its effect on lipids have shown that at low radiation doses, lipids in the presence of their natural protectors are not particularly sensitive to radiation-induced peroxidation. The effect of radiation on protein is related to their state, structure, and composition, whether native or denatured, whether dry or in solution, whether liquid or frozen, and to the presence or absence of other substances. However long-term feeding studies also concluded that irradiation of raw and prepared meat, to prolong shelf life, does

Table 10.2 Relative sensitivity of vitamins to irradiation.

High sensitivity	Low sensitivity
Vitamin C[a]	Carotene
Vitamin B1 (thiamin)[a]	Vitamin D
Vitamin E	Vitamin K
Vitamin A	Vitamin B6 (pyridoxine)[a]
	Vitamin B2 (riboflavin)[a]
	Vitamin B12 (cobalamin)[a]
	Vitamin B3 (niacin)[a]
	Vitamin B9 (folate)[a]
	Pantothenic acid[a]

[a] Water-soluble vitamins, Fat-soluble vitamin.
From J. F. Diehl, Food irradiation: Is it an alternative to chemical preservatives?, Food Additives & Contaminants, Volume 9, 1992 - Issue 5, Pages 409-416.

not lead to a reduction in their nutritional value (De Groot et al., 1973; Roberts, 2016). The amount of vitamin loss due to the irradiation is affected by several factors, including doses, temperature, presence of oxygen, and food type. Finally, radiation ($\sim$3.0 kGy) at low temperatures in the absence of oxygen prevents vitamin loss in foods, and the storage of irradiated foods in sealed packages at low temperatures also helps to prevent future vitamin loss. However, not all vitamins have the same sensitivity to irradiation (Fanaro et al., 2015; Roberts, 2016) (Table 10.2).

Irradiation for food safety and quality

Consumers, who have negative feelings toward nuclear power, perceive irradiated foods as lower in quality, perceived fewer benefits and more risks associated with food irradiation and exhibit lower overall acceptance of this technology (Bearth and Siegrist, 2019). The consumer attitude toward food is very complex as it is influenced by sensory and nonsensory attributes, as well as interactions between them. Recently studies have shown that food irradiation is a technology that addresses both food quality and safety because of its ability to control food spoilage and foodborne pathogenic microorganisms without significantly affecting the nutritional value of foods and sensory quality the foods (Maherani et al., 2016). Besides, many studies have shown that irradiation technology in combination with other treatments such as mild heat treatment can be used as an innovative and effective method to reduce or eliminate the growth of bacteria and parasites and subsequently extend the shelf life of food products with acceptable nutritional values (Maherani et al., 2016).

The constant demand of consumers for safer, "healthier," and processed food drives the development of technologies in food processing to achieve their needs. Food safety is one of the major challenges for technology, although many preservation processes and regulations are already available to control the microbiological and chemical integrity of food (Aguilera, 2018). Food irradiation is one among many of available technologies that contribute to improve the safety of food. Food irradiation is a physical method of food processing that involves exposing prepackaged or bulk foodstuffs to ionizing energy. This process is sometimes called "cold pasteurization" because the inactivation of microorganisms is achieved at low temperatures unlike the traditional heat pasteurization. Using irradiation, the microbiological safety of food can be improved and its shelf life prolonged without substantially changing, in most cases, its nutritional, chemical, and physical properties (Farkas and Mohacic-Farkas, 2011).

Finally, the effect of irradiation on foods depends on the absorbed dose, expressed in Gray (Gy). One Gy equals 1 J/kg of product. Low doses (0.05−0.15 kGy) are enough for inhibition of potato sprouting, disinfection (insects and parasites) of fruits, and delay of ripening in fresh fruits and vegetables. A medium absorbed dose (1.0−10 kGy) is sufficient for prevention of foodborne diseases through destruction and control of pathogens such as Salmonella spp., *Campylobacter jejuni*, *Escherichia coli* O157:H7, *Listeria monocytogenes*, and *Staphylococcus aureus*. Higher doses (10−50 kGy) are used for decontaminating food ingredients, like spices and herbs. Doses from 30 to 50 kGy are applied for sterilization of foods for space and hospital diets at an industrial scale (Ihsanullah and Azhar, 2017).

The elimination of pests in agricultural commodities can also be achieved, thus reducing food losses and the use of chemical fumigants and additives. Food irradiation up to an overall dose of 10 kGy has been considered a safe and effective technology since 1981 by several international food organizations (FAO/IAEA/WHO, 1981). Later on, doses above 10 kGy were also considered safe for some niche products and markets (FAO/IAEA/WHO, 1999). Nonetheless, food irradiation is not as widespread as other conventional technologies due to the high costs of irradiation units and, particularly, because of a negative perception of consumers relatively to its safety (Calado et al., 2014).

Irradiation should only be used in combination with good manufacturing and storage practices to prevent the proliferation of toxigenic fungi and the associated production of mycotoxins. Also important is that irradiation should never be used in commodities already molded or contaminated with mycotoxins with the intent of remediating the problem (Calado et al., 2014). The radiolytic process is influenced by many factors, such as absorbed doses, initial mycotoxin concentration or fungal load, the position in the irradiated system, the amount of moisture, and/or the presence of other matrix components. As already observed, molds are one of the main causes of postharvest decay problems. The presence of molds in food may result in not only a reduction in quality and in quantity but also contamination with mycotoxins, causing important health problems. Irradiation can be used for the direct purpose of eliminating or of reducing the presence of molds and mold spores in foods and in feeds, improving their shelf life and safety (Calado et al., 2014). Nonetheless, the application of this technology for other purposes can indirectly aid in the control of contamination with molds and, subsequently, with mycotoxins. For example, it is well known that grains damaged by insects are more susceptible to mold development and to mycotoxin accumulations because insects carry fungal spores and compromise the integrity of grains and plant tissues, facilitating the penetration and access to nutrients of fungal hyphae and, by consequence, fungal development and mycotoxin formation (Jouany, 2007). Thus, the elimination of insect pests from agricultural commodities through irradiation can indirectly have a positive effect on the reduction of fungal contamination and thereby reduce mycotoxin levels in treated commodities.

Radiosensitivity of fungi also depends on strain characteristics, mold forms (mycelium or spores), the moisture content of spores or commodities, spore age, commodity characteristics, the existence of periods of refrigeration or of heating before or after treatments, and on the combinations of radiation with other technologies. Fungi with melanized mycelia and spores are also more radioresistant than other structures. Commodities with higher moisture content may favor fungal recovery after irradiation if inactivation is not complete. Although there are several contrasting reports regarding the effect of gamma rays on fungi and mycotoxins in different foods, gamma irradiation can be generally considered to significantly improve the mycotoxicological safety of food and feed (Calado et al., 2014).

As can be observed from these studies, a substantial reduction of the fungal load in spices and in seasonings is only achievable with irradiation levels above 5 kGy. In this case, the high levels of irradiation do not seem to affect the quality of products because no losses of flavor compounds, changes in volatile oil compositions, and weakening of antioxidant properties at irradiation levels of 10 kGy or even 30 kGy were found by several researchers and reviewed by Alam and Abrahem (2010). Thus, the irradiation of spices is widely used as an excellent substitute to fumigation with gases, such as ethylene, propylene oxide, or methyl bromide, which leave chemical residues (for example, ethylene chlorohydrins and ethylene bromohydrin) that are suspected to be harmful. The dried nature of these products may be the factor that favors their greater resistance to the ionizing energy (Calado et al., 2014).

Since mycotoxins are highly toxic, it is imperative to reduce their levels both in food and in feed as low as technologically feasible. Ionizing radiation is one among many technologies that can contribute to this purpose. As we have observed, first, its action on mold viability contributes to the avoidance of fungal development and, consequently, to the production of mycotoxins in commodities (Calado et al., 2014). Second, because ionizing radiation can have a direct action on mycotoxins under specific conditions, contributing to their elimination, this subject has been widely investigated (Calado et al., 2014). Finally, dried mycotoxins are extremely radioresistant, whereas in solution, mycotoxins are sensitive to irradiation. The oxidative radicals that originate from water radiolysis are responsible for their degradation. Combining gamma irradiation with other treatments can improve the breakdown of mycotoxins (for example, using hydrogen peroxide, ammonium bicarbonate, or higher moisture conditions). Generally, more than 10 kGy doses are required to eliminate a significant amount of mycotoxins in food matrixes (Calado et al., 2014).

Future of food irradiation

The future growth of food irradiation depends in part in demonstrating to food producers and retailers that not only is the technology beneficial, it will be purchased by consumers. This would be assisted by a review and harmonization of labeling requirements. The food trade regards labeling as an extra cost and, perhaps more importantly, as a focus of the remaining opposition to food irradiation and consumer fears about the Technology (Roberts, 2016).

The key of changing the sluggishness of implementation of the manyfold potential use of food irradiation technology is a better appreciation of its potential role in controlling foodborne diseases and spoilage, as well as the willingness to pay for processing for food safety (Farkas and Mohacsi-Farkas, 2011). Further progress in food irradiation legislation, particularly in the European Union, should encourage a wider acceptance of the process by all relevant stakeholders. Consumer acceptance is a matter of education and proper communication diminishing the unfair image that food irradiation is a nuclear technology (Teisi et al., 2009). The challenge represented by consumer acceptance and regulatory approval requires the demystification of food irradiation (Crawford, 2001). Marketing trials showed that an increasing number of consumers are willing to purchase irradiated food if they are properly informed about the process and its effects on food (Eustice and Bruhn, 2006).

Further developments in design and adaptation of uses of machine radiation sources (e-beam facilities and X-ray machines) (Arthur et al., 2005; Cleland, 2006; Pillai et al., 2006) can also assist altering the image of the process into one kind of electrical technologies (see the success of household uses of microwave ovens, or the TV utilities). In the United States and in some other countries where health authorities actively encourage the use of this technology, commercial application has greatly advanced in recent years. In contrast, progress in the European Union is still slow (Diehl, 2002). Finally, there is also a need for radiation processors to recognize the difficulties that the food trade perceive when inserting an extra and unfamiliar technical step into the supply chain from farm to fork for highly perishable commodities (Roberts, 2016). Cooperation between irradiation processors and the food trade is necessary to make the irradiation step as uncomplicated and smooth as possible. Finally, one of the major challenges facing the global food sector in the use of irradiation is harmonization of regulations and equivalence of standards, dose, and labeling. Legislation needs to be harmonized and updated continuously to facilitate the effectiveness of global food chains and trade and respond to global food safety challenges. However, they can also add complexity and confusion if not harmonized globally (King et al., 2017).

Conclusions

Irradiation is an effective and safe method of food preservation, as it reduces spoilage, improves food hygiene, and extends shelf life. Decontamination of spices, herbs, and condiments used mainly as ingredients remains the single largest application of irradiation. The success at retail level of irradiated meats and fresh produce indicates that consumer acceptance of irradiated food is considerably greater than has been indicated in many surveys of consumer opinion.

There is a comprehensive and well-established framework of international standards, national regulations, and bilateral agreements for the irradiation of food and trade in irradiated products. Future growth of the technology will involve demonstrating the market successes to food producers and retailers. Greater cooperation between irradiation processers and the food trade to minimize disruption to the food supply chain would also be helpful. Labeling is an added cost to the food trade and is a focal point for opposition to irradiated foods. Rationalization and great consistency in labeling regulations and enforcement would be advantageous.

Acknowledgments

The authors would like to acknowledge the support they received from FONDECYT Project 1150146.

References

Aguilera, J.M., 2018. Food engineering into the XXI century. AIChE Journal 64, 1–10.

Alam, K., Abrahem, M., 2010. Effect of irradiation on quality of spices. International Food Research International 1, 825–836.

Arthur, T., Wheeler, T., Shackelford, S., Bosilevac, J., Nou, X., Koohmaraie, M., 2005. Effects of low dose, low penetration electron beam irradiation of beef carcass surface cuts on *Escherichia coli* O157:H7 and meat quality. Journal of Food Production 68, 666–672.

Bearth, A., Siegrist, M., 2019. "As long as it is not irradiated"—Influencing factors of US consumers' acceptance of food irradiation. Food Quality and Preference 71, 141–148.

Breidbach, A., Ulberth, F., 2016. Comparative evaluation of methods for the detection of 2-alkylcyclobutanones as indicators for irradiation treatment of cashew nuts and nutmeg. Food Chemistry 201, 52–58. https://doi.org/10.1016/j.foodchem.2016.01.032.

Calado, T., Venancio, A., Abrunhosa, L., 2014. Irradiation for mold and mycotoxin control: a review. Comprehensive Reviews in Food Science and Food Safety 13, 1049–1061.

Cleland, M., 2006. Advanced in gamma ray, electron beam, and X-ray technologies for food irradiation. In: Sommers, C.H., Fan, X. (Eds.), Food Irradiation Processing of Food. CAC/RPC 19-1979, Rev 1-2003. Codex Alimentarius Commission, Rome.

Crawford, L., 2001. Change and opportunities for food irradiation in the 21st century. In: Loahanaru, P., Thomas, P. (Eds.), Irradiation of Food Safety and Quality. Technomic Publ. Co, Lancaster, Basel, pp. 9–16.

De Groot, A., Mijll Dekker, V., Slump, P., Vos, H., Willems, J., 1973. New wholesomeness data on radiation-pasteurized chicken. Food Irradiation Information 2, 71–72.

Diehl, J.F., 1995. Nutritional adequacy of irradiated foods. In: Diehl, J.F. (Ed.), Safety of Irradiated Foods, second ed. Marcel Dekker, Inc., New York, NY, USA, pp. 241–282. 1995.

Diehl, J., 2002. Food irradiation — past, present and future. Radiation Physics and Chemistry 63, 211–215.

Eustic, R., Bruhn, C., 2006. Consumer acceptance and marketing of irradiated foods. In: Sommers, C.H., Fan, X. (Eds.), Food Irradiation Research and Technology. Blackwell Publ., Ltd, Oxford, pp. 63–83.

Eustice, R.F., 2017. Global status and commercial applications of food irradiation. Chapter 20. In: Ferreira, I.C.F.R., Antonio, A.L., Verde, S.C. (Eds.), Food Irradiation Technologies: Concepts, Applications and Outcomes, pp. 397–424.

Fanaro, G., Hassimotto, N., Bustos, D., Villavicencio, A., 2015. Effects of γ-radiation on microbial load and antioxidant proprieties in green tea irradiated with different water activities. Radiation Physics and Chemistry 107, 40–46.

Farkas, J., 2004. Charged particle and photon interactions with matter. In: Mozumder, A., Hatano, Y. (Eds.), Food Irradiation. Marcel Dekker, New York, pp. 785–812.

Farkas, J., 2004. Food irradiation. In: Mozumder, A., Hatano, Y. (Eds.), Charged Particle and Photon Interactions with Matter.

Farkas, J., Mohacsi-Farkas, C., 2011. History and future of food irradiation. Trends in Food Science and Technology 22, 121–126.

Hammad, A.A., Abo Elnour, S.A., Salah, A., 2006. Use of irradiation to ensure hygienic quality of minimally processed vegetables and fruits. IAEA-TECDOC 1530, 106–129.

Ihsanullah, I., Azhar, R., 2017. Current activities in food irradiation as a sanitary and phytosanitary treatment in the Asia and the Pacific Region and a comparison with advanced countries. Food Control 72, 345–359.

Jouany, J., 2007. Methods for preventing, decontaminating and minimizing the toxicity of mycotoxins in feeds. Animal Feed Science and Technology 137, 342–362.

Junqueira-Goncalves, M.P., Galotto, M.J., Valenzuela, X., Dinten, C.M., Aguirre, P., Miltz, J., 2011. Perception and view of consumers on food irradiation and the Radura symbol. Radiation Physics and Chemistry 80 (1), 119–122.

Kilcast, D., 1995. Food irradiation: current problems and future potential. International Biodeterioration and Biodegradation 36 (3–4), 279–296.

King, T., Cole, M., Farber, J.M., Eisenbrand, G., Zabaras, D., Fox, E.M., Hill, J.P., 2017. Food safety for food security: relationship between global megatrends and developments in food safety. Trends in Food Science and Technology 68, 160–175.

Maherani, B., Hossain, F., Criado, P., Ben-Fadhel, Y., Salmieri, S., Lacroix, M., 2016. World market development and consumer: acceptance of irradiation technology. Foods 5, 1–21.

Mittendorfe, J., 2016. Food irradiation facilities: requirements and technical aspects. Radiation Physics and Chemistry 129, 61–63.

Pauli, G.H., Tarantino, L.M., 1995. FDA regulatory aspects of food irradiation. Journal of Food Protection 58, 209–212.

Pillai, S., Braby, L., Maxim, J., 2006. Technical challegues and research direction in electronic food pasteurization. In: Sommers, C.H., Fang, X. (Eds.), Food Irradiation Research and Technology. Blackwell Publ, Inc, Oxford, pp. 279–287.

Roberts, P., 2016. Food irradiation: Standards, regulations and world-wide trade. Radiation Physics and Chemistry 129, 30–34.

Teisi, M., Fein, S., Levy, A., 2009. Information effects on consumer attitudes toward three food technologies: organic production, biotechnology and irradiation. Food Quality and Preference 20, 586–596.

Thayer, D., 1990. Food irradiation: benefits and concern. Journal of Food Quality 13, 147–169.

WHO, 1981. Wholesomeness of Irradiated Food. Report of a Joint FAO/IAEA/WHO Expert Committee. Technical Report Series 659. World Health Organization, Geneva.

WHO, 1999. High-dose Irradiation. Wholesomeness of Food Irradiated with Doses above 10 kGy. Report of a joint FAO/IAEA/WHO study group on high dose irradiation. WHO Technical Report Series. World Health Organization, Geneva (Food Irradiation Clearances).

Woodside, J., 2015. Nutritional aspects of irradiated food. Stewart Postharvest Review 3, 1—6.

Can irradiated food have an influence on people's health?

11

Joseph John Bevelacqua, PhD [1], **S.M. Javad Mortazavi, PhD** [2]

[1]*Bevelacqua Resources, Richland, WA, United States;* [2]*Diagnostic Imaging Department, Fox Chase Cancer Center, Philadelphia, PA, United States*

Introduction

Humans have always tried to find effective methods for food preservation. Sun drying, salting, and smoking were among the early methods while later canning, freezing, and the addition of chemicals were introduced. Food irradiation currently provides a substantially superior method for preserving food. It is becoming an increasingly popular way for fast food restaurants to protect themselves from food-poisoning litigation. Further, fast food corporations are beginning to irradiate the shredded lettuce, sliced tomatoes, and other condiments to extend their shelf life. The use of radionuclides and radiation-generating devices are important methods to preserve food, stabilize food supplies, and enhance nutrition throughout the world. Since food irradiation relies on nuclear technology, it has a number of unique aspects that can influence public acceptance and use. Accordingly, the topic of food irradiation is addressed in numerous publications (Walter, 1986; Sun, 2018).

A World Health Organization report (WHO, 2017) concluded that foodborne disease is a significant threat to human health and contributes to a reduction in economic prosperity. Food preservation methods include canning, chemical preservation, cooking, freezing, salting, smoking, and sun drying. A more recent addition is irradiation by exposing foods to safe, predetermined amounts of ionizing radiation. Decades of research and development demonstrate that irradiation retards food spoilage, reduces insect infestations, and eliminates the propagation and growth of other organisms that cause disease and illness (Walter, 1986; Sun, 2018). Although the traditional techniques are widely utilized and accepted, any association with ionizing radiation creates a negative bias toward food irradiation and limits its beneficial use. This phenomenon is another example of radiophobia that is an irrational response to the beneficial use of nuclear technology.

If society applied the radiophobia logic to cooking food, it would also be viewed as a negative technology. A hypothetical example illustrates applying the radiophobia mindset to cooking food with thermal radiation:

> Scientists have developed a new technology called thermal radiation (e.g., infrared radiation) as a method that is alleged to improve the taste and edibility

of foods. Thermal radiation proponents claim that it kills known pathogens and prolongs the food's shelf life. Unfortunately, thermal radiation has a number of negative side effects that suggest its use is potentially harmful. Thermal technology produces carcinogenic materials in meat, reduces the vitamin content of fruits and vegetables, and produces hazardous chemical compounds in eggs. Therefore, cooking foods with thermal radiation should be avoided and restricted by regulations until detailed research proves that it is not harmful to human health.

Scientists have developed a new technology called thermal radiation (e.g., infrared radiation) as a method that is alleged to improve the taste and edibility of foods. Thermal radiation proponents claim that it kills known pathogens and prolongs the food's shelf life. Unfortunately, thermal radiation has a number of negative side effects that suggest its use is potentially harmful. Thermal technology produces carcinogenic materials in meat, reduces the vitamin content of fruits and vegetables, and produces hazardous chemical compounds in eggs. Therefore, cooking foods with thermal radiation should be avoided and restricted by regulations until detailed research proves that it is not harmful to human health.

The fallacy of this logic illustrates the inherent bias against an ionizing radiation−based technology such as food irradiation.

Traditional methods to kill bacteria and other pathogens include pasteurizing milk and pressure-cooking foods that are subsequently canned. Food irradiation is just another technique that can be utilized to ensure food safety. Food irradiation kills bacteria, molds, and pathogens in food. Irradiation breaks chemical bonds to stop bacteria and other pathogens from multiplying but does not remove chemical toxins that may be present in food or make food radioactive (Walter, 1986; Sun, 2018).

Food irradiation has other benefits. As noted in by the US Environmental Protection Agency (EPA Report 402-F-14-016, 2014), irradiation preserves the nutritional value of the food and inhibits the aging of fruits and vegetables. Shelf lives of dry foods including grains and spices are significantly extended through food irradiation. Food irradiation does not make the irradiated material radioactive, which is a common misconception.

Radioactive material including ^{60}Co and ^{137}Cs and electron and X-ray beams has been utilized to irradiate foods (Walter, 1986; Sun, 2018). ^{60}Co is a radionuclide that is used in industrial radiography and selected medical applications. It has a half-life of 5.27 years and emits both photon (1.17 and 1.33 MeV) as well as beta-radiation (320 keV). ^{137}Cs also has medical and industrial applications and has a 30-year half-life. Its principle radiation emissions are a 662 keV photon and a 500 keV beta particle. The reader should note that X-rays are used (and have been used for a long time) to investigate patients. The units MeV and keV represent 1 million and 1000 electron volts, which are energy units.

Irradiation occurs when bulk or packaged food passes through a radiation chamber. The food does not come into direct contact with radioactive materials as it traverses the radiation field. As the food passes through the field, energy is deposited into the food and contained matter. Ionizing radiation deposits sufficient energy into bacterial or mold cells to either kill the pathogens or limit their capability to reproduce. This inhibits their capability to cause illness or spoilage.

The degree of irradiation is characterized in terms of the energy deposited per unit mass or the absorbed dose using the units of Gray (Gy = J/kg). Doses <1 kGy are used to control insects and parasites and delay the ripening of fruits, doses in the range of 1−7 kGy reduce foodborne pathogens, and extend shelf life, and doses >25 kGy are used for sterilization (EPA Report 402-F-14-016, 2014).

History of concerns about food irradiation

Universal acceptance of irradiated foods has yet to be achieved. As noted in Tauxe (2001), surveys conducted by the Food Marketing Institute suggest that about 50% of the population will purchase irradiated foods. Acceptance would increase if the cost is similar to an unirradiated product. The surveys suggest that if the public understands that irradiation minimizes harmful bacteria, then the acceptance rate would increase from 50% to 80%−90%.

The public tends to be hesitant to accept a new food processing technology. Historically, public concerns were expressed toward milk pasteurization and canning. Given its association with radiation and radioactive materials, food irradiation has created a number of unique concerns. One common concern is that the irradiation process creates induced radioactivity in foods and that the food becomes a radioactive material (Tauxe, 2001; Mostafavi et al., 2010; EPA Report 402-F-14-016, 2014). Although activation can occur in irradiated materials, the radiation types and energies that are utilized and the administered absorbed doses preclude these concerns (21CFR, 2018).

Concerns have also been raised that food irradiation compromises the nutritional content of the product (Tauxe, 2001; Mostafavi et al., 2010; EPA Report 402-F-14-016, 2014). However, the changes produced by irradiation are less severe than those caused by other processes including by canning and pasteurization. As with other food preservation techniques (e.g., pasteurization), some minor taste and smell changes may occur (Tauxe, 2001; Mostafavi et al., 2010; EPA Report 402-F-14-016, 2014).

The fear of radiation or radiophobia is cited as a common concern that affects the acceptance of the irradiation technology. Tauxe (2001) notes that most Americans are favorably disposed toward food irradiation if the benefits are clearly explained. In particular the improvements in safety following pathogen elimination are important considerations affecting the acceptance of a technology. This acceptance is facilitated when the public is informed that irradiation is commonly utilized to sterilize medical equipment and supplies. Population acceptance of other radiation types used in routine medical examinations (e.g., diagnostic X-ray examinations) and household products (e.g., microwaves) serves as a portion of the basis for public acceptance of food irradiation. The use of a distinctive logo denoting that the food product has been processed by irradiation informs consumers of the processing technology and permits them to make informed product choices.

Although microwaves and X-rays are accepted by the public, radioactive materials utilized in the food irradiation process are of greater concern because they are associated with nuclear power reactors. The gamma rays associated with ^{60}Co and ^{137}Cs create concern in some members of the public. This is particularly true following press reports that associated the releases of ^{137}Cs during the Chernobyl and Fukushima Daiichi accidents with contamination of food and water[18]. Although these are partially valid statements, they fail to consider the numerous radionuclides used in industrial applications and medical applications. For example, ^{60}Co is used in industrial radiography to verify weld integrity, oil and gas exploration to ascertain the extent of the deposit, and to measure densities of materials such as coal and grain (Bevelacqua, 2009, 2010). In medical applications, ^{137}Cs is used in brachytherapy and radiotherapy and as a calibration source for radiation detection equipment (Bevelacqua, 2009, 2010).

Associated with induced radioactivity concerns are issues involving the transportation of irradiated foods and their presence on store shelves. Since the absorbed doses used in irradiation do not create radioactive material, these concerns are also unwarranted.

Concerns have also been expressed (Tauxe, 2001) that the efficiency of food irradiation will allow current food industry sanitation standards to be relaxed, and that this relaxation will create a public health concern. From a safety perspective, combining irradiation with increased sanitation measures would permit lower absorbed doses to be utilized and that would decrease the possibility of taste or smell changes in a product. This issue will not be fully resolved until the public has confidence that the food industry will demonstrate that irradiation is only used in conjunction with existing sanitation methods to maintain food quality.

Unique concerns regarding the usage of irradiation to reprocess poor quality food or to salvage expired food has also been expressed (Tauxe, 2001). Irradiation will preserve foods but will not reverse the effects of aging or transform a poor quality product into a more acceptable version. Other concerns including the creation toxic chemicals and unique radiolytic products (EPA Report 402-F-14-016, 2014) are addressed in subsequent discuss.

Safety issues of food irradiation technologies

As noted in Tauxe (2001), food trials, nutritional assessments, and toxicity studies support the contention that food irradiation is safe and this food processing technology is approved by numerous national regulatory agencies (Walter, 1986; Sun, 2018). In the United States, food irradiation safety is ensured through compliance with the Code of Federal Regulations (CFR) (Title 21) (2018). 21CFR codifies accepted safety standards as part of the US regulatory basis. Compliance with the

10CFR (10CFR20, 2018; Bevelacqua, 2010, 2016) and 21CFR (2018) requirements ensures safety of workers employed in the food irradiation industry as well as consumers that utilize its products.

For example, the question of radiation safety is often raised since the food irradiation technology utilizes radiation and radioactive materials as an integral part of the processing technology. The safety of irradiation technology is well documented (Walter, 1986; Sun, 2018). Irradiation is also a well-established and extensively utilized method to sterilize medical products including surgical implants and instruments. Within the United States, regulatory oversight of nuclear technology and transportation of radioactive materials are provided by the Nuclear Regulatory Commission (NRC) and the Department of Transportation (DOT), respectively. The NRC (10CFR, 2018) and DOT (49CFR, 2018) regulations provide sufficient legal requirements for the safe use and transport of radioactive materials (e.g., gamma-emitting ^{60}Co and ^{137}Cs) and other sources of radiation (e.g., electron and X-ray beam facilities).

Gamma-ray irradiation technology (Tauxe, 2001) uses the photon (e.g., gamma) radiation emitted by fission or activation products, including the 1.17 and 1.33 and 0.66 MeV photons emitted by ^{60}Co and ^{137}Cs, respectively. ^{60}Co is a neutron activation product and ^{137}Cs is a fission product that are commonly produced in nuclear reactors with half-lives of 5.27 and 30.1 y, respectively. These half-lives are sufficiently long for use in commercial food irradiation facilities. The food or other products that are to be irradiated are transported into a shielded chamber and exposed to photon radiation for a specified time to deliver the desired absorbed dose. Photon radiation provides thorough material irradiation (Sterigenics, 2007) even at densities approaching 0.5 g/cm^3. Food processing is relatively simple and depends on the gamma source activity and irradiation time.

When the ^{60}Co or ^{137}Cs source is not in use, it is stored, typically in a shielded pit or pool of water that attenuates the photon radiation. The high-energy photons are penetrating which facilitates production-scale treatment of foods loaded onto shipping pallets. Worker safety is ensured using bulk shielding to attenuate the photon radiation and interlocks to prevent inadvertent entry into irradiation chambers (Bevelacqua, 2009, 2010). The source elevation and entry doors are interlocked to prevent personnel entry when the source is exposed (Bevelacqua, 2009, 2010). Warning signs, lights, and audible sounds are also used to indicate that the source is exposed. Radiation monitoring devices with alarm functions provide additional measures to ensure personnel safety.

Beam irradiation utilizes electrons generated by a source (e.g., gun device or accelerator) to irradiate materials. This technology is a flexible and high-speed process for sterilizing medical devices and pharmaceuticals. It is also used as a method of controlling contamination in packaging, cosmetics, and toiletries (Sterigenics, 2007).

Typical beam energies and food irradiation sources are provided in Table 11.1. Since electrons at the energies utilized in irradiation can only penetrate a few centimeters (Bevelacqua, 2009, 2010), foods that are to be irradiated are arranged in a

Table 11.1 Ionizing radiation safety limits for the treatment of foods.[a]

Radiation type	Production method/condition	Energy limit/radionuclide
Gamma rays	Sealed sources of the radionuclides	^{60}Co (1.17 and 1.33 MeV) and ^{137}Cs (0.66 MeV)
Electrons	Machine sources (e.g., electron guns and accelerators)	<10 MeV
X-rays	Machine sources	<5 MeV, except as noted in the next row[b]
X-rays	Machine sources using tantalum or gold as the target material	<7.5 MeV[b]

[a] *Based on 21CFR 179.26 (21CFR, 2018).*
[b] *Although 21CFR refers to these energies as X-rays, most sources would classify these upper limits as gamma rays. Typical X-ray sources operate in keV rather than MeV range.*

relatively thin slab geometry. Efficient penetration (Sterigenics, 2007) occurs at bulk densities between 0.05 and 0.30 g/cm^3. Processing is more complex than the gamma-ray approach. The delivered dose depends on the electron beam scan height, processing speed, number of passes, and orientation of the food with respect to the beam (Sterigenics, 2007).

Concrete or metal shielding is sufficient to protect workers from electrons after the food has been irradiated (Bevelacqua, 2009, 2010). The beam is only active when it is powered so the radiation source output ceases when power is terminated.

Residual radiation is limited because the electron energies are low. There will be minimal activation of the irradiation chamber, and production of secondary radiation including neutrons is also minimal. A detailed discussion of shielding electron sources is provided by Bevelacqua (2008, 2009, 2010, 2016). As with the gamma process, worker protection is enhanced through the use of shielding, interlocks, warning devices, and alarming radiation instrumentation to limit the worker's radiation dose (Bevelacqua, 2009, 2010).

X-ray irradiation is an additional technique for sterilization and contamination control. The production of X-ray radiation is achieved when electrons impinge upon a high-Z target (e.g., metal such as tungsten). The interaction produces X-rays through bremsstrahlung (e.g., the electromagnetic process that creates photon radiation when a charged particle is accelerated or decelerated) and characteristic radiation. Since X-rays are similar to gamma rays, but have lower energy, their interaction characteristics are similar (Bevelacqua, 2009, 2010). Given the energy limits noted in Table 11.1, the amount of shielding required by the X-ray beam strongly depends on its energy. Both electron and X-ray sources require electric power to function and their beams are terminated with the removal of power.

Materials processing depends on the speed of materials traversing the irradiation chamber, number of passes through the chamber, and the number of pallets on a conveyor transporting materials through the chamber (Sterigenics, 2007). X-ray irradiation applications include the sterilization of medical devices and the sanitization of packaging and toiletries[9]. As with the other processes, worker protection is enhanced by the use of shielding, interlocks, warning devices, and radiation instrumentation to limit the worker's radiation dose (Bevelacqua, 2009, 2010).

Do current regulations guarantee our safety?

The US Food and Drug Administration (FDA) is responsible for regulating the use of irradiation in the treatment of food and food packaging. Specifically, the FDA through the Center for Food Safety and Applied Nutrition evaluates food irradiation and its safety. As noted in Table 11.2, the FDA has approved food irradiation

Table 11.2 Ionizing radiation absorbed dose limits for the treatment of foods.[a]

Food treatment application	Absorbed dose limit (kGy)
Control of *Trichinella spiralis* in pork	0.3 (minimum) 1.0 (maximum)
Growth and maturation inhibition of fresh foods	≤ 1
Microbial disinfection of dry or dehydrated enzyme preparations	≤ 10
Microbial disinfection of dry or dehydrated aromatic vegetable substances (e.g., culinary herbs, seeds, spices, and vegetable seasonings)	≤ 30
Control of foodborne pathogens in fresh or frozen, uncooked poultry products	≤ 4.5 kGy (nonfrozen products) ≤ 7.0 kGy (frozen products)
Sterilization of frozen, packaged meats used solely in the National Aeronautics and Space Administration space flight programs	44 (minimum dose)
Control of foodborne pathogens and extension of shelf life of refrigerated or frozen, uncooked products that are meat, meat byproducts, and meat food products	≤ 4.5 (refrigerated products) ≤ 7.0 (frozen products)
Control of Salmonella in fresh shell eggs	≤ 3.0
Control of microbial pathogens on seeds for sprouting	≤ 8.0
Control of *Vibrio* bacteria and other foodborne microorganisms in or on fresh or frozen molluscan shellfish	≤ 5.5
Control of foodborne pathogens and extension of shelf life in fresh iceberg lettuce and fresh spinach.	≤ 4.0
Control of foodborne pathogens and extension of shelf life of chilled or frozen raw, cooked, or partially cooked crustaceans or dried crustaceans	≤ 6.0

[a] Based on 21CFR 179.26 (2008).

absorbed doses for a variety of foods (WHO, 1988; 21CFR, 2018). In the United States, irradiated foods are required by the FDA to have an irradiated food label that specifies that the product contain a logo and a statement that the food has been irradiated. In addition, the US Department of Agriculture coordinates with the FDA to promote the safe use of food irradiation. Detailed regulatory requirements are provided in 21CFR (2018).

The Food and Drug Administration approved irradiation as a treatment methodology because there are no conventional control measures to ensure bacteria-free food. As noted in Olson (1998), the FDA cited hundreds of studies that indicated there were no safety or health concerns from consuming irradiated food. Specific absorbed dose limits are noted in Table 11.2.

In 21CFR (2018), the FDA has approved a number of radiation types for the inspection of foods, inspection of packaged food, and controlling food processing. These activities may be safely performed under the following conditions (21CFR, 2018):

(1) X-ray tubes operating at ≤ 500 kVp,
(2) sealed sources emitting radiation types less than 2.2 MeV from one of the following isotopes: ^{60}Co, ^{85}Kr, ^{90}Sr, ^{125}I, ^{137}Cs, ^{226}Ra, and ^{241}Am,
(3) sealed ^{252}Cf sources to measure moisture in food,
(4) X-ray machines with energies ≤ 10 MeV, and
(5) monoenergetic neutron sources with energies in the $1-14$ MeV range.

These regulatory criteria are supported by research regarding appropriate absorbed dose values for food processing. Above 10 kGy, irradiation eliminates microorganisms in food products. Pasteurization or the elimination of a significant number of microorganisms occurs in the absorbed dose range of $1-10$ kGy (Walter, 1986; WHO, 1988; Olson, 1998). Lower dose levels are used to eliminate insect populations (<1 kGy), inhibit sprout formation technique in potatoes and onions (<1 kGy), delay the ripening of certain fruits (<0.3 kGy), and eliminate trichinosis in pork (<1 kGy) (WHO, 1988; GAO Report No. GAO/HUD-90-118, 1990; Olson, 1998).

Food irradiation can reduce available vitamins and minerals, but the reduction is not a serious loss of nutrition for individuals consuming a well-balanced diet (Walter, 1986; WHO, 1988; Olson, 1998). For example, the amount of thiamin may be reduced by a factor of 2 in irradiated pork, but this only represents about a 2% loss of the total intake of this vitamin. Since most thiamin intake is derived from cereal, bread, and pasta, the effect of food irradiation is insignificant.

The loss of thiamin is not unique to food-irradiated products. In canned beef, the thiamin retention in beef processed by canning, gamma irradiation, and electron irradiation is 21%, 23%, and 44%, respectively.

Sterile, stable products are produced by irradiation, and no harmful effects have been observed at absorbed doses at 60 kGy (Walter, 1986; WHO, 1988; Olson, 1998). At these absorbed doses, some vitamin losses occur, but the irradiated food is sterile and has a useful life that is similar to canned foods. The National

Aeronautics and Space Administration Space Program utilizes these higher doses for its astronaut foods, and this approach is also used for individuals with compromised immune systems (WHO, 1988; Olson, 1998; CFR, 2018).

How did fear of radiation affect public perception about food irradiation?

Acceptance of food irradiation has been hampered by the general perception that radiation and radioactive materials and their use are detrimental to public health and safety. These concerns are derived from the general lack of public understanding of radiological science and the risks of technology based on nuclear physics principles (Adler and Kranowitz, 2005; Bevelacqua, 2008). Concerns are reinforced by the fears of thermonuclear war and exaggerated press reports regarding commercial nuclear power accidents including the 1979 Three Mile Island (TMI) Unit-2 accident in the United States (Bevelacqua, 2008, 2009, 2010, 2016), 1986 accident at Chernobyl Unit-4 in the Ukraine (Bevelacqua, 2008, 2009, 2010, 2016), and the 2011 accidents at Fukushima Daiichi Units 1, 2, 3, and 4 in Japan (Bevelacqua, 2016). These accidents and associated evacuations create public fear and apprehension regarding nuclear technology and its application. The deaths associated with the Chernobyl-4 accident and public evacuations following the TMI-2, Chernobyl-4, and Fukushima Daiichi accidents serve as perceived validation of these fears. These accidents reinforce an inherent bias toward an agent that is invisible and perceived by the public to be deadly (Adler and Kranowitz, 2005; Bevelacqua, 2008).

Specific fears and their intensity vary with individual countries and their experience with nuclear technology. As a result of the Chernobyl-4 accident, many Ukrainian individuals are apprehensive about nuclear technology for any purpose (WHO, 1988). In areas where food irradiation has been proposed, elected officials, the media, and other individuals who influence public opinion may not be fully cognizant about the irradiation process and the effects of the irradiation on the food product.

Public apprehension is often based on radiophobia, lack of credible information, confusion regarding differences between the effects of the irradiation process and radioactive material contamination, and failure of the nuclear food processing industry to successfully communicate the risks and benefits of the food irradiation technology. Consumers provided with accurate food irradiation information and the opportunity to taste irradiated goods are more likely to accept the technology (Mostafavi et al., 2010). As discussed in this reference, consumers tend to be cautious and are reluctant to accept irradiated foods. It is important for government, professional organizations, the media, and scientific leaders to educate the public regarding the benefits and limitations of the food irradiation technology to facilitate informed decisions by the public (GAO Report No. GAO-10-309R, 2010; Mostafavi et al., 2010).

There are sound psychological reasons for the public fear of radiation that is explained by considering the risk communication process (Adler and Kranowitz, 2005; Bevelacqua, 2008). Risk communication is based on clear and accurate information, honesty, and trust. Individuals responsible for communicating risk information to the public face two key challenges. First, risk must be communicated in a manner that acknowledges its emotional aspect and provides sufficient information to alleviate the public concern. Second, communication must also engage the public to become an effective partner in addressing and understanding the food irradiation process.

Risk communication is complicated because the public does not have a complete understanding of radiation and radioactive materials and their associated biological effects. Radioactive materials and radiation also tend to be regarded negatively by the public. The public is more accepting radiation if it is received in a voluntary manner (e.g., through a medical procedure). Public reaction to radiation following a power reactor accident is much less acceptable since it is a nonvoluntary or imposed exposure situation. Voluntary and imposed situations are particular risk attribute types. Other risk attributes and associated risk types are illustrated in Table 11.3.

As summarized in Table 11.3, these risk communication factors contribute to the challenges associated with conveying risks associated with food irradiation. Nuclear technology is often characterized in terms of the undesired rather than preferred risk factors. For example, the public views radiation as an imposed, exotic man-made agent that is controlled by an outside organization and is imposed on individuals without their consent. It also has a negative impact on children. Given the public's level of knowledge, a degree of radiophobia is understandable.

Table 11.3 Risk communication preference types.[a]

Risk attribute	Risk communication type	
	Preferred	**Undesired**
Situation	Voluntary	Imposed
Required action	Controlled by the individual	Controlled by others
Benefit	Clearly positive	Little or none
Consequence	Distributed uniformly	Distributed unfairly
Event type	Natural	Man-made
Nature	Statistical	Catastrophic
Origin	Caused by a trusted source	Caused by a source that is not trusted
Hazard	Familiar	Exotic
Group	Adults	Children
Impact	Affects the individual	Affects others

[a] Derived from Adler and Kranowitz (2005) and Bevelacqua (2008).

The public is also more suspicious of communications coming from a representative of the nuclear food industry (not viewed as a trusted source) than a physician or university professor (trusted sources). The individual delivering the message is often as important as the message itself. However, food irradiation has numerous benefits and with sufficient understanding of the level of knowledge of the general public can be explained in a comprehensive manner that will foster acceptance and product use.

Why are not irradiated foods a real health concern?

To kill pathogenic bacteria, insects, and parasites, food products can be treated by exposing them to ionizing radiation. Given this consideration, National Aeronautics and Space Administration (NASA) astronauts use irradiated sterilized meat to prevent the risk of foodborne illnesses during space missions (Todar, 2006). However, prevention of foodborne illness (e.g., effectively elimination of bacteria such as Salmonella and *Escherichia coli*) is not the only reason for food irradiation. Preservation, control of insects, delay of sprouting and ripening, and sterilization are among the other applications of food irradiation.

To answer the question of food irradiation safety, we note that not only is safety a relative term, but other methods of food processing have not been subjected to as thorough an assessment of safety as food irradiation (Waltar, 2004). Many individuals asking about a health concern from irradiation have used or consumed food that has been irradiated (e.g., canned goods that cannot be sterilized by steam, such as condensed milk) and never knew it. While food irradiation has been used in some parts of Europe for increasing the shelf life of fruits and vegetables (up to 500% increase), this practice has not been approved in the United States. However, to control pathogens, the FDA has approved irradiation of poultry and pork and foods such as fruits, vegetables, and grains. Moreover, to control microorganisms, spices, seasonings, and dry enzymes used in food processing are allowed to be irradiated (U.S.FDA, 2016).

The public needs to understand that radiation cannot make the food radioactive, decrease nutritional quality, or significantly alter the taste, texture, or appearance of food. In fact, any changes made by irradiation are so minimal that it is not easy to tell if a food has been irradiated (U.S.FDA, 2016). The FDA has evaluated the safety of irradiated food for more than 3 decades and found it to be safe. Furthermore, the safety of irradiated food has also been endorsed by the World Health Organization (WHO), the Centers for Disease Control and Prevention (CDC), and the US Department of Agriculture (USDA) (U.S.FDA, 2016).

The concerns over the safety of irradiated food can be divided into 4 different areas (Fig. 11.1):

1. Having the right to know what foods are irradiated and what are not.

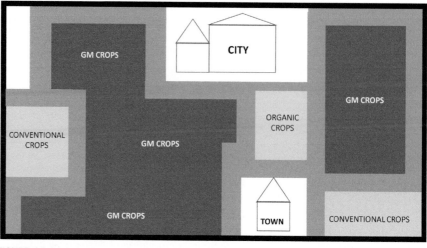

FIGURE 11.1

Current concerns over the safety of irradiated food.

Jean-Victor Balini, modified by Mortazavi.

2. Irradiation only stops food from putrefaction, but the free radicals produced during irradiation affect the safety of the food.

3. Irradiation destroys the essential vitamins and other nutrients and decreases the quality of food.

4. Irradiation will make foods radioactive.

To address these concerns, regulations mandate that labeling of irradiated foods is usually required. The international Radura symbol is being used for irradiated food. Moreover, it is worth noting that the free radicals (atoms or molecules with an unpaired electron) produced during irradiation cannot affect the safety of the food *"There is no evidence to suggest that free radicals, per se, affect the safety of irradiated food."* Although free radicals are generally very reactive, unstable structures, which react with substances to form stable products, they disappear by reacting with each other in the presence of liquids, such as saliva in the mouth. Therefore, WHO reports that their ingestion does not create any significant toxicological effects (Farkas, 2006). Despite attempts for isolating radiation-induced radiolytic products, no substances truly unique to irradiated foods have been identified. Furthermore, food safety tests include microbiological as well as other examinations. Based on a joint FAO/IAEA/WHO study, food irradiated at doses under 10 kGy poses no toxicological hazards (Farkas, 2006).

In addition, irradiation does not destroy the essential vitamins and other nutrients and hence it does not decrease the quality of food. It has been shown that food irradiation has no detrimental effect on essential amino acids, essential fatty acid,

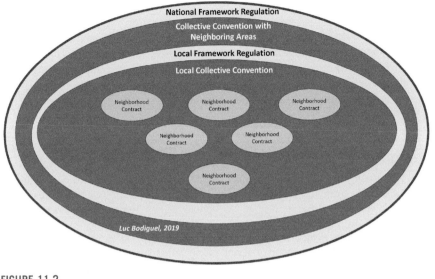

FIGURE 11.2

Different hydrogen isotopes (Blausen, 2014).

minerals, trace elements, and most vitamins as long as it is performed under conditions of actual or potential commercial applications (Farkas, 2006).

Another major concern regarding food irradiation is that radiation causes the food to become radioactive (Eller, 2014). By reviewing the basic nuclear physics, it is evident that when the binding energy of a particle is less than the absorbed energy of incident photon, that particle can be ejected from the nucleus and the remaining nucleus may become radioactive. The 5 major reactions, which can lead to photon-induced activation, are as follows:

1. Photoneutron reactions (γ, n) reactions
2. Photoproton reactions (γ, p)
3. Photodeuterium reactions (γ, ^{2}H)
4. Phototritium reactions (γ, ^{3}H)
5. Photoalpha reactions (γ, α)

Different hydrogen isotopes are shown in Fig. 11.2. As long as the incident energy is limited to about 10 MeV, the photo-neutron reactions are most likely. However, the emission of other particles would be significant at higher photon energies. Usually gamma rays emitted from ^{60}Co and ^{137}Cs sources are used for irradiating foods (Farkas, 2006). Some evidence shows that X-rays with energies up to 5−7 MeV can be used without concern about induced radioactivity in food (WHO, 1995). Therefore, by limiting the energy of electrons and photons, especially X-rays, the production of radionuclides would be insignificant (Findley et al., 1993).

Summary

Food irradiation represents a viable technology for preserving consumables. It has a sound regulatory foundation that is based on extensive research and verification of the technology and its ability to produce a safe product. Concerns regarding food irradiation are based on fears that are unfounded and can be readily alleviated once the public understands the technology and its appropriate usage.

References

Adler, P.S., Kranowitz, J.L., 2005. A Primer on Perceptions of Risk, Risk Communications and Building Trust, the Keystone Center. Available at: https://www.researchgate.net/publication/228383118_A_primer_on_perceptions_of_risk_risk_communication_and_building_trust.

Bevelacqua, J.J., 2008. Health Physics in the 21st Century. Wiley-VCH, Weinheim, Germany.

Bevelacqua, J.J., 2009. Contemporary Health Physics: Problems and Solutions, second ed. Wiley-VCH, Weinheim, Weinheim.

Bevelacqua, J.J., 2010. Basic Health Physics: Problems and Solutions, second ed. Wiley-VCH, Weinheim.

Bevelacqua, J.J., 2016. Health Physics: Radiation-Generating Devices, Characteristics, and Hazards. Wiley-VCH, Weinheim.

Balini, J.-V., 2019. Illustration of a Sandwich. http://www.freestockphotos.biz/stockphoto/15375.

Blausen, B., 2014. Figure Hydrogen Isotopes. https://commons.wikimedia.org/wiki/File:Blausen_0530_HydrogenIsotopes.png#filelinks.

10CFR20, 2018. Standards for Protection against Radiation. National Archives and Records Administration, US Government printing Office, Washington DC, USA.

21CFR, 2018. Food and Drugs. National Archives and Records Administration , US Government Printing Office, Washington DC, USA.

49CFR, 2018. Transportation. National Archives and Records Administration, US Government Printing Office, Washington DC, USA.

Eller, A., 2014. The Validity of Certain Myths About Food Irradiation. Physics 241. Stanford University, Winter 2014, Stanfort, USA.

EPA Report EPA 402-F-14-016, 2014. Office of Radiation and Indoor Air, Washington DC, USA.

Farkas, J., 2006. Irradiation for better foods. Trends in Food Science and Technology 17 (4), 148−152.

Findley, D.J.S., Parsons, T.V., Sené, M.R., 1993. Irradiation of food and the induction of radioactivity. Radiation Physics and Chemistry 42 (1), 417−420.

GAO Report 3. No. GAO/HUD-90-118, 1990. Food Irradiation-Federal Requirements and Monitoring. United States Government Accountability Office, Washington, DC, USA.

GAO Report No GAO-10-309R, 2010. Food Irradiation: FDA Could Improve Its Documentation and Communication of Key Decisions on Food Irradiation Petitions. United States Government Accountability Office, Washington, DC, USA.

Mostafavi, H.A., Fathollahi, H., Motamedi, F., Mirmajlessi, S.M., 2010. Food irradiation: applications, public acceptance and global trade. African Journal of Biotechnology 9 (20), 2826–2833.

Olson, D.G., 1998. Irradiation of food. Journal of Food Technology 52, 55–62.

Sterigenics, 2007. Sterigenics International Brochure (RevFS07). The Sterilisation of Spices, Herbs and Vegetable Seasonings: Understanding the Options, Oak Brook, IL with Additional Technical Data at. https://sterigenics.com.

Sun, D.W., 2018. Emerging Technologies in Food Processing, second ed. Academic Press, Cambridge, , MA, USA.

Tauxe, R.V., 2001. Food safety and irradiation: protecting the public from foodborne infections. Emerging Infectious Diseases 7, 516–521.

Todar, K., 2006. Todar's Online Textbook of Bacteriology. University of Wisconsin-Madison Department of Bacteriology Madison, Wis, USA.

U.S. FDA, 2016. Food Irradiation: What You Need to Know. U.S. Food and Drug Administration.

Waltar, A.E., 2004. Radiation and Modern Life: Fulfilling Marie Curie's Dream. Prometheus Books, Amherst, , New York, USA.

Walter, M., 1986. Urbain, Food Irradiation. Academic Press, Cambridge, MA, USA.

WHO, 1988. Food Irradiation A Technique for Preserving and Improving the Safety of Food. World Health Organization, Geneva, Switzerland.

WHO, 1995. The Development of X-Ray Machines for Food Irradiation (Proceedings of a Consultants' Meeting).

WHO, 2017. Technical Report Series No. 1007, Evaluation of Certain Food Additives: Eighty-Fourth Report of the Joint FAO/WHO Expert Committee on Food Additives. World Health Organization, Geneva, Switzerland.

Further reading

Molins, R.A., 2001. Food Irradiation: Principles and Applications. Wiley-Interscience, New York, USA.

Pillai, S.D., 2016. Introduction to electron-beam food irradiation. Chemical Engineering Progress 112 (11), 36–44.

Steele, J.H., 2002. Food irradiation: a public health opportunity. International Journal of Infectious Diseases 4, 62–66.

Yousefi, M.R., Razdari, A.M., 2014. Irradiation and its potential to food preservation. International Journal of Advanced Biological and Biomedical Research 2, 477–481.

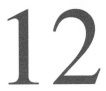

CHAPTER

Safety of irradiated food

Jun Nishihira, MD, PhD [1,2]

[1]*Department of Medical Management and Informatics, Hokkaido Information University, Ebetsu City, Hokkaido, Japan;* [2]*Professor, Health Information Science Center, Hokkaido Information University, Ebetsu, Hokkaido, Japan*

Background

With global trade in agricultural and foodstuffs continually on the rise, it is expected that incidents and hazardous situations related to the import and export of food will increase. The use of quarantine treatments or other mitigation approaches to prevent pest introduction in traded commodities raises many phytosanitary regulatory issues (Follett and Neven, 2006; Maherani et al., 2016). Food irradiation treatment is a robust method to solve this problem. Food irradiation is an efficient technology that can be used to ensure food safety by eliminating insects and pathogens to prolong shelf life. Unfortunately, irradiation has yet to be generally accepted as safe among customers. Standardized phytosanitary measures on food irradiation from country to country are required to gain consumers' trust in a globalized market.

In 1989, food irradiation was approved by the US Department of Agriculture (USDA) and US Food and Drug Administration (FDA). However, this technology is still controversial due to largely unwarranted fears of the modification of food properties, formation of dangerous substances, and the sense of its being a dangerous process with the possibility of accidents in association with the nuclear establishment. A number of researches have been reported, showing that all of these prejudices are misleading and overestimated (Maherani et al., 2016). However, more recent studies have shown that consumers remain reluctant to purchase irradiated food because of these prejudices. Their fears may be intimately related to the lack of information about the irradiation process and the natural human resistance to change. The acceptance of irradiated food by consumers depends on the degree of their knowledge about irradiation technology.

The growing number of recalls after food poisoning incidents offers a good opportunity to implement a revised marketing policy for irradiated food making consumers more aware of the benefits of this technology for consumers. Ironically, the fact that international organizations and the Codex Alimentarius have limited the dose level to 10 kGy (kilogray) has mistakenly been interpreted as meaning that this is a dose above which toxic substances could be introduced or the nutritional adequacy of foods could be negatively influenced (World Health Organization,

Genetically Modified and Irradiated Food. https://doi.org/10.1016/B978-0-12-817240-7.00016-4
Copyright © 2020 Elsevier Inc. All rights reserved.

1999). More than that, consumers are still confused and fail to differentiate irradiated foods from radioactive foods. In this review, the history of food irradiation is introduced at first, and then its usefulness and future application are discussed.

History of food irradiation

At first, the germination prevention effect of irradiation was reported in 1950 on potatoes, and the initiation of a chronic toxicity test by the US Army feeding irradiated potatoes, wheat, bacon, peaches, etc (Sparrow and Christensen, 1950). A process for approving legislation regarding food irradiation, similar to that for food additives, was introduced in 1958. As follows, irradiation to prevent the germination of potatoes was permitted in the Soviet Union in 1958 and in Canada in 1959.

A joint meeting of the Food and Agriculture Organization (FAO), the International Atomic Energy Agency (IAEA), and the World Health Organization (WHO) on the soundness of irradiated foods was held in 1961, and irradiation of bacon was permitted in the United States in 1963. The Joint Expert Committee on the Technical Foundation of Laws and Regulations of Irradiated Foods of FAO/IAEA/WHO was held in 1964, where it was decided to treat irradiated products as food additives. On this matter, "Food irradiation research and development of basic plan in Japan" was introduced in 1967 focusing on seven food items (Jaga potato, onion, rice, wheat, wiener—sausage, fishery products, and oranges).

The first meeting of JECFI (FAO/IAEA/WHO Joint expert committee on the wholesomeness of irradiated foods) was held in 1975, and the International Project in the Field of Food Irradiation (IFIP) was launched in the same year. At the second JECFI meeting in 1976, it was recommended to regard food irradiation as a physical processing technology rather than treat irradiated foods as food additives. The third JECFI meeting in 1980 declared there was no issue in terms of the food's wholesomeness when it is irradiated at levels of 10 kGy or less. An "international general standard on irradiated food" was adopted in the FAO-WHO Codex Alimentarius of 1983. In FAO/WHO/IAEA and ITC, international agreement documents were adopted on the acceptance, management, and trade of irradiated foods in 1988.

Irradiation of poultry meat at levels up to 3.0 kGy was permitted in the United States in 1992, which was followed by decisions to permit the irradiation of red meat by FDA in 1997. An FAO/IAEA/WHO Joint Study Group on High-Dose Irradiation in 1997 showed no undesirable effects of irradiation above 10 kGy. The EU enacted in 2000 the EU Directive that defines the framework of irradiated food. In the same year, the All Nippon Spices Association received permission from the Japanese government for sterilization of spice by irradiation by 10 kGy. The FAO/IAEA/WHO Joint Study Group on High-Dose Irradiation reached an agreement to allow irradiation at 10 kGy in 2003.

Present situation

Interest in introducing food irradiation technologies continues to increase because of persistently high food losses from infestation, contamination, and spoilage by bacteria and fungi, rising concern about foodborne diseases and a growing international trade in food products that must meet strict import standards of quality and quarantine. Thus far, food irradiation has demonstrated valuable and practical benefits when integrated within an established system for the safe handling and distribution of food products. It has been gradually accepted that food irradiation is efficient to eliminate insect pests before products are exported to remote areas where the pests do not occur. The technology of irradiation is also the most straightforward approach to overcome regulatory trade barriers and gain market access (Follett, 2014). As a particular example, the United States and Australia, as well as the International Plant Protection Convention, have approved the generic radiation dose of 150 Gy for quarantine treatment of tephritid fruit flies.

To date, several reports have confirmed that irradiated foods are nutritionally equivalent or even better than nonirradiated foods that are subjected to normal processing (Swallow, 1991; Diehl, 1995; Cetinkaya et al., 2006). Accordingly, under restrictive regulations or complete prohibition of the use of chemical fumigants for insect and microbial control, irradiation is becoming a much more effective alternative to protecting food against insect damage and spoilage. Irradiation is regarded as an effective quarantine treatment for fresh produce in the food industry, and at present, more than 60 countries have adopted the technology (Ehlermann, 2016). In addition, it has been confirmed that irradiation can help to ensure a safer and more plentiful food supply by extending food shelf life through the control of pests and bacterial pathogens. According to the WHO and FAO (Follett, 2014; Lacroix and Follett, 2015), irradiation is a safe technology for the processing of food commodities when the appropriate radiation dose is respected. To support this, several reports from international scientific and political bodies have resolved the misunderstandings, exaggerations, and conflicting claims regarding the safety of irradiation (Diehl, 1995). Commercially, relatively low-dose radiation has been shown to be an effective postharvest treatment and quarantine control for dried raisins, figs, and apricots (Cetinkaya et al., 2006).

In recent years, the use of irradiation for phytosanitary purposes is becoming practical and essential around the world. More than 50 countries worldwide have approved irradiation for over 60 products. Phytosanitary irradiation of fruits and agricultural products has recently increased, with six countries irradiating 18,500 tons in 2010 (Kume and Todoriki, 2013). The United States, China, Netherlands, Belgium, Brazil, Thailand, and Australia are the major countries that have adopted the technology commercially. In the EU, the quantity of irradiated foods was estimated to 9264 tons, especially for spice decontamination. More than 18,446 tons of food are irradiated worldwide for phytosanitary purposes, representing 5734 tons in Hawaii, 493 tons in Australia, 100 tons in India, 951 tons in Thailand, 850 tons in Vietnam, and 10,318 tons in Mexico, mostly for export to the United States. In the United States, the volume of irradiated meat and poultry sold is holding steady in the United States, and the amount of irradiated produce is growing rapidly (Eustice, 2011). Estimates are about 15,000 tons of irradiated fresh produce was consumed in 2010.

Safety of food irradiation

The adoption of food irradiation has differed from one country to another. The technology is a processing technique that involves exposing food to ionizing radiation such as gamma radiation and has multiple benefits in food preservation through several steps such as disinfection, delaying maturation, sprout inhibition, decontamination, and sterilization. In one case, the process can be applied to fresh or frozen products without affecting the nutritional value (Patil et al., 1999). In another case, irradiation induces specific alterations that can modify both the chemical composition and the nutritional value of foods (Crawford and Ruff, 1996). These changes can be observed in the case of vitamins, depending on the irradiation dose, and other factors such as temperature and presence or absence of oxygen. Despite these facts, irradiation offers a wide range of benefits to the food industry and the consumer by ensuring the hygienic quality of solid or semisolid foods through inactivation of foodborne pathogens.

The safety of irradiated food consumed by humans is a crucial issue for the development of food preservation methods and technologies. The potential benefits of food irradiation are yet to be realized due to slow progress in the commercialization of the technology, but now there is sufficient evidence that retail consumers will purchase irradiated food (Roberts, 2014). According to a comprehensive agreement between FAO of the United Nations, IAEA, and WHO, on the basis of knowledge derived from over 50 years of research, irradiated foods were considered generally safe. It is reported that a joint FAO/IAEA/WHO Study Group on High-Dose Irradiation (JSGHDI) stated that any food treated at any high dose is acceptable and healthy as long as it is palatable. This statement sends a strong message that any food subjected to inappropriate irradiation treatment may have lost its essential properties but is not hazardous for consumption (Filho et al., 2014).

Regarding the nutritional value, irradiation does not cause any significant loss of macronutrients. Proteins, fats, and carbohydrates undergo little modification in nutritional value through irradiation, even at doses over 10 kGy, although there may be some sensory changes. In a similar manner, the essential amino acids, essential fatty acids, minerals, and trace elements are unchanged. A decrease in certain vitamins (mostly thiamin) has been demonstrated, but these decreases are of the same order of magnitude as occurs in other manufacturing processes such as drying or canning (Mostafavi et al., 2012)

Regarding other foods, irradiation of fresh fruits, e.g., raspberries and beet leaves (Chen et al., 2016; Finten et al., 2017) and dried fruits, e.g., raisins, figs, and apricots, has been shown to result in elevated nutrient levels and good sensory acceptance (Cetinkaya et al., 2006). Indeed, irradiation processing of fruits and vegetables can increase the levels of quercetin, vitamin C, and phenolic compounds (Patil et al., 1999). Despite these benefits of irradiation, food processed with irradiation still encounters several barriers, one of which is the belief that consumers will not purchase irradiated food and a consequent caution among food retailers and producers. Providing evidence to food retailers and producers is critical to lowering barriers to wider use of the technology in the food industry (Roberts, 2014).

Appropriate irradiation dose

Appropriate dose of irradiation is well summarized in the report of the WHO (World Health Organization, 1994), showing the following examples: For prevention of microbial spoilage, levels of spoilage bacteria in poultry may be reduced sufficiently to prolong shelf life by as much as 1–2 weeks following exposure at 3 kGy. Many meats can tolerate relatively high doses of irradiation if appropriate precautions are taken. For example, blanching, freezing, and the exclusion of oxygen, together with doses in the 25–45 kGy range, can result in sterilized food with a long shelf life. Much of the raw poultry sold for human consumption is contaminated with *Salmonella* and *Campylobacter*, both of which can be effectively controlled by irradiation, as they are readily destroyed by doses in the range 2–3 kGy. Irradiation of pork at doses of 0.3 kGy or less can kill the larvae of the parasite *Trichinella spiralis,* and low-dose irradiation may also reduce the risk of cysticercosis caused by the pork tapeworm. Spices and related materials may contain large amounts of molds, bacteria, and their heat-resistant spores. Doses of 3–10 kGy can significantly improve the hygienic quality of spices, dehydrated vegetables, herbs, and other dry ingredients. Doses of 1 kGy or less can prevent losses from insect infestation in stored grains, pulses, flour, cereals, and coffee beans.

Concerning fruit and vegetable pests, including fruit flies, the mango seed weevil, the navel orange worm, the potato tuber worm, the codling moth, spider mites, and scale insects, may be controlled by doses of 1 kGy or less. Insect disinfestation of nuts and dried fruits can also be achieved, since most insects are killed by doses in the range 0.25–0.75 kGy.

As for retardation of postharvest issues, sprouting in root crops such as potato, sweet potato, and others tubors can be inhibited with irradiation doses of 0.05–0.15 kGy. Irradiation of tropical and subtropical fruits such as bananas, mangoes, and other fruits at doses of 0.25–1 kGy delays maturation and senescence. Ripening is suppressed in temperate-zone fruits such as apples, pears, and other fruits at doses in excess of 1 kGy. Strawberries are relatively resistant to damage by irradiation, and thus higher at 2–2.5 kGy may be needed.

Attitudes of consumers to irradiated food

As discussed above, irradiation technology has proved to be effective in reducing microbial contamination and providing sterile food. However, research has shown that the public still tends to take a negative attitude toward irradiated food even though it has been recognized as safe by authorities (Cardello et al., 2007). Multiple factors may explain these untoward attitudes, one of which may be the lack of proper knowledge about the technology employed to process the food. Public awareness of food irradiation is not high; many people do not even know what irradiation is (Frewer et al., 2011). It is of interest that a study showed that increased awareness of the nature and benefits of food irradiation led to positive changes in consumers' perception and influenced their decisions to buy irradiated food (Nayga et al., 2005). In this context, consumers are willing to pay for a reduction in the risk of foodborne illness once informed about the nature of food irradiation.

For this processing technique to become more widespread, it is essential to establish effective strategies to encourage consumers to buy irradiated food (Resurreccion et al., 1995). Positive and negative factors coexist in any food debate. Consumers generally value "freshness" more than increased shelf life, which is often seen as "unnatural." Therefore, it is important to establish a good partnership with less biased and reliable food retailers who promote the marketing of irradiated food. Labeling is not required for food irradiation, but showing the advantages of irradiation may be a good way to decrease consumer opposition to irradiated food. It is useful to explain the possible consequences of foodborne pathogens to create a consciousness of the importance of food safety. Because irradiation is a process that does not affect the physical aspects of the product, the role of the food industry and food retailers should be to inform the public either by labeling products or by telling consumers about the benefits of the irradiation.

It appears that consumers perceive most food risks to stem from farming practices and processing, while farmers, on the other hand, believe that the most significant food safety risks occur as a result of consumer and processor actions. Both the scarcity of knowledge of consumers on food processing and poor communication with farmers by food processing technologists or engineers may increase the misunderstanding between these two groups. In this respect, a joint meeting in 1997, involving the WHO, the FAO, and the IAEA, determined that food irradiated with an appropriate dose to achieve the intended objective was both safe and nutritious (World Health Organization, 1999). Indeed, mild food irradiation can be used to maintain both food quality and safety because of its ability to control spoilage and foodborne pathogenic microorganisms without significantly affecting the sensory attributes of the food (Xavier et al., 2014). Furthermore, there is an increasing demand from consumers concerning sensory and nonsensory attributes of foods, as well as by the interactions between them. In this matter, a study demonstrated the sensory acceptance of irradiated foods, in which the influence of food irradiation on consumer behavior has been reported using raspberries (Chen et al., 2016).

It is certain that the demand for irradiated food products depends on acceptance by consumers. Although public knowledge about irradiation continues to be limited, the demand for safety-enhanced irradiated food is increasing, especially after people receive information about potential benefits and risks (Eustice and Bruhn, 2006). Most studies on consumers' attitude toward irradiated food have shown that reliable information seems to be the key to consumer acceptance. Several studies on the perception of consumers clearly showed that they are not only willing to buy irradiated foods but also often prefer them over food treated by conventional means when given a choice and even a small amount of accurate information. Consistent with these studies, a variety of market research has demonstrated that the majority of consumers would choose irradiated products over nonirradiated ones after they learn the facts and understand the benefits (Marcotte, 1989).

Overall conclusion

It is concluded that irradiation will not change the composition of the food from a toxicological point of view. That is, the technology would not have an adverse effect on human health and not induce changes of the microflora of the food that would increase the microbiological risk to the consumer (World Health Organization, 1994). Even though, any novel food processing, involving irradiation process, poses a serious challenge to the purchasing behavior of consumers. Thus, researchers in the food industry and food retailers engaged in irradiated foods should focus more directly on questions and issues related to the needs of consumers. To improve the acceptance of these technologies by consumers, not only strong scientific evidence demonstrating the safety of irradiated food but also communication, labels, and education about this particular technology are essential (Maherani et al., 2016). New strategies based on positive messages of irradiation in the marketplace will thus encourage consumers to be more receptive to safety-oriented and high-quality irradiated foods.

Data collected from over half a century of research have established that foods irradiated at appropriate doses are safe and wholesome. The irradiated foods are generally nutritionally equivalent or more nutritious than nonirradiated foods subjected to normal processing. Irradiation will not lead to nutrient losses to an extent that would have an adverse effect on the nutritional status of individuals or populations. Taken together, irradiated food processed in accordance with established good manufacturing practice is considered safe and nutritionally adequate because of the process of irradiation.

Perspectives

Several studies have shown that irradiation technology in combination with other treatments can be used as an innovative and effective method to add values to food products. It is still difficult for consumers to differentiate irradiated foods from radioactive foods. When well informed, most of the consumers will not reject irradiated food. They are looking for products with good quality and a competitive price. When consumers are aware of the short- and long-term dangers of chemical additives as alternatives to irradiation, they are more willing to accept the application of irradiation to food products. In addition to informing customers, companies should update their quality system and implement new procedures to support risk management and the supply and distribution chains of irradiated foods.

References

Cardello, A.V., Schutz, H.G., Lesher, L.L., 2007. Consumer perceptions of foods processed by innovative and emerging technologies: a conjoint analytic study. Innovative Food Science and Emerging Technologies 8, 73–83.

Cetinkaya, N., Ozyardımci, B., Denli, E., Ic, E., 2006. Radiation processing as a post-harvest quarantine control for raisins, dried figs and dried apricots. Radiation Physics and Chemistry 75, 424–431.

Chen, Q., Caoc, M., Chena, H., Gaoa, P., Fua, Y., Liua, M., Wanga, Y., Huanga, M., 2016. Effects of gamma irradiation on microbial safety and quality of stir fry chicken dices with hot chili during storage. Radiation Physics and Chemistry 127, 122–126.

Crawford, L.M., Ruff, E.H., 1996. A review of the safety of cold pasteurization through irradiation. Food Control 7, 87–97.

Diehl, J.F., 1995. Nutritional adequacy of irradiated foods. In: Diehl, J.F. (Ed.), Safety of Irradiated Foods, second ed. Marcel Dekker, Inc., New York, NY, USA, pp. 241–282.

Ehlermann, D.A.E., 2016. Wholesomeness of irradiated food. Radiation Physics and Chemistry 125, 24–29.

Eustice, R.F., Bruhn, C.M., 2006. Consumer acceptance and marketing of irradiated foods. In: Food Irradiation Research and Technology. USDA, ARS, Eastern Regional Research Center, Wyndmoor, PA, USA, pp. 63–83.

Eustice, R.F., 2011. Food irradiation: a global perspective and future prospects. Available online: http://ansnuclearcafe.org/2011/06/09/food-irradiation-a-global-perspective-future-prospects/#sthash. YyeeMQ5M.dpbs.

Filho, L.T., Lucia, S.M.D., Limaa, R.M., Scolforoa, C.Z., Carneiroa, J.C.Z., Pinheirob, C.J.G., Passamai Jr., J.L., 2014. Irradiation of strawberries: influence of information regarding preservation technology on consumer sensory acceptance. Innovative Food Science and Emerging Technologies 26, 242–247.

Finten, G., Garrido, J.I., Agüero, M.V., Jagus, R.J., 2017. Irradiated ready-to-eat spinach leaves: how information influences awareness towards irradiation treatment and consumer's purchase intention. Radiation Physics and Chemistry 130, 247–251.

Follett, P.A., Neven, L.G., 2006. Current trends in quarantine entomology. Annual Review of Entomology 51, 359–385.

Follett, P., 2014. Phytosanitary irradiation for fresh horticultural commodities: generic treatments, current issues, and next steps. Stewart Postharvest Review 10, 1–7.

Frewer, L., Bergmann, K., Brennan, M., Lion, R., Meertens, R., Rowe, G., Siegrist, M., Vereijken, C., 2011. Consumer response to novel agri-food technologies: implications for predicting consumer acceptance of emerging food technologies. Trends in Food Science and Technology 22, 442–456.

Kume, T., Todoriki, S., 2013. Food irradiation in Asia, the European Union, and the United States: a status update. Radioisotopes 62, 291–299.

Lacroix, M., Follett, P., 2015. Combination irradiation treatments for food safety and phytosanitary uses. Stewart Postharvest Review 11, 1–10.

Maherani, B., Hossain, F., Criado, P., Ben-Fadhel, Y., Salmieri, S., Lacroix, M., 2016. World market development and consumer acceptance of irradiation technology. Foods 79.

Marcotte, M., 1989. Consumer Acceptance of Irradiated Food. Nordion International Inc.: Kanata, , ON, Canada, p. 17.

Mostafavi, H.A., Mirmajlessi, S.M., Fathollahi, H., 2012. The potential of food irradiation: benefits and limitations. In: Eissa, A.H.A. (Ed.), Trends in Vital Food and Engineering. INTECH, Rijeka, Croatia.

Nayga, R.M., Aiew, W., Nichols, J.P., 2005. Information effects on consumers' willingness to purchase irradiated food products. Applied Economic Perspectives and Policy 27, 37—48.

Patil, B.S., Pike, L.M., Howard, L.R., 1999. Effect of gamma irradiation on quercetin on onion. Subtropical Plant Science 51, 16—22.

Resurreccion, A.V.A., Galvez, F.C.F., Fletcher, S.M., Misra, S.K., 1995. Consumer attitudes toward irradiated food: results of a new study. Journal of Food Protection 58, 193—196.

Roberts, P.B., 2014. Food irradiation is safe: half a century of studies. Radiation Physics and Chemistry 105, 78—82.

Sparrow, A.H., Christensen, E., 1950. Effects of X-ray, neutron and chronic gamma irradiation on growth and yield of potatoes. American Journal of Botany 37, 667 (Abstract).

Swallow, A.J., 1991. Wholesomeness and safety of irradiated foods. Advances in Experimental Medicine and Biology 1, 11—31.

World Health Organization, 1994. Safety and Nutritional Adequacy of Irradiated Food. World Health Organization, Geneva, Switzerland.

World Health Organization, 1999. High-Dose Irradiation: Wholesomeness of Food Irradiatied with Doses above 10 kGy. World Health Organization, Geneva, Switzerland.

Xavier, M.P., Duber, C., Mussiob, P., Delgadob, E., Maquieirab, A., Soriab, A., Curuchetb, A., Márquezb, R., Méndeza, C., López, T., 2014. Use of mild irradiation doses to control pathogenic bacteria on meat trimmings for production of patties aiming at provoking minimal changes in quality attributes. Meat Science 98, 383—391.

Further reading

CMC Publishing, 2002. "On Radiation Irradiation on Food" Atomic Energy Commission Food. Items Irradiation Expert Group Added Information on September 26, 2006.

Lacroix, M., Ouattara, B., 2000. Combined industrial processes with irradiation to assure innocuity and preservation of food products—a review. Food Research International 33, 719—724.

Roberts, P., Hénon, Y.M., 2015. Consumer response to irradiated food: purchase versus perception. Stewart Postharvest Review 3, 1—6.

Turgis, M., Millette, M., Salmieri, S., Lacroix, M., 2012. Elimination of Listeria inoculated in ready-to-eat carrots by combination of antimicrobial coating and -irradiation. Radiation Physics and Chemistry 81, 1170—1172.

Novel processing technologies: facts about irradiation and other technologies

13

Ronald F. Eustice

Tucson, AZ, United States

Introduction

Many innovations, even those with obvious advantages, require a period of time between scientific discovery, commercial availability, and when they are widely accepted by the general public (Rogers, 1983).

Technologies such as pasteurization, immunization, and chlorination are now considered by health experts to be "pillars of public health," yet each of these lifesaving innovations was met with suspicion and resistance when first introduced. Even in this age of advanced learning, there are those who want to consume raw milk, avoid vaccination of their children, and refuse to drink water that has been chlorinated. In recent years the use of food irradiation has raised issues that consumers and the food industry have had to deal with. What is the truth about food irradiation? Is it safe; are there "unknown risks"?

In this, chapter I will use actual experience and scientific evidence to separate fact from fiction to answer questions and help clarify some of the concerns that are raised by critics food irradiation. I will compare the arguments raised by critics of highly beneficial technologies such as pasteurization, immunization, and chlorination with arguments currently raised by critics of food irradiation.

I will present statistics on preventable foodborne illness caused by contaminated food, summarize consumer acceptance studies at leading universities, and finally show that significant progress is being made in the introduction of irradiated food at supermarkets in the United States and many other countries.

Finally, I will provide suggestions for future actions that will help expand the use of food irradiation.

Resistance to "new" technology

While pasteurization, vaccination, chlorination, and irradiation are very distinct technologies used for different purposes, many, perhaps most, of the arguments raised by critics of these technologies are similar.

Genetically Modified and Irradiated Food. https://doi.org/10.1016/B978-0-12-817240-7.00017-6

It is human nature to resist change and to fear the "unknown." Critics who believed the earth is flat stifled exploration of the "new world." Arguments against constructive change take many forms. University of Houston economics professor and noted author Thomas R. DeGregori says, "One common argument against change is the search for a *risk less* alternative." DeGregori says, "Every change has its risks; some real, others imagined. Whether a change is political, scientific, or technological, a simple assertion of risk should not in and of itself be an argument against that change. We must measure the benefits of change against the risks of not changing" (DeGregori, 2002).

Christopher Columbus and other explorers faced a multitude of risks, but their ships did not drop off the edge of the earth.

Those who wish to maintain the status quo and convince others that the risks outweigh benefits often make impossible demands for a zero-risk society. Those who choose to believe that the earth is flat despite overwhelming scientific evidence to the contrary have every right to do so. In a free society, proponents of the "Flat Earth Theory" have a right to their own set of opinions, but those opinions do not alter the fact that the earth is demonstrably and unequivocally spherical.

Risk versus benefits

DeGregori says, "If we examine the many changes over the past century, changes that have reduced infant and child mortality by more than 90%, have given Americans nearly 30 years of added life expectancy, have recently caused an even more rapid growth in disability-free years of life, and have allowed comparable or greater advances in other countries, we will find that all those changes carried risks."

Technologies such as chlorination of water, pasteurization of milk, synthetic fertilizers, chemical pesticides, modern medicine, genetically enhanced organisms (GMOs), immunization, and irradiation, to name a few, all faced and continue to face various levels of opposition. Most cities use chlorine to purify their water, most parents want their children immunized against dreaded diseases, and very few people would consider drinking unpasteurized (raw) milk because of the known risks. Yet these lifesaving technologies all have their risks. Chlorine is toxic, and immunization can sometimes cause the disease it was intended to prevent. Pasteurized milk tastes different than milk straight from the cow, can be recontaminated, and will spoil if not refrigerated. By comparison, the risks of genetically enhanced crops and irradiation, if there are any, are "unknown" because after years of study, scientists have not found any (U.S. Food and Drug Administration, 2016). Weigh that against the known risks of contracting bacterial illnesses from the consumption of food that harbors unseen pathogens.

Food irradiation

Although food irradiation, sometimes called "cold pasteurization," has been described as the "most extensively studied food processing technology in the history of humankind" and is endorsed or supported by virtually every medical and scientific organizations, the process is still considered a relatively "new" technology. Despite widespread media attention from food recalls, serious illness, and death, food irradiation technology remains underutilized and sometimes misunderstood.

What is food irradiation?

Food irradiation (the application of ionizing radiation to food) is a technology that improves the safety and extends the shelf life of foods by reducing or eliminating microorganisms and insects. Like pasteurizing milk and canning fruits and vegetables, irradiation can make food safer for the consumer. In the United States, the Food and Drug Administration (FDA) is responsible for regulating the sources of radiation that are used to irradiate food. The FDA approves a source of radiation for use on foods only after it has determined that irradiating the food is safe (U.S. Food and Drug Administration, 2016).

Irradiation does not make foods radioactive, compromise nutritional quality, or noticeably change the taste, texture, or appearance of food. In fact, any changes made by irradiation are so minimal that it is not easy to tell if a food has been irradiated.

Why irradiate food?

Irradiation **is one process that** can serve many purposes.

- **Prevention of foodborne illness**—to effectively eliminate organisms that cause foodborne illness, such as Salmonella and *Escherichia coli* (*E. coli*).
- **Preservation**—to destroy or inactivate organisms that cause spoilage and decomposition and extend the shelf life of foods.
- **Control of insects**—to destroy insects in or on tropical fruits imported into the North America, Europe, or other nontropical countries. Irradiation also decreases the need for other pest-control practices that may harm the fruit.
- **Delay of sprouting and ripening**—to inhibit sprouting (e.g., potatoes) and delay ripening of fruit to increase longevity.
- **Sterilization**—irradiation can be used to sterilize foods, which can then be stored for years without refrigeration. Sterilized foods are useful in hospitals for patients with severely impaired immune systems, such as patients with AIDS or undergoing chemotherapy. Foods that are sterilized by irradiation are exposed to substantially higher levels of treatment than those approved for general use (U.S. Food and Drug Administration, 2016).

How is food irradiated?

There are three sources of radiation approved for use on foods.

- Gamma rays are emitted from radioactive forms of the element cobalt (Cobalt 60) or of the element cesium (Cesium 137). Gamma radiation is used routinely to sterilize medical, dental, and household products and is also used for the radiation treatment of cancer.

- X-rays are produced by reflecting a high-energy stream of electrons off a target substance (usually one of the heavy metals) into food. X-rays are also widely used in medicine and industry to produce images of internal structures.
- Electron beam (or e-beam) is similar to X-rays and is a stream of high-energy electrons propelled from an electron accelerator into food (U.S. Food and Drug Administration, 2016).

Safety of irradiated foods

The FDA has evaluated the safety of irradiated food for more than 40 years and has found the process to be safe. The World Health Organization (WHO), the Centers for Disease Control and Prevention (CDC), and the US Department of Agriculture (USDA) have also endorsed the safety of irradiated food.

There is virtually unanimous agreement by scientific and medical associations and scientific groups that irradiation is not only safe but also that its widespread use would dramatically improve the safety of our food. Food irradiation has the potential to dramatically decrease the incidence of foodborne disease and has earned virtually unanimous support or approval from international and national medical, scientific, and public health organizations, as well as food processors and related industry groups.

Labeling of irradiated food

In the United States, the FDA requires that irradiated foods bear the international symbol for irradiation. Each country has their own separate rules, but the international symbol is the Radura symbol along with the statement "Treated with radiation" or "Treated by irradiation" on the food label. Bulk foods, such as fruits and vegetables, are required to be individually labeled or to have a label next to the sale container. The FDA does not require that individual ingredients in multi-ingredient foods (e.g., spices) be labeled. It is important to remember that irradiation is not a replacement for proper food handling practices by producers, processors, and consumers. Irradiated foods need to be stored, handled, and cooked in the same way as nonirradiated foods, because they could still become contaminated with disease-causing organisms after irradiation if the rules of basic food safety are not followed.

Consumer acceptance of irradiated food

A growing number of consumers around the world have purchased and continue to purchase irradiated fresh produce, meat products, and other foods. Approximately, one-third of the commercial spices consumed in the United States are irradiated. Based on the fact that millions of pounds of irradiated food are consumed annually and this amount is increasing dramatically, the evidence is substantial that the majority of consumers will readily buy irradiated food (Eustice and Bruhn, 2013), Consumers buy a product as they want that particular food because they believe it is of higher quality, more affordable, or possibly safer. For most consumers, the fact that the product has been irradiated is of minimal importance, if even considered at all.

While a small fraction of consumers choose not to purchase irradiated foods, research shows that often the "doubters" (nonconsumers) avoid foods that have been irradiated but also reject foods produced with many other "new" technologies. Research shows that many who are neutral or slightly negative about food irradiation become more positive when they receive even a small amount of information on the purpose of irradiation and the widespread support of the technology by health and scientific organizations (Frenzen et al., 2001).

Communication regarding marketing success and benefits to consumers is more effective than providing technical details of the technology. Retailers that are offering irradiated foods know that once irradiated foods are on the shelves, consumer acceptance is high and "push back" is negligible. Both retailer- and consumer-perceived concerns can largely be addressed by ensuring retailers are prepared to offer accurate and timely responses to any potential consumer concerns that are raised. Political and/or commercially motivated issues such as eat local versus imports can be addressed through progressive in-store merchandising that offers multiple choices that empower the consumer with choices to meet their own unique needs and beliefs. Often irradiated products have a distinct advantage in either quality and/or price, which are both key consumer decision-making factors that create the attraction for consumers.

Organizations that support irradiation

The extensive list of medical and scientific organizations endorsing or supporting irradiation of food (Foodirradiation.org, 2014) should be used broadly to convince retailers and the public of the widespread support for food irradiation. Irradiation of food is already approved in the United States for most perishable foods and has been endorsed by the WHO, CDC, US FDA, USDA, American Medical Association (AMA), and European Commission Scientific Committee on Food (SCF). In fact, hundreds of credible groups support irradiation while a very limited number of special interest groups opposed to the technology rely on inaccurate and outdated information as well as half-truths to create unwarranted fear and suspicion. Unfortunately, because of a widespread lack of understanding of the risks and consequences of foodborne disease and of the effectiveness and safety of irradiation—and because of intense opposition from antinuclear activists and other special interest groups—irradiation of food as a public health measure has not yet reached its full potential and not yet achieved widespread consumer acceptance (Foodirradiation.org, 2014).

Food safety

Dr. Robert Tauxe of the US CDC estimates that if 50% of poultry, ground beef, pork, and processed meats in the United States was irradiated, the potential benefit of the irradiation would be a 25% reduction in the morbidity and mortality rate caused by these infections. This estimated net benefit is substantial; the measure could prevent nearly 900,000 cases of infection, 8500 hospitalizations, more than 6000 catastrophic illnesses, and 350 deaths each year (Table 13.1). Given the probable number of unreported and undetected foodborne illnesses, this reduction is likely to be even greater (Tauxe, 2001).

Insect control

Irradiation is widely considered the most effective and environmentally friendly phytosanitary technology available to prevent the importation of harmful insect pests that may hitchhike on imported produce. As a result, there is a significant increase in the amount of irradiated produce entering the international market. The list of countries marketing irradiated produce is growing rapidly as producers, importers, and consumers begin to understand the benefits of irradiation and that irradiation is often the most effective technology available to protect local agriculture. In many cases, irradiation is the only viable option to gain this market access. For example, irradiation is a mandatory treatment for at least 17 fruits from Hawaii to enter the US mainland. Irradiation is mandatory for import into the United States of a wide variety of fruit from at least a dozen countries. High on the list are litchis, mangoes, and guavas among others.

Table 13.1 Potential number of health problems prevented annually if 50% of meat and poultry are irradiated (Tauxe, 2001).

Pathogen	Cases	Hospitalizations	Major complications	Deaths
E. coli O157:H7 and other Shiga toxin–producing *E. coli*	23,000	700	At least 250 cases of hemolytic uremic syndrome (HUS)	20
Campylobacter	500,000	2,600	250 cases of *Campylobacter*-associated Guillain–Barré syndrome	25
Salmonella	330,000	4,000	6000 cases of reactive arthropathy (arthritis)	140
Listeria	625	575	60 miscarriages	125
Toxoplasma	28,000	625	100–1000 cases of congenital toxoplasmosis	94
Total	881,625	8,500	6660 catastrophic illnesses	352

Availability and acceptance of irradiated foods

While there has been a significant increase in the availability of irradiated foods in the marketplace, one still has to look very hard at the supermarket to find foods that have been irradiated. It is estimated that more than 1 million tonnes of various foods are irradiated per year (Eustice and Lynch, 2019).

Although the mention of the word *irradiation* still creates a certain amount of apprehension in the minds of a number of consumers, the volume of food that is irradiated is increasing dramatically. Recent growth has occurred in the use of irradiation for phytosanitary purposes to gain market access by eliminating the spread of harmful insect pests that may "hitchhike" on shipments of foreign produce. As the result of major outbreaks of Salmonella in ground beef, poultry, and many other foods in the United States and elsewhere, there is increasing interest in irradiation as a "kill step" to eliminate risk.

Many different foods that have been irradiated are available at major retailers in the United States and elsewhere. Asian specialty stores have been especially eager to offer fruits that were previously unavailable due to phytosanitary concerns. Consumer acceptance has been extremely good, and the volumes have increased every year. This trend is likely to continue. Irradiation is being used on pet treats in the United States and Europe; however these volumes are not included in this summary (Table 13.2).

Resistance to "new" technologies

Let us take a look at the gradual acceptance of several technologies that were controversial when first introduced but that are now commonplace. These include pasteurization, immunization, and chlorination each of which are now considered lifesaving and indeed have saved thousands of lives.

Pasteurization

The process of heating or boiling milk for health benefits was recognized during the early 1800s. During the 1850s, Louis Pasteur discovered that heating could eliminate bacteria. This process became known as pasteurization and was highly controversial at that time (Hall and Trout, 1968).

As society industrialized around the turn of the 20th century, increased milk production and consumption led to outbreaks of milk-borne diseases. Common milk-borne illnesses included typhoid fever, scarlet fever, septic sore throat, diphtheria, tuberculosis, and diarrheal diseases (U.S. Food and Drug Administration, 2016).

A century ago, milk products caused approximately one out of every four outbreaks due to food or water in the United States. Today, far less than 1% of all food- and waterborne illnesses can be traced to dairy products (Eustice, 2017a and 2017b) in fact, dairy products cause the fewest outbreaks of all the major food categories (e.g., beef, eggs, pork, poultry, produce, seafood). This drastic improvement in the safety of milk over the last 100 years is believed to be due

Table 13.2 Worldwide use of food irradiation (Eustice, 2017a and 2017b).

Country	Product	Approximate volume tonnes	Year	Purpose
China	Spicy chicken feet and many others	>950,000	2017	Food safety
United States	Ground beef, spices, condiments, fresh fruit	>100,000	2018	Food safety, phytosanitary
United States/ Hawaii	Boniato sweet potato, papaya	~8,000	2018	Phytosanitary (shipments to continental United States)
Mexico	Guava, mango, chili manzano pepper, etc.	17,200	2018	Phytosanitary (Export to United States)
Malaysia Vietnam	Dragon fruit, longan, fresh fruit, seafood, spices, herbs, etc.	>25,000	2018	Phytosanitary, food safety for export
Indonesia	Spices, cocoa	>5,000	2018	Food safety for domestic use
Australia	Mango, lychee, cherries, grapes, spices, etc.	>5,200	2018	Export/ domestic
Thailand	Fermented pork sausage, spices, herbs, mangosteen, etc.	~2,000	2018	Export/ domestic
South Africa	Spices, herbs, honey, dehydrated vegetables, egg products, garlic (fresh and dried)	~27,000	2018	Domestic
India	Mango, spices	>1,200	2018	Export
Japan	Potatoes	~6,000	2016	Domestic
European Union	Spices, condiments, herbs, frog legs	5,543	2015	Domestic
Miscellaneous	Spices, herbs, fruits	~5,000		
Total (approximate)		~1,000,000	2016	

primarily to pasteurization and improved sanitation and temperature control during the processing, handling, shipping, and storage of fresh milk products.

The controversy over banning raw milk sales has raged since pasteurization was first introduced well over a century ago. Throughout decades of debate, the public health and medical communities have remained steadfast in their support of pasteurization as a key measure to protect the public health.

Pasteurization became mandatory for all milk sold within the city of Chicago in 1908, and in 1947 Michigan became the first state to require that all milk for sale within the state be pasteurized.

As late as the 1930s, many in the dairy industry resisted widespread use of pasteurization. Even today, there is a movement by some to promote raw, unpasteurized milk. One of multiple concerns expressed was that the promotion of pasteurized milk would cast a negative shadow over the nonpasteurized product and force milk handlers to install "expensive" equipment to pasteurize milk. Antipasteurization activists continue to spread misinformation about pasteurization. Many of the arguments made have been around for more than a century.

During the 1920s, the US dairy industry and insurance companies were promoting so-called certified raw milk as a more acceptable alternative to pasteurization. It was only through the insistence of medical and scientific groups that the dairy industry abandoned its "good milk" versus "bad milk" concerns and embraced pasteurization as a lifesaving technology that would help to make all milk safe (U.S. Food and Drug Administration, 2016).

Pasteurization took nearly 70 years to be fully accepted in the United States, and the arguments against it were almost identical to those used today against food irradiation. Among some 70 concerns raised by the critics of pasteurization were the following (Eustice and Bruhn, 2013):

- "We must not meddle with nature."
- "This process changes the properties of the food."
- "Dangerous substances could be formed."
- "This process could be carelessly done and accidents could happen."
- "Pasteurization will increase the price of the product. We have a direct and prompt food distribution system."
- "It is not necessary."

None of these doomsday predictions turned out to be true; however, the campaign against pasteurization, including resistance from dairy producers and processors, significantly delayed its introduction, with the effect that thousands of people suffered chronic illness, developed long-term health consequences, or died. The question of legal responsibility for inflicting this suffering was never explored (Eustice and Bruhn, 2013).

Antivaccination movement

Vaccination is one of the most successful programs in modern medicine, reducing, and in some cases even eliminating, serious infectious diseases. Public support for the vaccination program remains strong; in the United States, the vaccination rates are high, e.g., more than 90% for polio (Hill et al., 2018).

Despite a long history of safety and effectiveness, vaccines have always had their critics: some parents and a tiny fringe element question whether vaccinating children is worth what they perceive as the risks. In recent years, the antivaccination movement, largely based on poor science and fear mongering, has become more vocal and even hostile.

Despite the growing scientific consensus that vaccines are safe, a stubborn vocal minority still claims otherwise, threatening the effectiveness of this public health program. A recent surge in Measles outbreaks in the Western United States has been attributed to failure of parents to vaccinate their children (Centers for Disease Control and Prevention, 2019).

Antichlorination movement

Science shows that adding chlorine to drinking water was the biggest advance in the history of public health, virtually eradicating waterborne diseases such as cholera. The majority of our pharmaceuticals are based on chlorine chemistry. Simply put, chlorine is essential for our health.

Despite science concluding no known health risks—and ample benefits—from chlorine in drinking water, some environmental groups have opposed its use for more than 20 years (Moore, 2008).

According to the WHO: "In a study on the effects of progressively increasing chlorine doses... on healthy male volunteers (10 per dose), there was an absence of adverse, physiologically significant toxicological effects in all of the study groups" (WHO, 2003).

World's safest food supply; safe enough?

Food safety is at the top of every food processor's list of priorities. The public demands safe food and the marketing of an unsafe product is a recipe for disaster. Recalls are expensive, damage brand image, and almost always result in litigation. A foodborne illness outbreak resulting in hospitalization or death is always a serious threat to a company's viability.

In the United States and other highly developed countries, we often hear "we have the world's safest food supply" The food industry has invested hundreds of millions of dollars in technology to make food safer. Any claim about producing the world's safest food is open to challenge. The CDC estimates that 48 million foodborne illness cases occur in the United States alone every year. At least 128,000 Americans are hospitalized, and 3000 die after eating contaminated food (Centers for Disease Control and Prevention, 2011).

Irradiation: a powerful tool to make food safer

Although irradiation cannot prevent primary contamination, it is the most effective tool available to significantly reduce or eliminate harmful bacteria in raw product and make sure that contaminated ground beef does not reach the marketplace. At doses that are commonly used to irradiate ground beef, we can expect the following levels of pathogen reduction (see also Table 13.1) (U.S. Food and Drug Administration. 2016).

E. coli O157:H7	99.99%−99.9999%
Salmonella	99%−99.9%
Listeria	99.9%−99.99%

Consumer acceptance of foods that have been irradiated

While the amount of food that has been irradiated has increased significantly in recent years, acceptance of irradiation has been slowed by several factors. First, the term "irradiation" is sometimes confusing or alarming to consumers because of its perceived association with radioactivity. Second, the general public poorly understands the causes, incidence, and prevention of foodborne disease. Third, health professionals and the media are largely unaware of the benefits of food irradiation. Finally, certain activist groups because of their beliefs about food production issues, nuclear power, international trade, and industrialization, as well as the introduction of technologies, have conducted an anti-irradiation campaign. These same groups and individuals oppose most other new technologies and in many cases are against even technologies such as pasteurization, immunization, chlorination, and other widely accepted technologies.

It is not hard to conceive why consumers originally thought food irradiation is not safe. Special interest groups and antifood irradiation lobbyists loudly declared that irradiated products were neither wanted nor needed. The public may often equate irradiated food with radioactivity, and any new technology involving radiation or radioactivity has been mistrusted despite the long-term use of such technologies in medicine and industry.

The literature on surveys of consumer opinions on food irradiation is extensive. Articles on the US consumers' perception of food irradiation and irradiated meat predominate and have been reviewed by Eustice and Bruhn (Eustice and Bruhn, 2013).

Besides the United States, there are now data from the European Union, Canada, Brazil, Australia, New Zealand, and a few developing countries. The methodologies, the size of the studies, and the rigor of the analyses vary widely but there are some clear trends. Most survey respondents have never purchased or consumed irradiated food. Their opinion is sought about an abstract concept. Generally, it is found that

- The majorities of respondents have not heard of irradiation or know very little about the process.
- The initial reaction of most consumers asked if they would purchase irradiated food is negative.
- When provided with factual evidence, the number of respondents willing to consider purchasing irradiated food increases, often then comprising a majority of consumers even if asked to consider paying a premium. Providing negative

information at the same time as positive information offsets the increase in acceptance.

- For fresh produce, irradiation is viewed more favorably than chemical treatments when a similar level of information is provided about the technologies.
- Irradiation is viewed much less favorably than other physical processes such as cold storage with which the respondents feel they are familiar. Social scientists have now examined consumer reactions to novel technologies in greater depth through studies in which genetic modification, nanotechnologies, or high pressure are assessed together with irradiation. These studies show that irradiation is not unique in engendering both general and organized opposition. A full discussion of these important recent findings is beyond the scope of this review, but the studies show clearly that:
- The issue of acceptance of a new food technology has much to do with trust in the systems in place to regulate and deliver the technology. The issues are greater than risk perception per se.
- Technologies that are not perceived as "natural" or which are thought to alter the character of the food generate greater opposition than technologies that are familiar or perceived as more "natural."
- Labeling can help to provide some degree of control, although one-third of respondents in a US survey would consider the word "irradiated" on a label to be a warning.
- Information can be valuable in increasing positive responses to novel technologies, but the information must be focused on the benefits to consumers. Technical details of the process often lead to consumers feeling they cannot understand the process and that it will be out of their control. New technologies, which are perceived as being of benefit mainly to the food industry, tend to be distrusted.

It is estimated that in 2018, US retailers sold approximately 15 million pounds of irradiated ground beef and approximately 80 million pounds of irradiated fruits, mainly lychees, persimmons, mango, papaya, purple sweet potatoes, and guava. Spices have been commercially irradiated since 1986. Approximately one-third of the commercial spices consumed in the United States, some 175,000,000 lbs, are irradiated annually (Eustice and Lynch, 2019).

Future directions

Food irradiation should contribute appropriately to safer food, a more secure food supply, and facilitated trade in fresh produce. As a result of the early marketing trials of irradiated food, several authors noted that the willingness of consumers to purchase irradiated food might be greater than indicated by their initial response to a general survey when irradiated food was not actually available at retail. Most recently, this willingness to purchase irradiated foods has been confirmed in thousands of supermarkets in the United States and several other countries (Eustice and Bruhn, 2013).

Johnson, Estes, Jinru, and Resurrection showed that consumer attitudes in the United States improved significantly between 1993 and 2003. This improvement can most certainly be attributed to the nationwide availability of irradiated ground beef, which began in 2000. Since then, millions of pounds of irradiated produce, nearly all imported, have been successfully marketed at retail. In the real world, consumers buy products because they want that product. The fact that an item has been irradiated (or processed with another technology) is not top of mind (Johnson et al., 2004).

Previously, the response of irradiation advocates has often been to stress the need to provide consumers with more information about the process. Numerous consumer studies have shown that when given a choice and even a small amount of accurate information, consumers are not only willing to buy irradiated foods but also often prefer them over food treated by other means. Dozens of them hear the facts and understand the benefits (Eustice and Bruhn, 2010). Market research studies have also shown (mostly in the United States), conducted over the past 3 decades, and repeatedly demonstrate that 80%—90% of consumers will choose irradiated products over nonirradiated after that no amount of information would convince those who generally reject any new product (Eustice, 2017a and 2017b). Most of these studies were done before irradiated food became commercially available.

The now overwhelming success of actual retail of irradiated foods and the evidence from sophisticated studies of consumer attitudes to novel food technologies suggest future strategies for increasing the use of food irradiation. Elements of a future strategy should include (Eustice, 2017a and 2017b):

- Regulatory authorities to provide information on a technology that is very unfamiliar to consumers. The role of regulatory authorities is crucial. The US and New Zealand cases benefited from the attitude of food authorities that make science-based rules. Wherever food irradiation is considered too sensitive an issue to make science-based decisions, the public debate is dominated by vocal opponents.
- Stress the benefits of irradiation that are focused on the food and the consumer rather than the technicalities of the process. For example, in the case of meat, giving consumers a guarantee that they will not be poisoned by a pathogen is what will matter most. Consumers can relate to a nonchemical phytosanitary treatment that protects local agriculture and the environment as well as providing produce that is exotic or out of season. However, extension of shelf life of fresh produce is not necessarily seen as a benefit by consumers who have become used to the notion of fresh (meaning just harvested) produce.
- Take into consideration that both positive and negative points of view will coexist in any public discussion on food irradiation. As time progresses and food that has been irradiated becomes more readily available, resistance will diminish and become negligible.
- Ensure that labeling of irradiated food is both consistent and fair. Labeling is a very difficult issue to balance. Consumers see mandatory labeling as

empowering them and providing greater control over what they buy. An assurance that irradiated foods would be labeled played a significant role in decreasing opposition to irradiated foods in Australia and New Zealand. Consumers are likely to perceive it as a warning given that competing technologies are usually not required to be labeled (for example, competing phytosanitary treatments) and it carries some extra costs. National regulations on the labeling requirements should be consistent. For example, requiring that the tiniest quantity of irradiated ingredient in a processed food be mentioned on the label is extreme.

Technical aspects of food irradiation:

- Food producers do not relate easily to irradiation processing. Contrast the likely reaction of a fruit grower who for years has used hot water treatment in the packing shed or an insecticide spray in the field with a new requirement to send his fruit to a distant facility that requires special authorization and has hazard signs. The sterilization of healthcare products can be a useful analogy for growers.
- Irradiation requires the shipment of products to a specialized contractor during which time they are out of the control of the producer with a transportation time and a cost that comes on top of the price charged by the irradiation company. Food generally being a perishable commodity, smooth operation of supply chain logistics is even more essential than for healthcare products.
- Affordable irradiation devices that could be placed on-line in, for example, a fruit-packing house or meat processing chain would go a long way to encourage the adoption of the process. Such equipment is a research concept at present but would be the ideal answer for the final step in a HACCP (Hazard Analysis and Critical Control Points) or quarantine system; it would also empower the user.
- The number of irradiation facilities is limited and since most are located to capture nonfood products, they are not necessarily in the right place for food manufacturers or traders. Also, these facilities are often optimized to treat at much higher doses than those required for food. These factors result in a lack of capacity to treat food at present and keep commercial volumes low. The result is to feed doubts about the potential for food irradiation to expand.
- Food generally involves high volumes. If only a fraction of a specific food can be treated, this creates problems for the trade. These include practical issues of having two production streams and can include perception issues. For example, meat produced under GMP is rightly regarded as safe, but what would be the issues for a dual market, one with safe meat and one for irradiated meat that is even safer?
- Gamma irradiation is currently the predominant technology for food irradiation. The food irradiation industry must continue to emphasize that gamma facilities are safe and able to irradiate up to pallet size of products of high densities. They will undoubtedly continue to have an important role for many years. It is important to point out that a gamma ray photon and an X-ray photon of the same

energy are, in every way, identical. In the past, food irradiation service providers have spent far too much time arguing about the benefits or shortcomings of gamma versus electron beam and vice-versa. Such discussion is nonproductive.

Barriers to acceptance

The most significant obstacle to increased consumer acceptance of irradiated foods may well be the lack of availability in the marketplace. A survey of retail and food-service beef purchasers in the United States was conducted in January and February 2004 by the National Cattlemen's Beef Association to measure awareness of, and attitudes toward, irradiation technology among foodservice and retail establishments that do and do not offer irradiated beef, measure the willingness to offer irradiated ground beef among those that do not offer it, identify barriers/issues to offering irradiated ground beef including researchable knowledge gaps, and both identify successful retailers and determine which practices help them sell this product (National Cattlemen's Beef Association, 2004).

The study showed that about 4 in 10 knowledgeable past users and nonusers of irradiated ground beef reported lack of availability as the main reason for not offering irradiated ground beef to their customers. This same study showed that respondents were relatively positive about purchasing irradiated ground beef. Almost half of past users were very (14%) or somewhat (33%) likely to purchase the product within the next year, and more than a fourth of the knowledgeable nonusers were very (4%) or somewhat (23%) likely to do so. In addition, a majority of the current purchasers (58%) indicated they would increase the amount of irradiated ground beef they would buy (vs. 23% intending to decrease the amount). These data show a growing rather than a shrinking market.

Conclusions

Louis Pasteur said, "To those who devote their lives to science, nothing can give more happiness than making discoveries, but their cups of joy are full only when the results of their studies find practical applications." Pasteur did not live long enough to realize the magnitude of the impact resulting from his efforts. Neither did Marie Curie, whose landmark research on radiant energy and radiation earned her a Nobel Prize in 1904 and set the stage for the use of irradiation of food and medical products.

The first successful marketing of irradiated ground beef took place in Minnesota in May 2000 when several retailers began to offer frozen ground beef that had been irradiated. Minnesota-based Schwan's, Inc., a nationwide foodservice provider through home delivery started marketing irradiated ground beef in 2000. Omaha Steaks of Nebraska has successfully marketed irradiated ground beef through mail order since 2000. Today, all noncooked ground beef offered by Schwan's and Omaha Steaks is irradiated.

Rochester, New York, based Wegmans, with over 90 supermarkets in New York, New Jersey, Pennsylvania, and Virginia, is a strong believer in the irradiation process and is one of the most visible marketers of irradiated ground beef. Although Wegmans takes every measure to ensure that all its ground beef products are safe, the retailer views irradiation as a value-adding process that offers the consumer an additional layer of food safety protection.

Defining moments in food safety

The successful commercial introduction of irradiated ground beef in the United States went largely unnoticed. According to food safety expert Morton Satin, when irradiated ground beef was introduced, consumers gained a reasonable expectation of buying products that offered much greater food safety and lower risk (Eustice and Bruhn, 2006). As a consequence, untreated ground beef acquired the character legally defining a product having a built-in defect.

Extensive evidence from several countries shows that labeled irradiated foods (fresh and processed meats, fresh produce) have now been successfully sold over a long period by food retailers. There is no record of any irradiated food having been withdrawn from a market simply because it has been irradiated. Although there are some consumers who choose not to purchase irradiated food, a sufficient market has existed for retailers to have continuously stocked irradiated products for years, even more than a decade.

Studies show that it is trust in the systems and institutions rather than perceptions of risk that dictates consumer attitudes and governs the adoption of a new technology. Retailers play an essential role in communicating the benefits of new products to consumers, and it is likely that positive messages on irradiated food from retailers and food producers will generate the most favorable response from consumers.

No one single intervention can provide 100% assurance of the safety of a food product. That is why meat and poultry processing plants use a multiple barrier (hurdle) approach utilizing several types of interventions such as thermal processes combined with chemical and antimicrobial treatment to achieve pathogen reduction. These technologies have successfully reduced, but not eliminated, the number of harmful bacteria in ground beef. Food irradiation does not eliminate the need for established, safe food handling, and cooking practices, but when used in combination with other technologies including an effective HACCP program, irradiation becomes a highly effective and viable sanitary and phytosanitary treatment for food and agricultural products. Irradiation is one of the most effective interventions available because it significantly reduces the dangers of primary and cross-contamination without compromising nutritional or sensory attributes.

Despite the progress made in the introduction of irradiated foods into the marketplace, many consumers and even highly placed policy-makers around the world are still unaware of the effectiveness, safety, and functional benefits that irradiation can bring to foods. Education and skilled marketing efforts are needed to remedy this lack of awareness.

Morton Satin says, "Pathogens do not follow political imperatives or moral philosophies, they simply want to remain biologically active. Strategies to control them, which are based on political ideals or myth-information, will not be effective. If we want to get rid of pathogens, we have to destroy them before they harm us. Food irradiation is one of the safest and most effective ways to do this. An international coordinated effort to develop effective knowledge transfer mechanisms to provide accurate information on food irradiation to policymakers, industry, consumers and trade groups are vital to meet today's food safety needs" (Satin, 2003). The Global Consensus document produced by the Global Harmonization Initiative (GHI) may help to convince authorities that there is no reason to doubt information provided by stakeholders that irradiated food is safe (Koutchma et al., 2018).

During the 20th century, life expectancy in the United States increased from 47 to 79 years (WHO, 2015). Many public health experts attribute this dramatic increase to the "pillars" of public health: pasteurization, immunization, and chlorination. Some of these same experts predict that food irradiation will become the fourth pillar of public health. Time will tell whether this prediction is correct and the trend toward widespread acceptance is positive.

References

Centers for Disease Control and Prevention, 2011. Burden of Foodborne Illness: Findings. https://www.cdc.gov/foodborneburden/2011-foodborne-estimates.html.

Centers for Disease Control and Prevention, 2019. Measles Cases and Outbreaks. https://www.cdc.gov/measles/cases-outbreaks.html.

DeGregori, T.R., April 24, 2002. The Zero Risk Fiction. American Council on Science and Health, New York, NY. https://www.acsh.org/news/2002/04/24/zero-risk-fiction-thomas-r-degregori.

Eustice, R.F., Bruhn, C.M., 2006. Consumer acceptance and marketing of irradiated foods (Chapter 5). In: Sommers, C.H., Fan, X. (Eds.), Food Irradiation Research and Technology, first ed. Wiley-Blackwell Publishing Amer, Iowa, USA.

Eustice, R.F., Bruhn, C.M., 2010. Consumer acceptance and marketing of irradiated meat (Chapter 19). In: Doona, C.J., Feeherry, F.E. (Eds.), Case Studies in Novel Food Processing Technologies. Innovation in Processing, Packaging and Predictive Modelling, first ed. Woodhead Publishing Limited, Cambridge, UK.

Eustice, R.F., Bruhn, C.M., 2013. Consumer acceptance and marketing of irradiated foods. In: Fan, X., Sommers, C.H. (Eds.), Food Irradiation Research and Technology, second ed. USA. Wiley-Blackwell Publishing, Ames, Iowa, pp. 173–195.

Eustice, R.F., 2017a. Global status and commercial applications of food irradiation. Chapter 20. In: Ferrira, I.C.F.R., Antonio, A.L. (Eds.), Food Irradiation Technologies: Concepts, Applications and Outcomes (Food Chemistry, Function and Analysis). Royal Science of Chemistry (RSC) Publishing.

Eustice, R.F., 2017b. Successful marketing of irradiated foods (Chapter 17). In: Ferrira, I.C.F.R., Antonio, A.L. (Eds.), Food Irradiation Technologies: Concepts, Applications and Outcomes (Food Chemistry, Function and Analysis). Royal Science of Chemistry (RSC) Publishing.

Eustice, R.F., Lynch, M., 2019. Personal Contact with Various Suppliers and Irradiation Service Providers.

Foodirradiation.org, 2014. US and International Agencies and Organizations that En Dorse and Support Food Irradiation. http://www.foodirradiation.org/pages/Learnmore-usinternation.html.

Frenzen, P.D., DeBess, E.E., Hechemy, K.E., Kassenborg, H., Kennedy, M., McCombs, K., McNess, A., 2001. Journal of Food Protection 64, 2020–2026.

Hall, C.W., Trout, G.M., 1968. In: Milk Pasteurization. Westport. AVI Publishing Company, Connecticut, USA.

Hill, H.A., Elam-Evans, L.D., Yankey, D., Singleton, J.A., Kang, Y., 2018. Vaccination coverage among children aged 19-35 months- United States, 2017. CDC Morbidity and Mortality Weekly Report 67 (40), 1123–1128.

Johnson, et al., 2004. Consumer attitudes toward irradiated food: 2003 vs. 1993. Food Protection Trends 24 (6), 408–418.

Koutchma, T., Orlowska, M., Zhu, Y., 2018. Fruits and fruit products treated by UV light (Chapter 17). In: Rosenthal, A., Deliza, R., Well-Chanes, J., Barbosa-Cánovas, G.V. (Eds.), Fruit Preservation, Novel and Conventional Technologies. Springer Science + Business Media, LLC. Part of Springer Nature, New York, NY 10013, USA.

Moore, P., 2008. 100th Anniversary of Water Chlorination.

National Cattlemen's Beef Association, 2004. Irradiation. Beef Industry Study. National Cattlemen's Beef Board, Centennial, Co.

Rogers, E.M., 1983. Diffusion of Innovations, third ed. The Free Press, New York.

Satin, M., 2003. Future Outlook: International Food Safety and the Role of Irradiation. World Congress on Food Irradiation: Meeting the Challenges of Food Safety and Trade. Chicago, Illinois, USA.

Tauxe, R.V., 2001. Food safety and irradiation: protecting the people from foodborne infection. Emerging Infectious Diseases Journal 7 (7), 516–521. https://wwwnc.cdc.gov/eid/articles/issue/7/7/table-of-contents.

U.S. Food and Drug Administration, 2016. Food Irradiation: What You Need to Know. https://www.fda.gov/Food/ResourcesForYou/Consumers/ucm261680.htm.

WHO, 2003. Chlorine in Drinking- Water. Background Document for Development of WHO Guidelines for Drinking- water, Geneva, 2003.

WHO, 2015. World Health Statistics 2015. Part II. Global Health Indicators. Table 1. Life expectancy and mortality, p. 50.

Conclusions

14

Veslemøy Andersen

GHI Association, Global Harmonization Initiative, c/o University of Natural Resources and Life Sciences (BOKU), Vienna, Austria

Because of the immense apparent confusion about genetic modification and food irradiation, there is a need for a book that in an unbiased way tries to explain what the differences are between conventional and genetically modified (GM) food and between irradiation and radioactivity. It is the intention of the book to discuss whether conventional food could be or would be safer than GM food and to discuss whether food preserved by traditional methods, e.g., using heat, could be or would be safer than food preserved by irradiation. Presumably the chapters in the book make this clear and remove undue concerns and scares from the minds of the readers. I hope that various chapters also removed skepticism about why new techniques have been developed, in particular, because the techniques may contribute significantly to solving the problem of feeding a still continually increasing number of people on the only conventional planet we have.

Discussing food produced with genetically modified seeds, it probably has become clear to the reader that nature modifies genes all the time and at random, in a trial-and-error way, to produce progeny that may cope better under new hostile conditions. Nature does not check if such progeny is safe for other living things, including humans. Nature uses what nature offers: natural radiation, natural mutagenic substances, and spontaneous mutations. Also, for thousands of years, farmers modified genes, be it unknowingly, in the Mendel way, by crossbreeding, long before Mendel discovered this and started to convince other scientists how it worked.

Nature is not caring about humans; every living thing is caring about itself and its own progeny and will do whatever is needed to protect it even if it means killing other living things. How some people have come to the conclusion or conviction that what is natural is safer and better is not based on facts but on emotional preoccupation. If mankind had not protected itself, driven by the same principle, there would be no mankind as we know it today or probably there would be no mankind at all. There is no tenable reason why genetic engineering, certainly with the progress in the past few years, would be a threat to food safety. None of the claims of antis that incidents have taken place and that GM food has adverse health effects has been substantiated by evidence. Almost all results of research, in particular research aimed at detecting adverse effects of GM food, shows that, with respect

Genetically Modified and Irradiated Food. https://doi.org/10.1016/B978-0-12-817240-7.00018-8

to food safety, there is no difference between GM and conventional food. On the other hand, modern genetic engineering today offers the possibility to accurately remove undesired traits and equally accurate introduce desired traits—without accidently introducing unwanted changes.

As shown in the second part of the book, any processing technique causes changes in the product processed, the main and intended change being the inactivation of microbes and pests that otherwise would multiply and ultimately make the food unfit for consumption or cause illness or even death if consumed. Generally, the changes caused by the heat treatment used to pasteurize food are more severe than those caused by irradiation. In the case of sterilization, this may be the reverse. Nevertheless, in both cases, the changes are of such nature that they do not make the resulting product harmful for the consumer. In general irradiation has less influence on color and flavor of the product than heat, delivering the same safety.

Some readers may feel more comfortable because they now understand that irradiation does not make the food radioactive. The predominant irradiation technology is exposing the food to gamma irradiation that has not enough energy to make the food radioactive. Therefore, after the treatment, no radioactive energy remains in the food and thus the food that has been irradiated is not radioactive. Food exposed to dust resulting from nuclear accidents does become radioactive, because they are contaminated with radioactive dust. Irradiation, however, does not involve contact between the food and any radioactive material.

Both food irradiation and genetic engineering that met much negative but evidently scientifically unfounded publicity, offer possibilities to solve problems without introducing unwanted traits. Irradiation enables preservation of food without heat-induced chemical changes, similarly to treatment with high-pressure, preserving flavor and color, and irradiation of packed food can prevent insects from spreading over the globe.

Food can be made insect resistant by genetic modification, and with modern techniques this can be done by very accurate gene editing. Genetic modification thereby prevents huge losses of harvested crops. Genetic modification moreover can make foods more nutritious, such as by introducing the capability to produce (pro-) vitamin A, saving the lives of millions of children. In addition, with gene editing, food plants can be made more resistant to environmental challenges such as high and low temperatures, extreme drought, and long-lasting exposure to excess water or flooding. Recent research also shows that gene editing can be used to make food plants resistant to infections from deadly viruses, such as the papaya ringspot virus that otherwise would wipe out entire crops.

Recommended literature

Blair, R., Regenstein, J.M., 2015. Genetic Modification and Food Quality: A Down to Earth Analysis. John Wiley & Sons Ltd., UK. ISBN: 978-1-118-75641-6.

The National Academies of Sciences, Engineering, and Medicine Report, 2016. Genetically Engineered Crops: Experiences and Prospects. The National Academies Press, Washington D.C., USA. ISBN: 978-0-309-43738-7.

International Consultative Group on Food Irradiation (ICGFI; joint FAO, IAEA and WHO), 1999. Consumer Attitudes and Market Response to Irradiated Food. Vienna, Austria. http://www-naweb.iaea.org/nafa/fep/public/consume.pdf.

Loaharanu, P., 2007. Irradiated foods. In: Kava, R. (Ed.), Michigan State University and Food and Environmental Protection Section, Joint FAO/IAEA Division, sixth ed. for the American Council on Science and Health, Vienna, Austria https://www.acsh.org/sites/default/files/Irradiated-Foods-ACSH-2007.pdf.

Index